LAWS AND LEGISLATION

FOCUS ON MENTAL HEALTH AND ILLNESS

LAWS AND LEGISLATION

Additional books and e-books in this series can be found on Nova's website under the Series tab.

LAWS AND LEGISLATION

FOCUS ON MENTAL HEALTH AND ILLNESS

ISAAC BANKS
EDITOR

snova
New York

Library of Congress Cataloging-in-Publication Data

ISBN: 978-1-53615-081-0

Published by Nova Science Publishers, Inc. † New York

CONTENTS

PREFACE

According to the Mental Health Services Administration, about one in five adults had a mental health condition in the past year. That's nearly 10 million adults with illnesses such as schizophrenia, bipolar disorder, or depression that interferes with a major life activity. Chapter 1 focuses on mental health issues in America and the role the Medicaid and Medicare programs play in addressing the needs of those with behavioral and mental health issues. Chapter 2 offers recommendations on how to address the mental health crisis. Chapter 3 presents prevalence estimates of any mental illness and serious mental illness based on surveys and ends with a brief discussion of how these prevalence estimates might inform policy discussions.

People with mental illness comprise a significant proportion of the population involved with the criminal justice system. Mental health courts were developed to respond to the large number of people in the criminal justice systems with mental illness as described in Chapter 4. Law enforcement encounters with individuals with mental illness may require special training and skills and can sometimes involve volatile situations, risking tragic injuries or even death as reported in Chapter 5. The Federal Bureau of Prisons (BOP) is responsible for confining offenders in environments that are safe, humane, cost-efficient, and appropriately secure. To do so, the BOP utilizes various forms of Restrictive Housing Unit (RHU) to confine certain inmates, including those with mental illness. However, according to chapter 6, confinement in RHUs, even for relatively short periods of time, can adversely affect inmates' mental health and can be particularly harmful for inmates with mental illness.

Chapter 1 - This is an edited, reformatted and augmented version of Hearing before the Committee on Finance, United States Senate, One Hundred Fourteenth Congress, Second Session, Publication No. S. HRG. 114–581, dated April 28, 2016.

Chapter 2 - This is an edited, reformatted and augmented version of U.S. Senate Hearing of the Committee on Health, Education, Labor, And Pensions United States Senate

One Hundred Fourteenth Congress, Second Session, Publication No. S. HRG. 114–719, dated Wednesday, January 20, 2016.

Chapter 3 - Determining how many people have a mental illness can be difficult, and prevalence estimates vary. While numerous surveys include questions related to mental illness, few provide prevalence estimates of *diagnosable mental illness* (e.g., major depressive disorder as opposed to feeling depressed, or generalized anxiety disorder as opposed to feeling anxious), and fewer still provide *national* prevalence estimates of diagnosable mental illness. This chapter briefly describes the methodology and results of three large surveys (funded in whole or in part by the U.S. Department of Health and Human Services) that provide *national prevalence estimates of diagnosable mental illness*: the National Comorbidity Survey Replication (NCS-R), the National Comorbidity Survey Replication Adolescent Supplement (NCS-A), and the National Survey on Drug Use and Health (NSDUH). The NCS-R and the NCS-A have the advantage of identifying specific mental illnesses, but they are more than a decade old. The NSDUH does not identify specific mental illnesses, but it has the advantage of being conducted annually.

Between February 2001 and April 2003, NCS-R staff interviewed more than 9,000 adults aged 18 or older. Analyses of NCS-R data have yielded different prevalence estimates. One analysis of NCS-R data estimated that 26.2% of adults had a mental illness within a 12-month period (hereinafter called 12-month prevalence). Another analysis of NCS-R data estimated the 12-month prevalence of mental illness to be 32.4% among adults. A third analysis of NCS-R data estimated the 12-month prevalence of mental illness *excluding substance use disorders* to be 24.8% among adults. The 12-month prevalence of *serious* mental illness was estimated to be 5.8% among adults, based on NCS-R data. Between February 2001 and January 2004, NCS-A staff interviewed more than 10,000 adolescents aged 13 to 17. Using NCS-A data, researchers estimated the 12-month prevalence of mental illness to be 40.3% among adolescents. Some have suggested that the current approach to diagnosing mental illness identifies people who should not be considered mentally ill. The 12- month prevalence of *serious* mental illness was estimated to be 8.0% among adolescents, based on NCS-A data. The NSDUH is an annual survey of approximately 68,000 adults and adolescents aged 12 years or older in the United States. According to the 2016 NSDUH, the estimated 12-month prevalence of mental illness *excluding substance use disorders* was 18.3% among adults aged 18 or older. The estimated 12-month prevalence of *serious* mental illness (excluding substance use disorders) was 4.2% among adults. Although the NSDUH collects information related to mental illness (e.g., symptoms of depression) from adolescents aged 12 to 17, it does not produce estimates of mental illness for that population. The prevalence estimates discussed in this chapter may raise questions for Congress. Should federal mental health policy focus on adults or adolescents with *any* mental illness (including some whose mental illnesses may be mild and even transient) or on those with *serious* mental illness? Should substance use disorders be addressed through the same policies as other mental illnesses? Members of Congress may approach mental health policy differently depending in part on how they answer such questions.

Chapter 4 - People with mental illness comprise a significant proportion of the population involved with the criminal justice system. The Bureau of Justice Statistics reports that at midyear 2005, over half of state prison and local jail inmates had a mental health problem. Mental health courts were developed to respond to the large number of people in the criminal justice systems with mental illness. The federal government provides funding to support mental health courts across the country through the Justice and Mental Health Collaboration program. The purpose of the program is to increase public safety by facilitating collaboration among the criminal justice, juvenile justice, mental health treatment, and substance abuse systems to increase access to treatment for offenders with mental illness. Authorized funding for this program expired at the end of FY2014, although, Congress has continued to appropriate funding for the program.

Chapter 5 - Law enforcement encounters with individuals with mental illness may require special training and skills and can sometimes involve volatile situations, risking tragic injuries or even death. The 21st Century Cures Act includes a provision for GAO to review the practices that federal first responders, tactical units, and corrections officers (for the purposes of this study, "law enforcement officers and agents") are trained to use in responding to incidents involving individuals with mental illness. This chapter addresses:

- challenges that federal law enforcement officers and agents face;
- applicable training, policies, and guidance; and (3) existing leading practices, relevant tools, and efforts to leverage information.

GAO selected the five DHS and five DOJ law enforcement components (e.g., Secret Service, Federal Bureau of Investigation) that represent the largest concentration of law enforcement officers within the two departments. GAO reviewed the training, policies, and guidance in place, as well as efforts to enhance them, and discussed these matters with knowledgeable officials. In addition, GAO held discussion groups with a nongeneralizable sample of law enforcement officers and agents, selected through component contacts, to discuss their perspectives. GAO also reviewed studies on law enforcement responses to individuals with mental illness to help identify leading practices and tools and interviewed stakeholders, selected through a structured process, to obtain their perspectives.

Chapter 6 - The Federal Bureau of Prisons (BOP) is responsible for confining offenders in environments that are safe, humane, cost-efficient, and appropriately secure. To do so, the BOP utilizes various forms of Restrictive Housing Unit (RHU) to confine certain inmates, including those with mental illness. However, according to recent research and reports, as well as the BOP's own policy, confinement in RHUs, even for relatively short periods of time, can adversely affect inmates' mental health and can be particularly harmful for inmates with mental illness. As of June 2016, of the 148,227 sentenced inmates in the

BOP's 122 institutions, 9,749 inmates (7 percent) were housed in its three largest forms of RHU: Special Housing Units (SHU) in 111 institutions; 2 Special Management Units (SMU) at the U.S. Penitentiaries (USP) in Lewisburg and Allenwood, Pennsylvania; and the USP Administrative Maximum Security Facility (ADX) in Florence, Colorado. The Office of the Inspector General conducted this review to examine the BOP's use of RHUs for inmates with mental illness, including trends in the use of restrictive housing and the screening, treatment, and monitoring of inmates with mental illness who are housed in RHUs. The authors found significant issues with the adequacy of the BOP's policies and its implementation efforts in this critical area.

In: Focus on Mental Health and Illness
Editor: Isaac Banks

ISBN: 978-1-53615-081-0

Chapter 1

MENTAL HEALTH IN AMERICA: WHERE ARE WE NOW? HEARING BEFORE THE COMMITTEE ON FINANCE, UNITED STATES SENATE, ONE HUNDRED FOURTEENTH CONGRESS, SECOND SESSION, APRIL 28, 2016*

Thursday, April 28, 2016
U.S. Senate, Committee on Finance,
Washington, DC.

The hearing was convened, pursuant to notice, at 2:31 p.m., in room SD–215, Dirksen Senate Office Building, Hon. Orrin G. Hatch (chairman of the committee) presiding.

Present: Senators Crapo, Roberts, Cornyn, Thune, Scott, Wyden, Stabenow, Cantwell, Carper, Cardin, Bennet, and Casey.

Also present: Republican Staff: Kimberly Brandt, Chief Health-care Investigative Counsel; Chris Campbell, Staff Director; and Jill Wright, Detailee. Democratic Staff: Ann Dwyer, Health-care Counsel; Michael Evans, General Counsel; Elizabeth Jurinka, Chief Health Policy Advisor; Joshua Sheinkman, Staff Director; and Beth Vrable, Senior Health-care Counsel.

* This is an edited, reformatted and augmented version of Hearing before the Committee on Finance, United States Senate, One Hundred Fourteenth Congress, Second Session, Publication No. S. HRG. 114–581, dated April 28, 2016.

OPENING STATEMENTS

Opening Statement of Hon. Orrin G. Hatch, a U.S. Senator from Utah, Chairman, Committee on Finance

The CHAIRMAN. The committee will come to order.

I apologize for being late. We had to finish up some Judiciary work, and Senator Grassley asked me to chair that matter. It is a pleasure to see everyone here this afternoon.

Today's hearing will focus on mental health issues in America and the role the Medicaid and Medicare programs play in addressing the needs of those with behavioral and mental health issues. Together, Medicare and Medicaid financed nearly 45 percent of mental health spending in the United States, which amounted to more than $75 billion—that is with a "b"—in 2014 alone.

As the Senate committee with jurisdiction over these programs, it is our responsibility to better understand the drivers behind the growing needs for and the costs of these services and to work together to develop better solutions for identifying and treating these issues. A report issued by the Medicaid and CHIP Payment and Access Commission in June 2015 indicated that the majority of Federal spending on mental health comes out of Medicaid. That same study found that Medicaid is the single largest payer in the United States for all behavioral health services, including mental health and substance abuse. In fact, Medicaid accounted for 25 percent of nationwide spending on behavioral health in 2009, the year with the most recent data.

One of the many difficulties we face in addressing these issues is that Medicaid enrollees with behavioral health diagnoses have varied physical and behavioral health needs. Patients often range from young children who need screening, referral, and treatment for autism or depression to chronically homeless adults with numerous diagnoses involving severe mental illness. In 2011, only one in five Medicaid beneficiaries had a behavioral health diagnosis, but they accounted for almost half of total Medicaid expenditures.

Needless to say, these types of behavioral health issues can seriously impair a patient's quality of life, cause disability, and significantly decrease life expectancy. These types of issues are associated with significantly higher rates of chronic disease, substance use disorders, and inpatient hospitalization among Medicare beneficiaries.

In Medicaid, patients with behavioral or mental health diagnoses are more than twice as likely to be hospitalized as those without such diagnoses. The number is drastically higher if the patient also has a substance use disorder. These high hospitalization rates are major drivers in the cost of our Federal health programs. However, what is more unfortunate is that all too often, people with mental or behavioral health issues get no care at all.

According to the 2012 National Survey on Drug Use and Health, nearly 40 percent of adults diagnosed with severe mental illness, such as schizophrenia or bipolar disorder, received no treatment for their illness in the previous year. When you broaden that scope to include all adults with any mental or behavioral illness, 60 percent went untreated for the prior year.

It gets worse. Every year, suicide claims the lives of 38,000 Americans, more than car accidents, prostate cancer, or homicides, and about 90 percent of suicides are related to mental illness, according to the National Institute of Mental Health.

Utah is not immune from this preventable tragedy. Suicide has been the greatest threat to our young people in recent years, and it is time for everyone to take notice. This is absolutely tragic. However, the tragic pattern expands beyond the suicide rate, as overall, people with serious mental illness have an average life expectancy that is 23 years shorter than the nationwide average.

Patients and their advocates say the country's mental health system has been drowning for a long time—not from flood waters, but from neglect. As we talk about solutions, we need to note that the distinction between mental health, mental illness, and severe mental illness is crucial, because each group requires different clinical and policy prescriptions. For example, the current system, proportionately speaking, provides far more support for mental health than severe mental illness. We need to review these priorities and find an equitable solution to ensure that all needs are being met.

Today's panel will give us an opportunity to hear from witnesses who can speak to these issues from almost every perspective. We have an advocate who has suffered with these issues firsthand. We also have experienced professionals who will share their experiences providing care at the local, State, and Federal levels and who can speak to the successes and limitations of providing care in each of those environments.

I look forward to hearing the testimony of today's witnesses and beginning a dialogue with my colleagues on these important issues that hopefully will lead to better solutions. With that, I am going to turn to our ranking member, Senator Wyden, for his opening statement.

[The prepared statement of Chairman Hatch appears in the appendix.]

Opening Statement of Hon. Ron Wyden, a U.S. Senator from Oregon

Senator WYDEN. Thank you very much, Mr. Chairman, and thank you for scheduling this important hearing.

The Finance Committee is responsible for the programs—Medicare and Medicaid—that spend more on mental health than any others in America. That is why this committee, working in conjunction with other Senate committees—the Health, Education, Labor, and Pensions Committee and the Judiciary Committee—now have to develop a fresh approach for protecting and caring for Americans with mental illness. The focus of that approach should be breaking health care, social service programs, and law enforcement out of their individual silos and bringing them together in a coordinated system that deploys their strengths to help people dealing with mental health issues.

The Wyden family knows a little bit about this subject. My brother struggled with schizophrenia for decades, and he had a lot of his health-care bills covered by Medicaid. In and out of halfway houses, confrontations with law enforcement officers, problems securing funds for services or treatments—it was certainly something that has confronted millions of families and demonstrates the need for a fresh approach to helping those with mental illness. Like so many families across the country, you went to bed at night constantly thinking that your loved one might the next day hurt themselves or somebody else.

Because of the lack of appropriate places to meet the needs of those with these mental health challenges, we so often have patients boarded in emergency rooms or in fights with police, sometimes deadly, winding up in prison, where more than half of all inmates suffer from mental health problems and minorities are vastly overrepresented.

Now, I would be the first to say that mental health is not an issue that falls neatly and precisely under just one Senate committee's jurisdiction. A lot of different members with different areas of expertise are going to have to pull the same end of the rope to make progress on this front.

Now, fortunately, Senator Stabenow is here. She has been a champion on these mental health issues. She is our leader here on the Finance Committee, working to build a bipartisan approach. We so appreciate her leadership. Senator Murray, the Democratic leader on the HELP Committee, is also right at the forefront.

In my view, the biggest challenge on mental health is to focus on three priorities. First, there needs to be a sharp new focus on preventing—preventing—mental illness. Patients need better care earlier on to keep the illnesses from escalating.

Furthermore, there are nearly 2 million low-income, uninsured Americans suffering from mental health or addiction in States that have not expanded their Medicaid programs. Those are 2 million Americans who, without treatment or help, are far more likely to go homeless, far more likely to be incarcerated, far more likely to face addictions, far more likely to commit suicide. The choice to expand Medicaid and give new hope to those 2 million individuals and their families, in my view, ought to be an easy one to make.

Second, services from health care to social work need to be better coordinated. It does not make much sense to tell a person struggling with an illness that they are on their own managing treatments, figuring out what specialist to see, scheduling appointments, and handling medications.

Even outside the doctor's office, there are a lot of areas where people with mental illness often need help that they are not getting today: paying the bills, making it to appointments, maintaining a home. Taxpayer dollars need to reach deeper into our communities and improve the coordination of mental health services to help those whom today the system largely overlooks.

Third and finally, there needs to be a better link between mental health and law enforcement. In many cases, that is going to mean more training on what to do when responding to a person with mental illness. Too many individuals who should be in proper health-care facilities are winding up in jail cells instead.

In my hometown, Portland, the police bureau has recently put a lot of work into building a team of specially trained officers to handle these challenges safely. And I can tell you, in my hometown, at least in the early going, this is paying off big. In my view, more agencies around the country ought to pick up on some of these Oregon lessons with respect to law enforcement.

Of course, and I will close with this, the big challenge is funding. Each year, mental illnesses cost the United States $450 billion, only a third of which is actually spent on medical care, with roughly $75 billion, combined from Medicare and Medicaid, making up the biggest portion of the pie.

Those are huge numbers, and a lot of the overall total goes to emergency room visits and jail time. In my view, if you can begin to shift some of that funding to the three priorities I have mentioned—preventing mental illness, better coordination of services, and linking law enforcement with mental health—you will see many more Americans being in a position to manage their mental illness and living healthier lives. Big challenge.

Once again, as you and I have talked about, Mr. Chairman, with our colleagues, this is going to take bipartisan teamwork, the kind of bipartisan approach that Senator Stabenow is working on. But I think that the members here want to come together. We have been talking about this for a long time, and it is time to move forward and actually put in place these new priorities.

I thank you, Mr. Chairman. I also want to welcome all our witnesses and thank them very much for being here.

[The prepared statement of Senator Wyden appears in the appendix.]

The CHAIRMAN. Thank you, Senator.

I have to say that Senator Stabenow and the Senator from Missouri, Roy Blunt, have met with us this morning on precisely these issues, and we are going to see what we can do.

But before we begin this very serious discussion, I would like to bring to everybody's attention that May 3rd is our distinguished ranking member's birthday. Now, I personally hate birthdays, because when I was a kid, they never had a birthday party for me, and all the other neighborhood kids—we were so poor, we could not afford one, and I just blow them out of mind. It affects me even to this day, although I am getting over it. [Laughter.]

But we just want to mention that Oregon's soccer team, the Timbers, were national champions in 2015 [handing Senator Wyden a wrapped gift box]. [Applause.]

Senator WYDEN. Mr. Chairman, thank you.

The CHAIRMAN. That is a soccer ball.

Senator WYDEN. I can tell. [Laughter.]

The CHAIRMAN. I know you would not know what it is. He only played basketball. But it is a signed soccer ball from the Timbers on your birthday, and we hope you have many more really great birthdays.

Senator WYDEN. Mr. Chairman, thank you. This is above and beyond, and I look forward to coming to your office and throwing the ball around with you. [Laughter.]

The CHAIRMAN. His wife owns the leading bookstore in the country, so I let him get away with anything. [Laughter.]

Let me take a few minutes here to introduce our witnesses. I am very pleased to introduce our first witness, Mr. Brandon Marshall, an all-pro and six-time Pro Bowl receiver with the New York Jets.

In 2011, Brandon was diagnosed with Borderline Personality Disorder and spent 3 months in intensive treatment after struggling with his mental health for years. Since then, he has become a dedicated advocate for mental health issues. His main platform is an organization called Project 375, which he founded to bring awareness to mental illness and to eradicate the stigma.

Brandon regularly produces PSAs, gives interviews and speeches, and partners with other organizations that are dedicated to improving mental health. The list of organizations that he has worked with includes the National Alliance on Mental Illness, Glenn Close's Bring Change 2 Mind, the Kennedy Forum, the National Council for Behavioral Health, and the Linehan Institute, just to mention a few. In addition to speaking arrangements through those organizations and his own, he has given interviews on his mental illnesses on national networks, including CBS, NBC, MSNBC, ESPN, and Fox.

I think I speak for all of us when I say you are an inspiration, Brandon—an inspiration to everyone with mental illness and to all of us here today. I am just very grateful to have you here, and we look forward to hearing your testimony.

Our second witness will be Dr. Margaret Bennington-Davis, the chief medical officer at Health Share of Oregon, which coordinates physical, dental, and mental health benefits for 240,000 Medicaid- enrolled Oregonians.

Prior to coming to Health Share, Dr. Bennington-Davis served as the chief medical and operating officer at Cascadia Behavioral Healthcare, Oregon's largest mental health and addictions provider. Before that, she served as psychiatry medical director for Salem Hospital, as well as the hospital-wide chief of staff.

Dr. Bennington-Davis also served as faculty for the Sanctuary Institute. She has coauthored a book, published articles and chapters, and has done numerous consultations and presentations regarding organizational change, trauma-informed engaging environments, and leadership.

Dr. Bennington-Davis completed her M.D. and psychiatry residency at Oregon Health Sciences University, where she remains on faculty, and received her master's of medical management degree at Tulane University School of Public Health.

Next, we will hear from Mr. Doug Thomas, the Director of the Division of Substance Abuse and Mental Health for the State of Utah. We are grateful to have Mr. Thomas here. He also serves on the board of directors of the National Association of State Alcohol and Drug Abuse Directors, as well as the Utah Substance Abuse Advisory Council.

Additionally, Mr. Thomas serves as a member of the Utah Commission on Criminal and Juvenile Justice. He has worked in the mental health and substance abuse disorder field for over 20 years as a direct service provider and administrator. Mr. Thomas has worked in both urban and rural settings and previously oversaw county services, implementing evidence-based service delivery models.

Mr. Thomas graduated from Brigham Young University, my own alma mater, with a bachelor of science in psychology, and from the University of Utah with a master's degree in social work.

Finally, we will hear from Ms. Linda Rosenberg, the president and CEO of the National Council for Behavioral Health. The National Council for Behavioral Health represents and serves 10 million adults, children, and families served by the National Council's 2,700-member organization.

Prior to joining the council, Ms. Rosenberg was the Senior Deputy Commissioner of the New York State Office of Mental Health. She has over 30 years of experience in designing and operating hospitals, community and housing programs, and implementing New York's first mental health court.

Ms. Rosenberg serves on an array of boards of directors and is a really valued person in this area and a member of the executive committee of the National Alliance for Suicide Prevention.

I want to thank all of you for coming. I just want to mention that each of your experiences and perspectives is incredibly important on these sensitive issues—or set of issues, I think we should say. We will hear the witness testimonies in the order they were introduced.

So, Mr. Marshall, if you will, we will have you proceed with your opening statement. We look forward to hearing from you.

WITNESSES

Statement of Brandon Marshall, Executive Chairman and Co-Founder, Project 375, Chicago, Il

Mr. MARSHALL. Thank you, Mr. Chairman. Ranking Member Wyden, happy birthday.

Senator WYDEN. Thank you.

Mr. MARSHALL. I am grateful and thankful that you guys invited me out to speak before the U.S. Senate and the Finance Committee.

My name is Brandon Marshall, wide receiver for the New York Jets, and I just finished up my 10th year in the National Football League. In 2011, I was diagnosed with Borderline Personality Disorder. The best way to describe it is, it is an emotional disorder. Some people do not have the skills and tools to be able to cope and deal with some of the day-to-day stress of just life. So I had to spend 3 months in an outpatient program at McLean Hospital learning those tools. I sat in groups and dialectal behavioral therapy, learning those tools and skills; cognitive behavior therapy, where we studied the frontal lobe and tried to understand how to live a healthy and effective life; also, mentalization therapy, self-assessment.

But it was at McLean Hospital where I found my purpose. A lot of times, athletes think that their purpose is to catch a ball, shoot a basket, run fast, but I think we are here for something better. And it was at McLean Hospital where I learned that my purpose is to help bridge the gap in the mental health community.

At McLean Hospital, I was walking out of self-assessment, and one young lady was self-harming herself. Another young lady tried to commit suicide the night before. Another young lady, the week before, in the 3East program, named Sasha, from Canada, committed suicide.

I walked out of that group very sad, and I walked into a parking lot to go to Reebok's headquarters to work out and I saw 200 cars. I looked at those cars as patients. I asked myself, how many more people out there are suffering or suffering in silence and do not even know it?

It cost me $150,000 to get the treatment that I needed, and 3 months. Reimbursement, it was so bad that I did not even bother to deal with the insurance. My mother, a recovering alcoholic—and she gave me permission to tell her story—also deals with some things. It cost us $30,000 a month to get my mom the help that she needs. She is now 4 years sober, an amazing woman.

My sister—the same story. My younger brother, who is facing 30 years in prison, actually goes to court on the 28th, it cost us $150,000 to send him to Yellowbrick in Evanston, IL.

I say that because I truly believe that where we are at today is where the cancer and HIV community was 20–25 years ago, and it is time for us to galvanize the community, stand together, and make a change.

My wife and I, in 2011, also founded Project Prevent. Project 375 is our foundation project. Prevent is a program where we are trying to put on-site behavioral health-care services in our schools to also be preventative and intervene early, because we think that is the key.

I noticed, when I first got my diagnosis at McLean Hospital, I was 50 percent better. I was able to be in group and be validated by people who understood what I was going through. The other 50 percent came from the work.

The call to action is, we need to develop and support programs that are affordable, accessible, and scalable. We need to reimburse mental ailments the same way we do physical. I also think our call to action should be to adopt technology. There are 320 million Americans, and over 100 million are affected by mental illness. We need technology to be able to stand in the gap to help our professionals, our doctors, our government to get the people the help they need.

Last, this is the last great stigma in our country, and it is a civil rights issue.

Thank you.

[The prepared statement of Mr. Marshall appears in the appendix.]

The CHAIRMAN. Thank you, Mr. Marshall. That means a lot to us, and we appreciate you taking time to come see us.

Mr. MARSHALL. Thank you.

The CHAIRMAN. Dr. Bennington-Davis?

Statement of Margaret Bennington-Davis, MD, Chief Medical Officer, Health Share of Oregon, Tualatin, OR

Dr. BENNINGTON-DAVIS. Chairman Hatch, Ranking Member Wyden, honorable members of the committee, thank you for this opportunity to offer testimony on the state of mental health services, particularly those provided in the Medicaid program.

For the record, I am Dr. Maggie Bennington-Davis, an Oregon psychiatrist and chief medical officer of Health Share of Oregon.

Before I begin, I would like to thank you, Mr. Marshall, for your remarks about your own experience. Your presence here today is more important than you know.

I would like to begin by describing Oregon's recent innovations in Medicaid. Health Share is the State's largest Medicaid Coordinated Care Organization, or CCO, serving approximately a quarter of Oregon's Medicaid enrollees as the backbone in a collective impact organization of local health plans, health systems, providers, and community organizations.

CCOs were created through a Medicaid waiver in 2012, with the basic premise being that we would coordinate all Medicaid benefits for our members—physical health, mental health, dental health, addictions, even transportation—using a fixed, global budget.

The model is showing early signs of success both in holding down costs and in improving care. As a mental health provider myself, I can tell you this model of collaboration with other parts of the health-care system and even outside the health-care system that are serving the same individuals is remarkable. For the first time, we are able to work across systems of care and address the problems of having thought and planned and built services in silos. What is more, Oregon is predicted to save the Federal Government $1.4 billion over the first 5 years of implementation of the CCO model.

Oregon's CCO design has brought new attention to and appreciation of the roles of mental illness and addictions in costs and in poor health outcomes. I think of it as us finally discovering the neck—that there is, indeed, a link between the brain and the body.

People with serious mental illness die, on average, nearly a quarter-century sooner than the general public. That statistic is even worse in Oregon, where people with serious mental illness and addictions die, on average, in their mid-40s. These early deaths are almost always because of chronic physical illnesses that are modifiable with the right supports.

The financial impact is also striking. People with chronic physical conditions and mental health and substance use disorders have triple the cost of people with the same physical health conditions, but without mental illness or substance use.

The CCO model compels us to do a much more thorough job of connecting the brain and the body. Much of mental illness, like physical illnesses, is preventable, and the CCO model encourages us to look upstream toward prevention.

Trauma and chronic stress play an important role in all of our lives, in our society, and certainly in the context of the other social disparities of health and poverty in people who are Medicaid members. When Health Share of Oregon first analyzed the people who use the most services and were the highest-cost members, we asked them to describe what had happened to them throughout their lives. The results caught our attention. Often, these folks were born as a result of unintended pregnancy into unstable housing and chaotic families.

Some had been in and out of the foster child system early in life. Many had been neglected or sexually or physically abused as children. Most did not have the kind of childhoods that helped them to develop the emotional regulation skills to prepare them to be successful in school. Most had various erratic behaviors or depression or suicidal tendencies that led them to require services in specialty mental health, if they could get access, or in jails or hospitals if they could not. That is exactly what the Adverse Childhood Experiences Study, published in 1998 by Drs. Felitti and Anda, showed: that adversity and toxic stress during childhood led to significantly more physical and emotional problems in adulthood.

Knowing that mental illness and substance use disorders, along with other ill effects of childhood trauma, can be prevented, Health Share of Oregon felt we had to move upstream in our efforts to improve health. We are focusing on helping our members avoid unwanted pregnancies; get social, physical, and mental health supports during pregnancy; have basic needs met in order to successfully be able to attach to their new babies; and get the support and guidance they need to be effective parents.

My last example is Health Share's foster child initiative. We know from our own data, which mirror national data, that children in the foster child system have a much higher incidence of asthma, Attention Deficit Disorder, obesity, Post-Traumatic Stress Disorder, even hypertension and schizophrenia. What was news to us, though, was that these differences persist and are even higher in children who are no longer in the foster child system, but were once upon a time. So we at Health Share are developing coordination among mental health, physical health, and dental health providers to describe what are the right supports for these children in these health arenas.

Community mental health services, where I spent much of my career, have traditionally focused on people who have already developed chronic and severe mental illness. By adding emphasis to early childhood supports and the social disparities of health, by partnering with early intervention programs in schools, and by paying attention to the mental health supports within a community, all things CCOs can do, perhaps we can mitigate the tragic long-term effects of the toxic stress described in the Adverse Childhood Experiences Study.

In closing, thank you for this honor and opportunity to comment on our work in Oregon to bring attention to mental health and its inseparability from physical health and overall health, and to emphasize the importance of raising our children in safe and nurturing communities. CCOs are an early promising model for integrating and coordinating care, drawing attention to the health and economic impacts of mental illness and addictions, and clearly point to the need for mental health to include better awareness of the impact of toxic stress in childhood.

Thank you.

[The prepared statement of Dr. Bennington-Davis appears in the appendix.]

The CHAIRMAN. Thank you.

Mr. Thomas, we will take your testimony.

Statement of Doug Thomas, Director, Division of Substance Abuse and Mental Health, State of Utah, Salt Lake City, UT

Mr. THOMAS. Chairman Hatch, Ranking Member Wyden, and members of the committee, my name is Doug Thomas. I am the Director of the Division of Substance Abuse and Mental Health in the State of Utah, and I am honored to be here with you today along with these distinguished guests.

Medicaid saves lives and is the backbone of the public mental health system in Utah and throughout the United States. It provides the infrastructure and economy of scale necessary for States to standardize evidence-based practices to provide high-quality care to individuals with serious mental health needs.

The various Medicaid waivers and alternative benefit plans available to States allow them needed flexibility to customize plans to fit the unique challenges, needs, and resources of each State. Case management, peer support services for individuals and families, psychosocial rehabilitation, and respite services are all great examples of Medicaid reimbursable services that help people stay in their homes and communities despite serious illness and allow people the opportunity to reintegrate in place of being alienated from their families and communities of origin.

In 2009, the Institute of Medicine, IOM, issued a lengthy publication about the prevention and early intervention of mental, emotional, and behavioral disorders. The report highlights that almost one in five young people has such a disorder at any given time and that among adults in the United States, half of all these disorders were first diagnosed by age 14 and three-fourths by age 24.

The first symptoms usually precede a disorder by 2 to 4 years, giving us a window of opportunity. Narrowing the gap between the onset of symptoms and evidence-based intervention is critical, as the research is showing us that this early intervention preserves executive functioning and allows people, especially young people and people suffering from the first episode of illness, to recover more quickly with less life disruption. This allows them to accomplish and maintain important developmental tasks, such as establishing healthy interpersonal relationships, succeeding in school, and making their way into and succeeding in the workforce.

For people with Medicaid, we are able to intervene early with positive outcomes, showing that people can and do recover from mental illness. Treating a person's mental illness improves physical health outcomes and reduces overall health-care costs as well.

There have been various Medicaid and other health-system studies which show that collaborative physical and mental health care lowers costs and improves health outcomes. Prevention and early intervention can help us get upstream and bend the cost curve.

In Utah, 3 years ago, with a new State legislative appropriation and county matching funds, we began to act on the IOM report with what we call Mental Health Early Intervention. This consists of three programs: school-based behavioral health, Mobile Crisis Outreach Teams for Youth in four of our five most populous counties, and Family Resource Facilitation With Wrap-Around to Fidelity, which is a peer support program.

Over the last 3 years, we have increased services to almost 5,000 additional youth, the majority with Medicaid funding. Office disciplinary referrals are down, literacy scores are up, symptoms of mental illness are being reduced, often to the community norm, and families are receiving the supports they need to keep their children safely at home, in their own school, and enhancing their family's natural support system through peer support.

Utah recently passed limited Medicaid expansion, designed to target people with the lowest income and the greatest need: parents with dependent children already on Medicaid, people who are chronically homeless, people with mental illness and substance use disorders involved in the criminal justice system, and people with mental illness and substance use disorders.

We must have Medicaid work with us to find a way to approve a waiver allowing Utah to extend Medicaid coverage to those people in need. People want to be served in the safest, least restrictive environment, and providers want to provide these types of services.

Sometimes children and adults need care beyond what can be provided appropriately in an outpatient or home-like setting. Allowing Medicaid residential services the ability to bill and be paid for room and board would be a great step in the right direction. Room and board is covered during a more costly inpatient hospital stay, but not covered during a more economical residential stay. This disincentivizes lower-cost, short-term residential services in lieu of more costly inpatient hospital care.

With the Patient Protection and Affordable Care Act, the Mental Health Parity and Addiction Equity Act, and more integrated care being provided, there is a need to modernize the Medicaid Institutes for Mental Disease (IMD) Exclusion.

I applaud the efforts of the Substance Abuse and Mental Health Services Administration, Centers for Medicare and Medicaid Services, and the Department of Health and Human Services to modernize this rule, including the option of State waivers around the IMD exclusion.

It must be done cautiously and systematically to ensure we are not re-institutionalizing people but that we are providing a short-term crisis intervention meant to help people stabilize and rejoin us in our communities where we all work and play and live.

Thank you for the opportunity to testify before you today.

[The prepared statement of Mr. Thomas appears in the appendix.]

The CHAIRMAN. Thank you for your testimony.

Ms. Rosenberg, we will take yours now.

Statement of Linda Rosenberg, MSW, President and CEO, National Council for Behavioral Health, Washington, DC

Ms. ROSENBERG. Thank you, Chairman Hatch, Ranking Member Wyden, and members of the committee. I am honored to be here with my very eloquent colleagues.

There is attention to mental illnesses and addictions everywhere we look, from presidential elections to the *New York Times* feature on the Portland police; from the 600,000 Americans who have taken a mental health first-aid course to last week's CDC data showing a 25-percent increase in suicides in the last 15 years.

But attention is not enough. It is not enough for the more than 28,000 who die from an opioid overdose. It is not enough for the more than 41,000 who committed suicide, and it is certainly not enough for their families.

It is not enough—and not because we do not know what works. It is not enough because of the limited availability of what works.

Respectfully, the question before you is not, where are we now but, where do we need to be? If we are serious about moving from pockets of excellence that you heard about from my colleagues to the widespread availability of effective interventions, we need to stop depending upon grants and then wondering why good practices do not spread.

When we have cancer or heart disease, getting access to chemotherapy or a stent does not depend upon a local clinic having a grant. Why are mental illnesses and addictions different?

The answer to where we need to be is the Excellence in Mental Health Act demonstration, a bipartisan initiative led by Senator Stabenow and Senator Blunt. The Act enables and sustains treatment systems that increase access, deliver evidence-based care, and integrate services.

Discussions of access often focus only on increasing beds. Beds can never be effective in a vacuum. Only community-based services prevent readmissions. At a time of Accountable Care Organizations and medical homes, beds alone are not enough. Neither, for that matter, is crisis care. Standing alone, it just is not enough.

The Excellence Act establishes criteria for Certified Community Behavioral Health Clinics, CCBHCs, that provide mental health and substance use services and primary care screening. CCBHCs deliver 24-hour crisis services, coordinating with law enforcement, criminal justice, and veterans' organizations.

But it is not just access. We need uniformly high-quality services. Unfortunately, the adoption of research-based practice is limited. An example is the successful NIMH RAISE study that improved outcomes for youth experiencing a first psychotic episode.

Most communities will be unable to implement this program. Block grant funds and philanthropic grants will not be enough, and thousands of young adults will be relegated to a life of disability.

CCBHCs can move the needle. They are required to offer evidence-based practices and are paid a rate inclusive of these activities. With outcome tracking and quality bonus payments, clinics will be held accountable for patient progress, a step in our move to value-based purchasing.

A key challenge to delivering science-based services is our shortage of professionals. Clinics all over the country struggle to recruit and retain staff. The fundamental barrier is that most clinics cannot afford skilled staff or investments in technology to extend staff's reach.

Those of you who have ever run a business know this is unsustainable. The Excellence Act offers certified clinics Medicaid payments based on the cost of treatment. They can hire critical staff and leverage new technologies, and even those historically opposed to prospective payments, like the National Association of Medicaid Directors, acknowledge there is not a better solution.

The average age of death, as we have heard, for Americans with serious mental illness is 53. The culprits are heart disease, lung disease, and cancer. And people with chronic physical illnesses, as you have heard, often have co-morbid depression and anxiety.

CCBHCs represent a foundational opportunity to advance the way care is integrated and coordinated. Shining a spotlight into the shadows of mental illnesses and addictions is not enough. The Excellence in Mental Health Act is where behavioral health needs to be.

Twenty-four States are now planning their participation in the demonstration, yet the law sets an 8-State limit. Every State that wishes to create and sustain quality systems should be able to do so. We urge you to allow all 24 States to participate and to open the planning process to the remaining 26 States. CCBHCs will transform services in this country, and that is what I call reform.

Thank you.

[The prepared statement of Ms. Rosenberg appears in the appendix.]

The CHAIRMAN. Thanks to all of you. This has been compelling testimony. I am very grateful to you.

Mr. Marshall, the stigma around mental health is very, very important. I want to thank you for sharing your personal story and perspective on living with Borderline Personality Disorder, and I want to also thank you for your courage in taking a leadership role to end the stigma surrounding mental illness.

You have spoken at length about the importance of proper treatment for all people, regardless of whether they are a parent in the suburbs of Salt Lake City, a single adult trying to make ends meet, or a wide receiver in the NFL who is admired by millions.

Can you expand on your work through your organization, Project 375, to end the stigma around mental health?

Mr. MARSHALL. Yes. First, like I said in my testimony, where we are at today is where the cancer and HIV community was 20–25 years ago. One of the first things they did was, they galvanized the community. They came together, they changed the narrative in the media, they broke down the stigma. Back in the day, it was called the Big C. So that is where we find ourselves.

So we spend a lot of our time telling stories, similar to what Glenn Close does. I think it is important for influencers in our country to stand up and say, “This is who I am, and this is what I have been dealing with.” It could be them or it could be a loved one.

So that is number one: breaking down the stigma. And I think it is important, because there are a lot of people out there suffering—and suffering in silence. Some people do not even know that they are suffering. That is their norm.

The second thing, which I always call the tangible, is preventative and intervention work. We want to put onsite behavioral health-care services into every single school. But to be honest with you, I am now realizing that that is really hard to do. So that is why I mentioned one of the calls to action is adopting technology to not replace, but help our professionals, our government, our doctors, stand in the gap. And so we are fighting hard for that, and we are looking for your support in any way we can get it.

The CHAIRMAN. Thank you. I am very proud of you for being willing to stand up on these issues.

I want to thank each of you witnesses for your work in this very important area. To the extent that each of you is involved in developing policies to address mental illness, what factors do you consider for changes to the mental health delivery system? If you would, I would like you to highlight any successes you have seen in mental health delivery as well.

We can start with you again, Mr. Marshall, and go from there. Mr. MARSHALL. I will pass it to you, Doctor.

The CHAIRMAN. That would be fine. Let us start with you. Dr. BENNINGTON-DAVIS. Thank you, Mr. Chairman.

I would like to mention a very particular initiative that Health Share of Oregon is partnering in with several delivery system parts in Portland, called Project Nurture.

Project Nurture is a program that is specific for women in Medicaid who are pregnant and who are addicted. This program encourages women to seek prenatal care as early as possible. We have a partnership with the Department of Human Services to make sure that there is an understanding that we are, in fact, giving the woman the support she needs to successfully get through the pregnancy. And during the prenatal period, the woman is also getting addictions treatment, she is getting peer support, and she is getting therapy, and her baby is also being taken good care of.

The program has staff who stay with the woman throughout the delivery period and then even postpartum to help her attach to her baby and learn the right parenting skills to give that baby a good start, all the while getting addiction treatment.

It is that kind of coordination and collaboration across mental health and physical health and that kind of multidisciplinary approach that I think is going to change outcomes, reduce mental illness, reduce addictions, and give people a better start, and we can do that because of our Coordinated Care Organization structure.

The CHAIRMAN. Thank you.

Mr. Thomas, let me just ask you this. The mental health workforce is an issue about which I care deeply. You have dedicated a great deal of your career to increasing peer support services in the State of Utah. Could you please share the impact of that model and ways in which it has spread to different States to make meaningful local impacts?

Mr. THOMAS. Having peer support is important, paraprofessionals—they are people who have lived experience, who have had a mental illness or a substance use disorder and are in recovery— and/or family members who can go in and do the same thing for families who are struggling with a child, who have been through the child welfare system or the juvenile justice system.

And they go in and they—just like Mr. Marshall—bring a lot of credibility with them. They are someone who has been through the system and has recovered and flourished. And so what they do is, they help other peers and are able to link them to services. But also, I think the main ingredient is, they give them hope. They give them hope and a vision of a better future, and many times, people really struggle to maintain that hope.

So we have done that in Utah and had great success. We now have family resource facilitators in some of our juvenile courts, in child welfare with the 4(e) waiver that is happening in Utah, which we appreciate your work on in that regard as well, to provide more home and community-based services in lieu of residential and in- patient. It means a lot and makes a big difference in people's lives.

The CHAIRMAN. Thank you.

My time is up. Senator Wyden?

Senator WYDEN. Thank you very much, Mr. Chairman.

Just for you, Mr. Marshall, your work to deal with the stigma associated with mental health is appreciated. I have been really struck by how negative perceptions about serious mental illnesses are actually growing and that one in three people say that they would not want their kid to be friends with another child who is diagnosed with depression. So a big, big thanks. I think that is enormously valuable work that you are doing to highlight the stigma issue.

My first question will be for you, Dr. Bennington-Davis. We are so proud of the work that you all are doing at home.

I want to focus on a group that is really getting left out in this debate, and that is kids. Children suffering from mental illness often are sort of given short shrift here, and research shows that half of all lifetime cases of mental illness begin by age 14.

So it would seem to me that screening and treating mental health disorders is especially critical for children. Again, this just seems to be an area that is being missed, and it is not some partisan thing, it is just being missed.

If you could make one recommendation with respect to children with mental illness, what would it be? I think my first choice, again, is that prevention issue that Mr. Marshall has highlighted and I have been interested in, which is screening and treatment.

What do you think would be your top priority in terms of trying to get kids help early?

Dr. BENNINGTON-DAVIS. You stole my answer, Ranking Member Wyden. One of the pushes that we have in the Coordinated Care

Organization setup in Oregon is to meet certain incentive metrics— so outcomes that are incentivized by the program—and one of those incentive metrics is to ensure that children get developmental screenings at the correct times.

Another one in the foster child system is to coordinate physical health and mental health—and dental, for that matter—screening as soon as the child enters DHS custody.

I think things like that that actually structure, require, and then incentivize and reward the provider system for doing the right things at the right times, are going to make a big difference in the lives of our kids as they go through the system.

Senator WYDEN. Let me bring our other panel members into the next question.

We are obviously not the Judiciary Committee, and that is why I indicated that several committees are going to have to be involved here. But there are several pieces to this issue. There is prevention, better coordinating the services, and obviously—again, in Oregon, we have tried to highlight the relationship between law enforcement and mental health services, and it is surely about time.

Of people who were shot and killed by police officers in 2015, 25 percent displayed signs of mental illness, and more than half of all prison and jail inmates have a mental health problem. So in Oregon, we sought to try to break some new ground here in terms of trying to define different relationships between law enforcement and mental health.

I would be curious—maybe we will work our way the other way. We can start with you, if we might, Ms. Rosenberg.

What would be your top priority in building a new, better coordinated relationship between mental health practitioners on the health side and law enforcement?

Ms. ROSENBERG. I think one of the biggest problems you will hear from law enforcement is, what do they do with someone who clearly has a mental illness? I hear that over and over again.

When you read my bio, you talked about my being involved actually in the first mental health court in New York City. I think they get someone clearly having a problem, maybe picked up on the street, maybe the family calls, there is nowhere to go, and I think that is one of the reasons we are so interested in fundamental change and ensuring that everybody knows where to go.

Those services are available 24/7. People who are professionally trained can intervene and the police are not left alone, and that is before anyone gets either booked or arraigned.

Senator WYDEN. Mr. Thomas, do you want to take a crack at that?

Mr. THOMAS. Sure. Crisis intervention training for police officers, mental health, first aid for first responders, are great models on the law enforcement side. And we have had a great justice reinvestment initiative in Utah with help from the Pew Foundation, building it based on risk, needs, and responsivity and having it very clear what the criminogenic risks are and then what the substance use and mental health needs are, and then targeting programs that help people who are low criminogenic risk, who have high mental health or high substance use disorder needs, and getting them into treatment programs that work and that keep them from the recidivism cycle.

Senator WYDEN. I am going to have to be on the floor in a few minutes, but I want to thank all of you. You have just been a superb panel.

Senator Stabenow, who, of course, has championed this cause for us here, will serve as our ranking minority member.

Mr. Chairman, I very much look forward to working with you and our colleagues.

The CHAIRMAN. Thank you so much.

Senator Roberts, you are next.

Senator ROBERTS. Well, thank you. Before Senator Wyden leaves, a special happy birthday to you, sir.

Senator WYDEN. Thank you.

Senator ROBERTS. We have worked together for quite a few years. I used to give you every extra 5 minutes that you needed on the Intelligence Committee.

Senator WYDEN. Always. [Laughter.] And we are Kansans.

Senator ROBERTS. Yes, we are both Kansans. I had the feeling that if you took that soccer ball and kicked it over to Ms. Rosenberg, Brandon would leap across there and catch it——

Ms. ROSENBERG. You have no faith in me——

Senator ROBERTS [continuing]. Laying out. [Laughter.]

The CHAIRMAN. Could I interrupt you for just a second? I have to leave for a few minutes. So the next one will be Senator Stabenow and then Senator Cornyn. So if you will follow up yourselves, I have to go speak to a group, and I will be right back.

Senator ROBERTS. So you are not leaving me in charge, is that right?

It is a coup. All right.

Mr. Chairman and Senator Wyden, thank you for holding this hearing. It is our committee's commitment to reviewing and finding ways to improve our mental health system.

Mr. Marshall, I did not know when we were having a good discussion back in the back room here that you held the record for most receptions, 21, in an NFL game. I thought that was Art Monk of the Redskins. [Laughter.]

One of five players in NFL history to have at least 100 receptions in three seasons—I thought that was probably Lynn Swann of Pittsburgh, whom you are familiar with. The NFL record for most receiving touchdowns in a single Pro Bowl game, I thought that was Jerry Rice. But that is you.

Mr. MARSHALL. Yes, sir.

Senator ROBERTS. And it is you who is sitting there who has really provided a beacon of hope for an awful lot of people. That is really special. That is even more special than going over the middle and getting popped by a linebacker and still holding onto the ball.

I really appreciate your testimony, and on the back page, if I can find it, you say, "As an NFL wide receiver, I have caught hundreds of passes during my career. Today, I am throwing one to you." "You" is us.

I still have good hands. I will not fumble it. [Laughter.]

I have a little bit different kind of questioning here. Last month, the Center for Medicare and Medicaid Innovation, CMMI—it is a brand new outfit, and we already have a brand new acronym—they proposed sweeping changes to how we pay for prescription drugs under Medicare Part B. This is under the heading, "we need to do good things on behalf of mental health, but we have to also prevent bad things from happening," and I am concerned about this center.

I know many of my colleagues on this committee share my concerns with how this demonstration, quote, "could affect patients' quality of and access to care."

As the president of the Kansas Medical Society described to me in a letter just yesterday, this demonstration, quote, "will force Kansas Medicare beneficiaries with serious, sometimes life- threatening conditions to participate in a CMS innovation initiative, disrupt their treatment processes, and impede their access to needed medications, with no evidence of improved health outcomes or financial gains for the Medicare system."

Most concerning for the purpose of our hearing today is the proposal's impact on those suffering from severe mental illness: schizophrenia, schizoaffective disorder, or bipolar disorder with psychosis. It is often extremely difficult for patients with these conditions to adhere to oral medications, and, as a result, many rely on long- acting injectable antipsychotics, which would fall under Medicare Part B.

Phase one of the demonstration would reduce reimbursements for all new second-generation long-acting injectables. Let me repeat that: it would reduce reimbursements. In phase two, CMS could decide—probably would decide—some of these medications are now deemed, quote, "high-value" and limit access to them.

This could result in the patient going to a hospital, which could be a lot further away, especially in rural Kansas, Texas, or Michigan, where we may end up paying more for the same treatment, or these patients could be switched to products that are less effective or have more side effects, which is where I get particularly concerned about the government coming between you and your doctor. This is particularly concerning for a patient with schizophrenia, as switching treatments impacts the likelihood of relapse, increasing the debilitating and lasting adverse effects on a progressive condition.

So my question to all of you on the panel would be this. Have you heard about this proposed demonstration, number one? Do you share these concerns about access to appropriate medications for those with mental illness?

We will start with you, Doctor. Pardon me—Ms. Rosenberg.

Ms. ROSENBERG. Yes. Thank you for promoting me. It feels very nice.

Senator ROBERTS. I just bestowed that upon you.

Ms. ROSENBERG. But I do feel strongly about this, particularly about reducing the price or the payment for injectables. As a country, we use less injectables than any other place in the world.

It is a highly effective treatment. Patients and their families are interested in it, and it is harder to administer than giving someone a script.

So the minute you make reimbursement lower, you are going to lower utilization even further. That is a very big mistake.

Senator ROBERTS. Mr. Thomas?

Mr. THOMAS. Before I became the State Director, I was the lead on a team that worked with people who struggled with schizophrenia and bipolar disorder—in and out of the hospital and State hospital for many years—and we did a lot of outreach to them in their homes and watched them take their medication to help them, because often that was one of their major things that led to their hospitalizations.

When the long-acting injectables, the new generation, came along with much less side effects than the old injectables, it was a godsend for a lot of people. They were able to get their shot and then not worry about it for a month and not have the daily reminder or the daily struggle to take the medication.

For me, this is deeply personal, and I think anything that gets in the way of that is dangerous for people.

Senator ROBERTS. Dr. Bennington-Davis?

Dr. BENNINGTON-DAVIS. Senator Roberts, Health Share, the company I work for, does not deal with Medicare, and I was unaware of the proposal. So I have learned from you today. Thank you.

Senator ROBERTS. Brandon Marshall?

Mr. MARSHALL. Yes. This is my first time hearing it, but I will say that I agree with Ms. Rosenberg and Mr. Thomas.

I speak a lot from experience. My first charity event after relaunch, after I spoke and said that I was diagnosed with borderline personality disorder and I spent 3 months at McLean Hospital, we had a charity event soon after, and there was a young lady and her family who came in, and we stayed in contact over the years.

Last year, she introduced me to injectables, and her experience is night and day. She was someone who was heavily sedated with medication, and this past year, she has just been amazing.

Senator ROBERTS. I appreciate that. I apologize to my colleagues for going way over my time. Let me just point out that over 300 organizations are asking that this rule be withdrawn. I agree.

This is another case of rationing health care. There are four rationers. This is one. My fears are coming home to roost, because we have a proposal which, if implemented by CMS, could ration health care.

That is where we fumble the ball, Brandon.

I recognize the distinguished Senator, my colleague and friend, Senator Stabenow.

Senator STABENOW. Thank you very much. Thank you, Senator Roberts. I share your concern about this issue and have written a letter, as well, expressing concern about this policy.

Welcome to all of you. It is terrific to have each of you here and share your experiences, and thank you for what you are doing.

I do want to make note that the last Finance Committee hearing on mental health was in 1999. So we are overdue.

I think it is also important to stress that President Kennedy signed the last law he ever signed on October 31, 1963, when he signed the Community Mental Health Act, and we have yet to fully implement the vision of the law that was enacted in 1963.

For me personally, in 1963, I was the eldest child in a family where my dad was suffering with mental illness. All of us have in one way or another been affected by mental illness.

Mr. Marshall, I can tell you that I am so grateful that you are here. I understand what it is like with the stigma for a family in a small rural town in northern Michigan, where folks do not understand, even though my mom was a nurse and it was a medical family, trying to understand what was happening with my dad: misdiagnoses, lack of services.

I also know what happens when you get the right diagnosis. At the time, my dad was diagnosed as a lot of things, but finally, accurately, manic depressive, which we now call bipolar, which is a chemical imbalance in the brain. He finally got the services he needed, the medication he needed, and lived the rest of his life healthy and productive.

So that is what fuels my commitment to this, both from a family as well as from a professional standpoint.

We also know that one out of five adults has mental illness—I hear one out of five, I hear one out of four; we are all affected by this—and 60 percent of them do not get the treatment they need in a year now, today. So you fast-forward from what happened to my father.

It is also, I think, interesting to note that the Cook County jail and the Cook County sheriff has hired a psychiatrist to be the head of the jail, and he said, "This is not surprising, because over a third of the people I house have mental illnesses."

So we know the impacts of this, whether it is a hospital emergency room, whether it is the jail. What we need is people to get the services that you have described today, and get them when they need them, get them early and be able to go on and have productive lives.

So I have worn a lot of different hats on this one, chairing at the State level in Michigan the mental health committee, and I have seen what works and what does not work. I have lived what works and does not work.

I am very excited about the fact that we have a moment now where we have wonderful bipartisan interest in behavioral health, mental health, and substance abuse. They are all connected. We have wonderful work going on in a bipartisan way, and it is time to seize this to be able to structurally change what we do so that, as Ms. Rosenberg has said, we are not depending on grants that come and go.

We do not depend on that if you have heart disease or kidney disease or you have a broken back. We do not go, well, you know, the grant ran out this year, so you will have to wait.

But yet, if it is a disease above the neck, if it is a disease in your brain, we have a very different system. And that is the challenge, I think: to integrate our health-care system so that brain diseases do not rely on grants when every other kind of disease relies on a healthcare system with full reimbursement. That is why I am so grateful to all of you. I am always saying that health care above the neck needs to be the same as health care below the neck.

Before asking a question, I do want to just say that we have begun that process. The exciting thing is, 2 years ago, on the last SGR patch that we did, we passed something that Senator Blunt and I worked on for some time to set up a requirement for quality behavioral health standards, 24-hour psychiatric emergency care, integrated care with primary care, help for families, all the things—substance abuse, mental health.

So we have these standards now and know what it looks like. We need to fund it, and we were able to get funding for eight States to be able to meet that, and 24 States stepped up. Now we are saying we need to provide the opportunity for every State that meets quality standards to be able to receive the funding and get the reimbursement, and I am very grateful for Senator Blunt's working with me so closely on this for so long now.

So I want to start with Dr. Bennington-Davis. I know Oregon is one of the States that has received a planning grant, one of the 24 States. Could you talk a little bit about why you applied for the planning grant and what you would hope for if you were able to fully provide services, quality services, and get reimbursed for it? What would that mean?

Dr. BENNINGTON-DAVIS. Thank you, Senator Stabenow. I just have to remark that I think your legislation is the most important legislation to emerge regarding mental health since President Kennedy signed that act. So thank you very much for your efforts along those lines, and I am really excited about it.

For 10 years, I worked for a community mental health provider agency, and we served about 15,000 people a year, most with serious and persistent mental illness, and the one thing that was missing was, as you said, the below-the-neck part. Even though so many of the people that we served had very serious chronic physical conditions, they either could not or would not get access around their primary care needs.

In the agency where I was, we were not set up to provide those services. So the CCBHC gives us an opportunity to really up our game and to connect the brain and the body and to understand the person as a whole person.

Ever since becoming an M.D., I have understood that that is the big gap. You cannot be a psychiatrist without thinking about the whole person, and certainly you cannot be a person in community mental health services without worrying about the rest of your health. They just impact each other so constantly.

So it was a no-brainer to apply for the CCBHC grant. I am thrilled that Oregon got it. It fits very nicely into the context of all of the other innovative things we are interested in in terms of integration. We need to integrate both ways, though, not just behavioral health into primary care; we have to integrate primary care into community behavioral health services.

Thank you again.

Senator STABENOW. Thank you.

I would just ask one quick question of Ms. Rosenberg. There are lots of things that I would love to ask all of you, but you touched on helping veterans. And one of the things we worked on as we looked at integrated care is integrating with veterans who may not live near a VA facility but maybe someplace in the community around their State.

We know that 22 veterans commit suicide every day. We know all the numbers. More than 25 percent of veterans have a psychiatric diagnosis.

How does providing fundamental reimbursement for community care make a difference for veterans?

Ms. ROSENBERG. It is going to make a tremendous difference for veterans and for their families. You know, one of the things we sometimes forget is, when someone comes home from service and comes home with a disability—traumatic brain injury, PTSD—it affects not only their spouse, but their children.

So we are going to create opportunities for treatment in every community, with your leadership, and we thank you so very much. It will make a tremendous difference.

Once someone is no longer involved in the VA, now is working with their families, those problems do not go away, and now they will have community capacity, and people will know where to go.

I think that is the other issue. Brandon Marshall—and, of course, I am a hero now to my grandson because I am sitting at this table with him—in addition to that, has brought attention to this. Now for people who are telling their story, it is, "Where do I go?"

The calls I get personally are from family members and from friends across the country who have someone with a mental illness, a child, an adult, and they really do not know where to go.

We have to create that vision you described from 1963, that there is a place in your community you can go and that, if your primary care physician who has someone on their staff who is a behavioral health specialist, if they feel you need more than they can provide, they have someplace to send you.

So I think we want to be a community resource. We know what to do. It is not that we do not. The grants have been very successful. They have proven it. Now, it is about how we systematize it so that every community has the resources they need, including the substance use resources.

Let me also say that both Mr. Thomas and Dr. Bennington-Davis worked in the past at member organizations of the National Council. It is no surprise they are in the positions they are in now. They were stars then.

Senator STABENOW. Thank you very much.

I think I am turning to Senator Cornyn.

Senator CORNYN. Thanks to each of you for being here today, and I appreciate your contribution to the discussion.

Actually, there has been a discussion going on for a while now, and I applaud Senator Stabenow and Senator Blunt, whom I know work very closely together bringing mental health services to the community, Federally Qualified Heath Centers, which I have always been a supporter of. But recognizing that these are existing health-care facilities, if we are able to enhance access to mental health services at those existing facilities, that is a pretty efficient and pretty effective way of dealing with this issue.

I come at this from a law enforcement perspective, as a recovering judge and Attorney General, but principally what I have been struck by is the successes at local levels in dealing with things like—Senator Wyden talked about training for law enforcement to deescalate confrontations between police and a person who is suffering a mental health crisis, but that takes training to know how to deal with it.

Also, our jails often become the mental health provider of first resort, or maybe it is of last resort. I actually met the other day through a friend of mine—the sheriff of Barrett County, San Antonio, TX—someone she introduced to me as the largest mental health provider in America. Meet the sheriff of the Los Angeles County jail.

So that speaks volumes for what our law enforcement community needs to do in order to become better-informed and better-trained. And I think there are some great models at the local level, and we need to identify those best practices and then scale those up and make those available across the country.

Here is an interesting statistic, or it was to me. The Federal Government provides $2 billion a year, $2 billion a year, in assistance to State and local law enforcement, but less than 1 percent of that is directed toward mental health issues. To me, that just seems like it cannot possibly be right. Since the Federal Government does not have limitless access to resources and we are going to have to find ways to pay and live within our means, it just seems to me that if we are already spending $2 billion a year, that maybe, just maybe, we ought to look at the allocation of some of those funds and direct them toward training and other things that the Federal Government can do in terms of highlighting best practices that already exist across the country.

The other thing is, I was struck by Pete Earley's book, "Crazy," and had the honor of meeting Pete. Pete has been courageous to talk about his family's experience, Mr. Marshall. He had a son who had a mental illness, but the biggest problem he had, his family had, is his son simply would not cooperate with his health-care treatment, would not take his medication, for example, and ended up in jail.

As we have seen, that is where many people end up, either that or homeless, living on the street. One of the biggest problems, it seems to me, is not about reimbursement, it is not about access to the best drugs necessarily, but it is, how does a family member get the cooperation of a loved one who happens to be mentally ill?

I think about somebody like Adam Lanza's mother in Connecticut, the shooter at Sandy Hook. His mother knew he was mentally ill and he kept getting sicker and sicker and sicker, and she did not know what to do. She could have had him involuntarily committed, but that is not forever. That is just for a short-order treatment. You can imagine the tension and friction in their relationship if she were to get an order for him for involuntary commitment.

So there are a lot of really interesting things that are happening, as I have said, across the country, including things like assisted outpatient treatment, which does not require an involuntary commitment, but it is a civil court order requiring people to comply with their doctor's orders.

Right now, the courts have the authority of probation, or parole even, and the control that comes along with that, but unless you have those tools, unless you are a drug court or some other judicial office, you do not really have the resources to require people to comply with their doctor's orders and take their meds.

My understanding is that a lot of what we see happening resulting in people ending up in jail, living on the street, or crowding our emergency rooms—if we could just do a little bit better in terms of getting people not only access, but ensuring better compliance with their doctor's orders, they could do a lot.

We have an effort that I know of. In addition to what Senator Stabenow and Senator Blunt have been doing, Senator Alexander and Senator Murray in the HELP Committee—Health, Education, Labor, and Pensions Committee—have a bill. Dr. Bill Cassidy I know is working with the Senate version of the House bill, along with Chris Murphy, on the larger mental health package that Tim Murphy has been proselytizing on quite a bit. I have a bill called the Mental Health and Safe Communities Act bill, which is from the Judiciary Committee jurisdiction.

So to the ranking member's point, we have all these different committees, and because of the silos we create here in terms of how we look at things, I think what we need is a better-coordinated effort, even internally within the Senate, to try to come up with a consensus package that we can actually act on, because I think there is a lot we can do in this area.

Mr. Marshall, I think you are right. This seems to be kind of a magic moment when people finally realize this is pretty important and we need to act on it.

So thanks, all of you, for being here. We look forward to continuing to work with you, and we ask for your continued advice and support.

Thank you.

Senator STABENOW. Senator Casey?

Senator CASEY. Thank you very much. I want to thank the chairman and ranking member for calling the hearing, and I also want to commend you, Senator Stabenow, for your work on this legislation over time.

I want to thank the panel. This is a panel that brings a lot of personal and professional expertise to this, and I am grateful to Brandon for being here. He has roots in Pittsburgh and I wanted to note that for the record.

Folks in New York and around the country know Brandon well, but he does have roots in Pittsburgh. I want to make sure—you grew up in East Liberty?

Mr. MARSHALL. East Liberty, yes.

Senator CASEY. Sometimes they pronounce it as one word in Pittsburgh.

Mr. MARSHALL. Correct.

Senator CASEY. But we are so grateful. I wanted to thank Brandon Marshall for his testimony, and I will excerpt just a few lines from his written testimony, talking about accepting mental illness as a disease, saying, number one, that it needs better research, better screening, better funding. You also say that we need to have better recognition of new therapeutic treatments proven to work. I guess if I were making a list, I would say number five would be education in schools.

So you have given us an assignment—to use your words: throwing us a pass. So we have an obligation to catch it and do our best to run with it. So I want to thank you for that.

I want to start with, and I may only have time for one broader question, but, Dr. Bennington-Davis, so much research, which is part of your testimony, shows the connection between childhood poverty and outcomes as adults. One of the ways to thwart that or prevent it from happening is early intervention.

I guess one kind of broad question—and you may have addressed this more broadly in your written testimony. But we know that early intervention works. I guess it is a corollary to "good treatment works," and we are having a lot of discussion on the opioid crisis. But we know that in this context, early intervention works.

What can you tell us about, in your professional opinion, the best method of early intervention? Is there one strategy that works, or two, or is it more than that?

Dr. BENNINGTON-DAVIS. Well, thank you for the question, Senator Casey. I think it has to be a complex answer because it is a complex set of issues, and poverty is complex, and the stresses that go along with poverty are complex, and the social disparities of health that are part and parcel of people's lives are extremely complex. But if I were to try to boil down what I think scientifically we are aiming at, I think what we are aiming at is to decrease the overall toxic stress that a young brain is experiencing both before birth and after birth.

If we can figure out how to decrease the overall stress, the adversity, if a child can be in a safe and nurturing relationship with a caretaker, in a safe and nurturing home, and in interactions that help that child's brain develop robustly, then I think humans are incredibly resilient and can overcome most things.

So I would aim at that, and there are a lot of ways to do that. There are parent supports, there are community supports, there certainly are programs in schools and so forth, but that would be the thought in my head as I set about trying to think of an array of programs.

Senator CASEY. I guess not to put too fine a point on it, the earlier we do early intervention, the better.

Dr. BENNINGTON-DAVIS. Yes. I think James Heckman, the Nobel Prize economist, says the earlier you intervene, the way more payoff that there is, and I think we in health care have to grasp that concept as well.

Senator CASEY. I may just have one more question.

Ms. Rosenberg—I could call you all doctors; you have a lot of experience. Psychological services in our State are not covered by Medicaid, and that is, obviously, a hurdle we have to overcome. What is the best way to expand that kind of access, access to mental health services generally?

Ms. ROSENBERG. CCBHCs are excellent. Actually, your State is a grantee. It just so happens that the chairman of our board is from Pennsylvania. Her name is Susan Blue. We have members all over your State, a very active association, and I think they are very committed to it.

I think what we need is a standard that does not exist now in terms of competence. That includes psychological treatment. I think right now what has happened is, for most community-based behavioral health organizations, they cannot afford skilled staff, believe it or not. So you have a physician who can do many things sitting and writing scripts all day. You have peers who do many important things. But in between, you really lack staff that can deliver cognitive behavioral therapies that are very effective for both depression as well as for more serious severe depression and other illnesses.

So I think we have to raise the floor, and this is your opportunity. And that is why we are so grateful that you have so many committees interested in this, and that is why, if there was one thing I could ask based upon my years of experience, it would be: do something that is systematic.

We do not necessarily need more grant programs. We know they work. There are great things going on out there. You heard it from the panelists. Now, it is about taking it to scale.

Senator CASEY. Great. Thank you very much.

The CHAIRMAN. Thank you.

Senator Thune?

Senator THUNE. Thank you, Mr. Chairman. And thank you to the panel for all your great insights today.

I just want to ask, Mr. Thomas, according to the Utah Department of Human Services' website, suicide was the leading cause of preventable death in Utah in fiscal year 2014. As you may know, South Dakota has experienced high rates of suicide, particularly among young people, and particularly on our reservations and in our tribal communities.

So my question is, what strategies has your department employed in order to reduce the high suicide rate in your State, and what are some of the other traits that you have noticed in successful suicide prevention programs? And maybe, if you could, talk a little bit about tele-health as an early intervention technique that might help or if it has been used in your success out there.

Mr. THOMAS. Thank you, Senator Thune.

We have a State Coalition for Suicide Prevention, and what we have done is, we have taken that State coalition and we have built up some of the substance use disorder prevention coalitions and had them add in suicide prevention as one of the things that they are addressing at the local level.

So we have over 40 coalitions that are attacking this problem at the local level throughout our State. We have had people from Zero Suicide, which is a national effort to lower the suicide rate and to have us look at comprehensive care; we have had experts come in. We have done surveys and studies with our workforce to find out gaps in their knowledge.

We have brought in training for them. Many people even in our field do not have the training that they need to address suicide specifically. So we have brought in evidence-based training to our State to target suicide-specific actions, behaviors, thoughts.

Another thing that we have done is, we have worked with all of our health-care providers, our health-care system, as well as our local mental health and substance abuse authorities, to have a standardized language and a standardized screening and risk assessment process.

So we are using the Columbia Suicide Severity Rating Scale. IHC, Intermountain Healthcare, our largest provider, has already implemented that into their health-care record, their electronic health record, as well as in their emergency room, crisis, and outpatient settings.

Then our local authorities—they are also the county providers— are implementing that. So everyone will be talking about risk the same way. Our crisis lines, they are doing the same training, and then we are also using the same safety plan, the Stanley Brown safety plan, which is top-of-the-line and really gets at five different factors to try to keep people safe. We have done a lot of campaigns and had a lot of legislators, local legislators, who have helped us pass some bills to target this issue as well, and we feel like we are making progress.

As you have said, we have had a really high suicide rate, along with the other intermountain States, and for the first year, a year ago, our data showed that we have actually dropped that rate a little bit. One person dying from suicide is too many, which is why we are part of the Zero Suicide initiative, and I feel strongly and passionately about this issue.

Tele-health for rural Utah—we have two counties that are over 7,000 square miles. One has 15,000 people, another has 60,000 people in it. Tele-health is definitely part of the solution, part of the answer, but we need to develop local resources as well, and have local trained staff to be able to help families and communities.

It does not always have to be professionals, but we do need professionals involved in the care, and tele-health has been used in our State to try to address this. It is not to scale. It needs more infrastructure, but it is definitely something that is part of the solution.

I believe it is good in South Dakota, and your Health and Human Services has been a great partner in this. We have had a Region 8 meeting with all of the States in our region to discuss suicide prevention because of the high rates in our region.

Senator THUNE. Thank you.

Mr. MARSHALL. Can I add to that?

Senator THUNE. Yes. Yes, please.

Mr. MARSHALL. I think Ms. Rosenberg was right when she said it needs to be systematic. Sometimes we do too much. As a patient and going through it and now on being a provider, so to speak, one thing I know for sure is, if we start the conversation early—we are talking about intervention in our adolescence—one thing I know for sure is, if we have this conversation in our schools, 50 percent of our problems would go away, because what happens is two things.

One, we have an invalidating environment, and, two, our professionals, our teachers, our parents, they do not know how to identify and deal with it. So that is the first step: being able to start the conversation early and being able to equip our professionals with the things they need to be able to identify it.

You talk about tele-health. There are companies out there, like Lantern and Enjoyables and the X2AIs, where you can deploy resources to those neighborhoods that may not have professionals or a clinic, where we all have telephones. How cool would it be if we are in school and we may not have counselors, because we do not have the budget for it anymore, or a professional, but you can do CBT with a clinician or dialectal behavior therapy or just self- assessment, where you are just talking about a day, instead of invalidating a kid and putting him in isolation, which turns to suicide.

Senator THUNE. I appreciate that perspective on that. I wanted, by the way, to say, Mr. Marshall, as a recognizable professional athlete, how much we appreciate your advocacy for people who struggle with mental illness, and especially for those who have not yet sought treatment.

Since you are a high-profile individual who is known for successfully pursuing treatment for mental illness, if you were going to suggest for somebody where they should start if they need help, particularly young people in some of those examples that you just mentioned where you have kids whose parents do not know how to identify it and teachers do not, where would you suggest they go?

Mr. MARSHALL. Mr. Thomas hit it. They have a program, Peer- to-Peer. The first place our children go to is their friends. So that is why we need to start the conversation, because when my son goes there—he is in elementary School—if he is having issues, if his friend is having an issue, they go to each other. Then what happens?

So I think there are many solutions, but one of the things that I always talk about is educating our kids. Project 375, we are working with this three-tiered program where we are teaching our children how to identify and how to talk about it, because that is what happens.

Even when you go to our young adults, the first outbreak is from the age of 18 to 24. That is on campus. That is peer-to-peer. The first person you go to is a friend or a loved one.

So that would be my answer. It is to start with the conversation. We threw around mental health first aid. I think that is really important not only in our school systems, but also when we talk about our police departments. How do we identify it? How do we deal with it? That is the first step.

Senator THUNE. Thank you for sharing your story. Thank all of you. By the way, we will be optimistic and say that when you play the Packers in the Super Bowl next year, take it easy on their secondary. [Laughter.]

Thank you.

Mr. MARSHALL. Thank you.

The CHAIRMAN. Senator Scott?

Senator SCOTT. Thank you, Mr. Chairman.

The CHAIRMAN. Senator, I have a whole office-full down there that has been after me, and I have been interrupted a few times. I apologize to you, because this is personally a very, very important hearing, and I definitely will pay attention to everything you have said.

I just want you to know this committee takes it seriously, and we are going to do some things here this year that hopefully will get us down the road a bit more. But I am fully aware of how much we need to do.

So we are going to turn it over to the last questioner, unless somebody else walks down, and if you will shut down the committee, I would appreciate it.

If I can just wave to you guys and just say how deeply appreciative I am that you could be here. I am sorry I have had so many conflicts, but the testimony I have heard has been just great.

Senator Scott?

Senator Scott [presiding]. Thank you, Mr. Chairman.

Thank you to all the panelists for being here this afternoon. It certainly is a very important issue that we are seeing, and there is a steady increase in interest around the country, which I think is really good news.

In South Carolina, we really have been on the cutting edge in the use of tele-psychiatry in our State. We have had, since 2009, about 27,800 mental health consultations that occurred using tele-psychiatry.

We think it is the future, frankly, in a number of areas in the medicine field, especially as you look throughout the States like South Carolina where the rural opportunities for access to health care and to mental health services are dwindling. They sometimes seems to be nonexistent.

I would love for the panelists to perhaps comment on the success and the opportunity for more innovation and creativity in the tele-health field, but specifically tele-psychiatry.

When you think about the fact that—my understanding is, when you are looking at it from an emergency standpoint, that the price point is about $3,000 less per episode, which is an important part of a State's consideration. When you think about the individual, there is no doubt that providing access to quality health care when the person needs it the most, especially if you are living in a rural area, is so important that you need to think about tele-medicine.

So I would love to hear your comments on the use of tele-psychiatry and using the whole next iteration of the opportunities from a mental health and a health-care perspective.

Mr. MARSHALL. Well, it is funny, because Tuesday I actually spoke at Collision in New Orleans. It is a tech conference, one of the largest out there. And a couple weeks ago, I spent some time in San Francisco really trying to study this market, because I have been pounding the pavement for a couple years—and I know you guys have been working longer than me—but I have been really frustrated, because my goal is to put a clinician in every single school in America, but now I am finally realizing that that is almost impossible.

So a few mentors of mine have been telling me for a few years that we have to adopt technology. I will say this. It is not to replace, but to assist and also help stand in the gap. There is some amazing technology out there, and I think the reason why it is the solution, part of the solution, a big part of the solution, is because it is accessible, affordable, and scalable.

When you look at our problems now, we are having problems just getting our youth to take up psychology in school. So it would be impossible for us to take one human being and take on a workload of 200 patients, where we can take one tool—and I love what you just threw out there and what you guys are doing in South Carolina—but you can take one tool and that one tool can treat or assist 2,000.

Senator SCOTT. Thank you. Are there any other comments? Then I have a couple more questions and only about 2 minutes left, according to—no longer according to the chairman, but according to the clock. Thoughts?

Dr. BENNINGTON-DAVIS. Senator Scott, I just would echo what Mr. Marshall said. I really like the way that he said assist, not replace. There is something about a human-to-human interaction that, in psychiatry, is particularly powerful.

That said, there are tremendous uses of tele-health. We are seeing it in dermatology, we have seen it in radiology for a long time, and it turns out that the next generation of people really like interacting through technology. So I think we are just seeing the tip of the iceberg.

Senator SCOTT. Thank you. I am going to move on to my next question to try to stay somewhat close to my 5-minute limit.

I would say that one of the areas where we are seeing a lot of emphasis is on our veterans. We have so many men and women who have donned the uniform, willing to sacrifice their lives on behalf of this country, on behalf of freedom, and sometimes they get back and it feels like our VA is failing so many of our veterans.

I know that at home, Scott Isaacks, who runs the Ralph Johnson VA location, has been one of the outliers, frankly, from my perspective. He has done a really good job of using tele-medicine and tele-psychiatry in a positive and powerful way to treat so many of our veterans.

Both of my brothers have served in the military, and my older brother, the unattractive one, has 32 years, has just retired from the Army, a command sergeant major, and focused on the war transition process.

Have you seen a collaboration between the VA and States on addressing some of the issues that our veterans have?

Ms. Rosenberg?

Ms. ROSENBERG. I was hoping you would not ask me.

Senator SCOTT. I am going to ask Mr. Thomas as well. So you can decide who goes first.

Ms. ROSENBERG. I will start. It is complicated.

Senator SCOTT. Yes, ma'am.

Ms. ROSENBERG. Is that a good way to say it? I think the VA often gets a bad rap. I think they do some very excellent things and some very fine work. Often, people are interested in the VA money more than they are interested in veterans, unfortunately. I am being very honest and very direct.

But that said, the VA is also a single-payer system and likes to keep control. So I think collaborations are difficult for them. I think they have made tremendous headway, and I think community organizations have worked very hard to create those partnerships.

I have seen some very good evidence, particularly in the area of the treatment of addictions, where there are some very good partnerships.

Senator SCOTT. Mr. Thomas?

Mr. THOMAS. With our VA, we also have Hill Air Force Base and then a large National Guard contingent in our State. We have worked with all three really well around, in particular, suicide prevention and peer support and outreach.

Those have been the areas where we seem to be able to share a lot of the same ideological and policy directions with them. Our VA, the folks that we interact with, try hard to get—there is some of the stigma that Mr. Marshall talked about in that system, and if I say that I have a problem and get my services through the VA, what will that do to my career?

So I think the clinics that they have started out in the communities, where it does not go on your record, have been really helpful and a step in the right direction.

Senator SCOTT. Perhaps not for right now, but perhaps you can submit it for the record, if you have any shining examples of States where you believe that that coordination is occurring in the most effective way, I would love to hear from you. If you want to respond now, you can, but if you do not mind including that in perhaps a follow-up later, that would be wonderful.

My final question for the panel would be one of the economic impact of the untreated person. I think so often we think about the cost associated with care, the cost associated with treatment. Too often, I believe that we forget that there is a cost to not treating.

I am not quite sure how we monetize and/or figure out how to effectively figure out that cost, but I think we would be remiss if we did not spend a few minutes on the fact that without treatment, the human cost is incredible, and without treatment, the economic cost is measurable, but it is pretty dismal.

Final thoughts?

Dr. BENNINGTON-DAVIS. I will chime in, Senator Scott. We have already mentioned today the early death of people who have mental illness and substance use disorders. I would add the school dropout rates and the tremendous economic and human impact of not being able to be successful in school, and I think those are probably a good start.

Ms. ROSENBERG. I would add to that. If you look at children who have been diagnosed with a serious emotional disturbance, what you see is up to 25 percent of them wind up in jails and prisons. So we then have that cost.

I think additional to that, if you look at Social Security Disability and SSI, the biggest driver is mental illness. So you have lost income, lost taxes, lost wages.

I think it is quantifiable. Lack of treatment does cost us a lot of money as a country.

Senator SCOTT. Yes, ma'am.

Mr. Thomas?

Mr. THOMAS. I would just add, I think those are all the big economic costs, but I think the biggest cost is the tear in the fabric of our families and society, that that is the devastation that occurs when a family member loses someone, whether it is to jail or suicide or early death because of not getting treatment.

Senator SCOTT. Absolutely. Well, thank you.

Mr. MARSHALL. I was going to say Mr. Thomas took all of my words verbatim.

Senator SCOTT. Excellent. I would add that coming out of South Carolina, approximately 38 percent of those between the ages of 18 and 20 are unemployed and 53 percent between 21 and 64 are unemployed. So the impact of mental challenges, mental health and mental illnesses, when you quantify it, it is drastic.

Thank you all for being here and participating in the process of engaging members of Congress, as well as the public, on such an important issue. I want to thank you all for taking the time. As we have heard, this is an incredibly important topic, and frankly, one that we need to spend more time on.

I will continue to work with our colleagues on and off of this committee to address mental illness.

As for our witnesses, once again, please keep us informed on the great work that you all are doing. Thank you for the courage and the commitment to making a difference not only in our own lives and the lives of your community, but of our Nation. We thank you for that.

I would ask that any questions for the record be submitted by Thursday, May 12, 2016.

With that, this hearing is adjourned.

[Whereupon, at 4:20 p.m., the hearing was concluded.]

APPENDIX

Additional Material Submitted for the Record Prepared Statement of Margaret Bennington-Davis, MD, Chief Medical Officer, Health Share of Oregon

Chairman Hatch, Ranking Member Wyden, honorable members of the committee, thank you for this opportunity to offer testimony on mental health services provided through the Medicaid program and Oregon's innovations in service delivery.

I have spent the better part of 30 years as a leader in the mental health services provider community in Oregon and abroad. I have worked as a mental health provider in the community and hospital settings, as a program administrator, and as a leader in organizational change. I have performed hundreds of consultations, both nationally and internationally, on trauma-informed care and the elimination of seclusion and restraints in psychiatric care settings. What I have learned in this time is that behavioral health—stable mental health and freedom from substance use disorders—is simply health. In other words, "health" requires not merely the absence of physical disease but a state of wellbeing in physical, dental, social, and mental health.

Currently, I serve as Chief Medical Officer for Health Share of Oregon, the State's largest Coordinated Care Organization (CCO). Health Share is a transformative model of Medicaid managed care that brings together local health plan, provider, and community organizations to coordinate physical, dental, mental health, and substance use disorder benefits for more than 25 percent of Oregon's Medicaid enrollees.

The CCO model was created by a Medicaid 1115 Demonstration Waiver 4 years ago, and Health Share was a new organization created specifically to fit that model. Even in this short time, the CCO model, which provides financial incentives for improving health care delivery, has allowed us to uncover data to support a simple truth about the population we serve: the most frequent and costly utilizers of Medicaid services are adults who experienced childhood trauma.

This discovery, and the CCO model in general, has brought new attention to and appreciation of the roles of mental illness and addictions in costs and poor health outcomes. As a result, there are initiatives in communities across the State to increase access to mental health and addictions services, integrate behavioral specialists into primary care, and ensure better primary care supports to people with serious mental illness.

In this testimony, I will: explore the promise of the CCO model; describe the impetus of Health Share of Oregon's decision to focus on access to services and promotion of early life health; provide examples of upstream interventions that Health Share believes will bend the cost curve in the long-term; describe the extant mental health system challenges that communities are addressing in Oregon and across the country; and comment on Federal policy challenges in the mental health and substance use disorder space.

Medicaid Coordinated Care Organizations: The Promise of Oregon's Health System Transformation

Oregon's CCOs are regional Medicaid managed care contractors, each with a governance model that reflects its community and health services marketplace. Each CCO has at least one Community Advisory Council that is made up of a majority of CCO enrollees. All 16 CCOs have 2 things in common: they are all different because they each reflect the community they serve, and they share the goals of better care, smarter spending and healthier people. There are a number of programs and incentives designed to help CCOs obtain those goals, including but not limited to:

- Integration of physical health, mental health, oral health, non-emergency medical transportation, addiction residential services, and children's wrap around services into each CCO;
- Withholding 5 percent of CCO budgets to be paid based on performance on robust set of incentive metrics;
- Requiring development of alternative payment methodologies and hosting "learning collaboratives" to spread successful models;
- Requiring CCOs to cover some "flexible services," which are non-covered services that may be more cost effective alternatives to covered services (e.g., vacuums for families whose children suffer from severe asthma; healthy meal vouchers); and
- Requiring CCOs to conduct regular community health needs assessments and implement community health improvement plans.

The CCO model is already showing signs of success. This program is expected to save the State and Federal governments $1.7 billion on Oregon's Medicaid program over the first 5-year demonstration.

Oregon made a significant promise to CMS when it signed the current Medicaid waiver agreement—that through the CCO model, our State would decrease the expected Medicaid spending trend by 2 percent over 5 years, not by cutting the number of individuals served or reducing provider payment rates, but by improving the way Medicaid services are delivered. CCOs did not have much time to make good on this promise, so we began with addressing the highest utilizing and most costly members.

The Need to Work Upstream: What We Learned from the Adverse Childhood Experiences Study (ACES)

When Health Share analyzed those among our 240,000 members who used the most services and led to the highest costs, we began by asking them to describe their lives. The results were compelling. Very often these members were born into unstable housing and chaotic families, and to parents who did not intend to have children and were not ready or able to parent. Some had been in and out of the foster child system early in life; many had been sexually or physically abused. Most did not have childhoods that prepared them to be successful in school. There was often drug use and other high-risk behavior during adolescence. Often their drug use had led to brushes with the criminal justice system. Many became parents themselves when they were not yet ready or able to parent. Most had various erratic behaviors, depression, or suicidal tendencies that led them to require services in specialty mental health if they could get access, or to jails or hospitals if they could not. Many had never finished school, and many had more than one chronic physical condition.

This is exactly what the Adverse Childhood Experiences Study (ACES), published in 1998, revealed: there is a powerful relationship between adversity and toxic stress during childhood and our physical and mental health as adults, as well as the major causes of adult mortality in the United Stated.

We know that almost half of children in the United States grow up in poverty, which is an important social determinant of health and contributes to child health and developmental disparities. Growing up in a stable and healthy home, in a language rich environment, and having access to quality preschool and regular well visits to a medical home are all critical for developing social and emotional competencies in children as they prepare to enter school. Evidence also shows that kindergarten readiness and success is linked with later educational success, which in turn is associated with better health and economic outcomes.[1] In other words, if children are prepared mentally, emotionally, and physically for kindergarten, they are more likely to be healthy adults. To be effective parents, adults need to be healthy themselves. To be healthy, they need access to physical, mental, and dental services. The cycle of poverty is one that we, in the health care community, have a role in ending.

Health Share of Oregon, in the face of such evidence, determined that if we are to move the dial on curbing Medicaid costs, we needed to move "upstream" in our efforts to improve health. We needed to build systems and communities that create effective parents and

[1] Jones, D, et al. (2015). Early Social-Emotional Functioning and Public Health: The Relationship between Kindergarten Social Competence and Future Wellness. *American Journal of Public Health*. Vol. 105, No. 11, pp. 2283–2290.

healthy, stable environments for children. To that end, Health Share is focused on helping our members: avoid unwanted pregnancies; access social, physical, and mental health supports during pregnancy; have their basic needs met in order to successfully be able to attach to their new babies; and get the support and guidance they need to be effective parents.

What the Decision to Move Upstream Means for Mental Health Services

Community mental health services have traditionally focused on people who have already developed chronic and severe mental illness. By adding emphasis to early childhood supports and the social determinants of health, focusing on early intervention, partnering with schools, and paying attention to the availability of mental health supports within a community, perhaps we can mitigate the tragic long term effects of the toxic stress described in the ACE study.

Nationally, people with serious mental illness die on average 25 years sooner than the general public;[2] this statistic has been even more severe in Oregon.[3] These early deaths are almost always because of chronic physical illnesses that are modifiable, with the right supports. Oregon's CCOs are working hard to identify those "right supports."

Senator Stabenow's Excellence in Mental Health Act is key to identifying those "right supports" and is, in my view, one of the most important legislative initiatives addressing mental health since the 1960s. This legislation builds on the original Community Mental Health Act, which described the continuum of services required to move from institutional care for people with serious mental illness to the community. Senator Stabenow's legislation now brings us to the important recognition that community mental health services also need to be providing or coordinating primary care because people with serious mental illness may not get health care anywhere else. Oregon is one of the eight pilot States, and improving care in community mental health centers fits in very well with the overall CCO model.

Moving Upstream for Special Populations: Creating Medical Models for Children in Foster Care and Addicted Mothers

Designing Health Care Systems That Work for Children in Foster Care

Through analysis of our population data, which mirror national data, we know that children ages 0–6 in the foster care system have a much higher incidence of asthma, attention deficit disorder, PTSD, and obesity than children in Medicaid who are not in the foster care system. These differences persist in older children, with the addition of much

---

[2] Parks, J., et al. (2006). *Morbidity and Mortality in People with Serious Mental Illness*. Alexandria, VA: National Association of State Mental Health Program Directors (NASMHPD) Medical Directors Council.

[3] (2008). *Measuring Premature Mortality Among Oregonians*. Salem, OR: Oregon Department of Human Services Addictions and Mental Health Division.

higher incidence of depression, and by late teens/early adulthood, the addition of higher incidence of schizophrenia and hypertension. The most surprising finding for us was that these differences persist, and are even higher, in children who were in the foster care system at one time but are no longer involved in the child welfare system. In other words, the experience in the foster care system was not healing, and did not provide a safe way to ensure healthy development, either physically or emotionally. We as a society need to address the root of this issue by ensuring the right supports to parents in the first place, so they keep their children in safe and nurturing families. In the meantime, we at Health Share are also focusing on developing coordination among mental health, dental health, and physical health providers for these kids, and describing what the right supports are for them in those health care arenas.

In October 2015, Health Share launched the Foster Care Advanced Primary Care Collaborative with seven of our area's clinics and clinic systems. The Foster Care APC is a year-long learning collaborative to explore and implement Foster Care Medical Home Models and interventions to better support the health needs of foster children. The collaborative consists of six half-day learning sessions held every other month that are focused on key population dynamics, such as identifying children in foster care, working with victims of abuse, neglect and trauma, understanding child welfare systems and processes, working with foster parents and biological families, coordinating with the mental health system of care, and more. Teams of four to eight staff from each clinic participate in each learning session. On the off months between learning sessions, a Steering Committee meets to help tailor the next session topic to meet needs identified by the clinics as they implement their models. The Steering Committee includes one representative from each clinic system along with a small group of local clinical and population champions from various organizations. These seven clinic systems together provide primary care to more than 1,000 foster children in Health Share's three counties and look to play an integral role in developing a system of care that meets the unique needs of this vulnerable population.

Project Nurture: Serving Pregnant Women with Substance Use Disorders

Another example of a special population that requires our immediate attention if we want to improve the health of future generations is pregnant women with substance use disorders. There are obvious fetal development risks involved with pregnant women battling addictions. These risks can be mitigated with proper treatment, but these women need to feel safe accessing appropriate medical care. To that end, Health Share funded the development of, and continues to support, a program called Project Nurture.

Project Nurture provides prenatal care, inpatient maternity care, and postpartum care for women who struggle with addictions, as well as pediatric care for their infants. Women who are enrolled also receive Level 1 outpatient addiction treatment by certified alcohol and drug counselors (CADCs), and Medication Assisted Therapy (MAT) using methadone or buprenorphine when indicated. Project Nurture's model is to engage women in prenatal care and drug treatment as early in pregnancy as possible, provide inpatient care for their delivery and follow them and their infants for a year postpartum providing case management and advocacy services throughout. Women who participate in Project Nurture are informed of policies regarding Child Welfare reporting and we believe that this transparency facilitates a trusting relationship with providers and allows us to advocate for women and their families whenever possible.

The Importance of Health Coverage to Improving Mental Health in America

Oregon was also an early adopter of Medicaid expansion under the Affordable Care Act (ACA). This was crucial for people with serious mental illness in our State. Without insurance coverage, people could not access community mental health services except for crisis, ERs, and hospitals—the least efficient and effective times and ways to aid recovery, and the most expensive. Nearly everyone in Oregon now has better access to services, and sooner. Things are looking up for people best served in community mental health settings, but we still have a long way to go.

Mental Health System Issues: Levels of Care and Workforce Challenges

One Size Does Not Fit All: Levels of Care in Community Mental Health

Even with nearly universal health coverage in Oregon, access to specialty mental health services is still not necessarily smooth or easy, and the array of services are not as broad and varied as is necessary for optimal health. A contributing factor is glaring holes in availability of certain types of mental health services along the spectrum of levels of care for people with mental illness.

Most community mental health services are office-based outpatient programs. Many people with serious mental illness need more intensive supports initially, and then episodically thereafter.

Intensive outpatient and assertive community treatment (ACT) models offer to literally meet the person where they are, at whatever hour works best for them (a lot of people served in community mental health centers are homeless or without transportation). ACT teams, sorely lacking in many States, including Oregon, are multidisciplinary teams that are on call to the individual 24/7, and help with myriad social supports in addition to psychiatric support. Although these teams require significant up-front investment, it is clear that they are extremely effective and ultimately cost-saving for people who otherwise cannot engage in traditionally administered clinic-based services, and who end up using the most expensive settings—EDs, jails, and hospitals—as their default service systems. Health Share is proud to have funded for our community what we believe to be the first forensic ACT team in the United States—designed specifically for people with high engagement with the criminal justice system.

Independent housing, supportive housing, supported education, and supported employment are also key components of a highly functioning community mental health system. The CCO model was intended to allow Medicaid managed care entities to expand payment for these types of services, which are not traditionally covered health care services. Oregon's CCOs are still learning how to best provide access to these necessary services without reducing payment rates that are largely based on utilization of traditional medical services.

Provider Workforce Challenges

There is a shortage of psychiatrists nationally, including in Oregon; 59 percent of psychiatrists are 55 or older, and not enough physicians are being trained. Federal health authorities have designated 4,000 areas in the United States as having insufficient access to psychiatry—areas with more than 30,000 people per psychiatrist. We need to train more psychiatrists.

In community mental health, workers are often entry-level and overworked. Once experienced, they move on to private practices or hospital settings for better pay and better working conditions. We need to make community mental health more attractive workplaces.

In addition to training more psychiatrists and improving working conditions in community mental health centers, we need to broaden our idea of who provides care (including peers and community health workers) and what that care looks like. The mental health provider community is only just beginning to understand the tremendous power of peer supports in mental health treatment. People with lived experience of mental illness and recovery are often the best coaches and system navigators; they expand the workforce, give relief to over-taxed professional teams, and are extremely effective and well-liked by those they serve. Our systems are working to integrate peers into treatment settings and teams, but there is work to do. Specifically, CCOs and other payers need to develop payment models to support these types of workers.

One program that Health Share has implemented in an attempt to address workforce challenges is Project ECHO. This is a tremendously successful "tele-mentoring" model developed by Sanjeev Arora, M.D. at the University of New Mexico to upskill primary care providers to be able to provide treatment to people with Hepatitis-C. Health Share, in cooperation with one of our founding organizations, Oregon Health and Science University (OHSU), brought the ECHO model to Oregon. Instead of using the model to train PCPs in treatment of HCV, we began by using the technology to train PCPs in psychiatric medication management. Oregon, as noted above, suffers from a shortage of psychiatrists. We used the ECHO model to bring teaching and consultation from psychiatrists to PCPs serving our members and, eventually, across the State. Building on that success, we started a second ECHO model this year, which is upskilling PCPs in developmental pediatrics, teaching them to screen for and treat developmental issues, such as trauma, ADHD or autism.

Medicaid Payment and Policy Issues: The IMD Exclusion, Mental Health Parity, and 42 CFR Part 2

IMD Exclusion

Experts agree that limiting institutionalization is an important policy goal. Oregon remains a national leader in providing long-term care services in home and community settings. However, it seems that the "IMD Exclusion"—the part of the Medicaid rules that prohibits use of Medicaid dollars for adult stays in "institutes for mental disease"—has lost its utility, at least in the context of limiting institutionalization.

The Supreme Court decision in *Olmstead v. L.C.* makes it clear that under the Americans with Disabilities Act (ADA), States are generally required to provide care in a community-based setting provided that the "State's treatment professionals have determined that community placement is appropriate, the transfer from institutional care to a less restrictive setting is not opposed by the affected individual, and the placement can be reasonably accommodated, taking into account the resources available to the State and the needs of others with mental disabilities." Repeal of the IMD Exclusion would not be expected to adversely impact efforts to establish community based care for, but rather to assure appropriate treatment for, those individuals needing care in an IMD.

In its recently released final Medicaid managed care rules, CMS partially lifted the exclusion for certain brief lengths of stay (15 days within a calendar month, up to 30 consecutive days over 2 months). CMS reasons the increased flexibility is warranted by a decline in the number of inpatient psychiatric care facilities and concerns about access issues for those who need inpatient care, and psychiatric boarding in emergency rooms. The limited length of stay, CMS reasons, would preclude the use of IMDs for long-term care, indicating that Medicaid is trying to balance the need for inpatient psychiatric beds with a desire to limit institutionalization.

For consumers, this provides more options if hospital-based care is needed. For provider organizations, this change would offer the opportunity for acute care programs with 16 or more beds to participate in the Medicaid program—and to offer more robust crisis response programs and alternatives to hospitalization.

A full reversal of the IMD exclusion is likely not fiscally practical, but revising the law even further could give providers better incentives to ensure access to the right level of care at the right time.

Allowing States to apply for waiver authority to exclude substance use disorders facilities from the IMD exclusion was a step in the right direction. The length of stay in an acute setting that is necessary for effective treatment of substance use disorders is typically longer than that needed for treatment of mental illness in an acute setting.

Allowing Medicaid payments for IMDs with average inpatient stays that exceed the current 15 day limit, such as 30 or 60 days, would be a stepwise approach to ensuring better access for Medicaid enrollees. Congress could also narrow the definition of IMDs to facilities with more than 30 or more psychiatric beds. These approaches would leave the IMD exclusion itself in place while making access to short- term inpatient care more accessible.

Mental Health Parity

Oregon was very early to ensure parity in access to mental health benefits. Part of what makes Oregon's Medicaid program unique is that in times of economic hardship for the State, rather than limiting the number of eligible Oregonians Medicaid can serve, we choose to use a public, deliberative, and evidence-based process to limit the benefit package, which we call the Prioritized List of Services. For more than 20 years, mental health conditions have been ranked amongst physical health conditions on the prioritized list. However, there are still non-quantifiable issues of parity—the need to be quite advanced in symptoms before getting access to specialty mental health and a high threshold for Medicaid enrollees to access hospitalization (dangerous to self or others). Truly effective parity still needs definition.

42 CFR Part 2: Privacy Protection and Sharing Information in a Coordinated Care Environment

Sharing pertinent health care information about our members is fundamental to providing truly coordinated care. We appreciate the concerns that lingering stigma about behavioral health issues, and substance use disorders in particular, raises for our members. Patients' trust is fundamental to their acceptance of treatment, so privacy is a particular concern for people receiving treatment for addictions. That said, SAMSHA's regulation, 42 CFR Part 2, which prohibits providers and health plans from sharing information about substance use disorder diagnoses and treatment plans with each other—and goes well beyond the privacy protections afforded to other health services through the Health Insurance Portability and Accountability Act (HIPAA)—restricts the sharing of information in a way that is detrimental to the people receiving treatment. As the greater health care community has shown through HIPAA, we are capable of limiting the sharing of information to what is absolutely necessary to provide the best possible care. We are encouraged by SAMHSA's current proposed regulations and hope to move to a regulatory environment where substance use disorder diagnosis and treatment information is treated like any other personal health information.

The Future of Mental Health in America Looks Bright, but We Have Work to Do

I am proud of what we have already accomplished at Health Share of Oregon, and I believe that this regional, collective impact model could work in any community and with other health care payer types. Looking upstream to social determinants of health, including poverty, and preventing trauma and chronic stress in childhood will reduce the incidence of all illness—both physical and mental. I encourage Congress to continue to support the kind of flexibility in the Medicaid program that allows States like Oregon to improve the health of our population and lower costs by focusing on prevention rather than the volume of services used to treat people once they are already ill.

Prepared Statement of Hon. Orrin G. Hatch, a U.S. Senator from Utah

WASHINGTON—Senate Finance Committee Chairman Orrin Hatch (R–Utah) today delivered the following opening statement at a hearing to examine various options on how to address mental health issues in the American health care system:

It is a pleasure to see everyone here today.

Today's hearing will focus on mental health issues in America and the role the Medicaid and Medicare programs play in addressing the needs of those with behavioral and mental health issues. Together, Medicare and Medicaid finance nearly 45 percent of mental health spending in the United States, which amounted to more than $75 billion in 2014 alone.

As the Senate committee with jurisdiction over these programs, it is our responsibility to better understand the drivers behind the growing needs for and costs of these services and to work together to develop better solutions for identifying and treating these issues.

A report issued by the Medicaid and CHIP Payment and Access Commission in June 2015 indicated that the majority of Federal spending on mental health comes out of Medicaid. That same study found that Medicaid is the single largest payer in the United States for all behavioral health services, including mental health and substance abuse. In fact, Medicaid accounted for 26 percent of nationwide spending on behavioral health in 2009, the year with the most recent data.

One of the many difficulties we face in addressing these issues is that Medicaid enrollees with behavioral health diagnoses have varied physical and behavioral health needs. Patients often range from young children who need screening, referral, and treatment for autism or depression to chronically homeless adults with numerous diagnoses including severe mental illness.

In 2011, only one in five Medicaid beneficiaries had a behavioral health diagnoses, but they accounted for almost half of total Medicaid expenditures.

Needless to say, these types of behavioral health issues can seriously impair a patient's quality of life, cause disability, and significantly decrease life expectancy. These types of issues are associated with significantly higher rates of chronic disease, substance use disorders, and inpatient hospitalization among Medicare beneficiaries.

And, in Medicaid, patients with behavioral or mental health diagnoses are more than twice as likely to be hospitalized as those without such diagnoses. The number is drastically higher if the patient also has a substance use disorder.

These high hospitalization rates are major drivers in the cost of our Federal health programs. However, what is more unfortunate is that all too often people with mental or behavioral health issues get no care at all.

According to the 2012 National Survey on Drug Use and Health, nearly 40 percent of adults diagnosed with severe mental illness—such as schizophrenia or bipolar disorder—received no treatment for their illness in the previous year. When you broaden that scope to include all adults with any mental or behavioral illness, 60 percent went untreated for the prior year.

It gets worse.

Every year, suicide claims the lives of 38,000 Americans—more than car accidents, prostate cancer, or homicides. And, about 90 percent of suicides are related to mental illness, according to the National Institute of Mental Health. Utah is not immune from this preventable tragedy. Suicide has been the greatest threat to our young people in recent years, and it is time for everyone to take notice.

This is absolutely tragic. However, the tragic pattern expands beyond the suicide rate as, overall, people with serious mental illness have an average life expectancy that is 23 years shorter than the nationwide average.

Patients and their advocates say the country's mental health system has been drowning for a long time—not from floodwaters but from neglect.

As we talk about solutions, we need to note that the distinction between mental health, mental illness, and severe mental illness is crucial, because each group requires different clinical and policy prescriptions. For example, the current system, proportionally speaking, provides far more support for mental health than severe mental illness. We need to review these priorities and find an equitable solution to ensure that all needs are being met.

Today's panel will give us an opportunity to hear from witnesses who can speak to these issues from almost every perspective. We have an advocate who has suffered with these issues firsthand. We also have experienced professionals who will share their experiences providing care at the local, State, and Federal levels and who can speak to the successes and limitations of providing care in each of those environments.

I look forward to hearing the testimony of today's witnesses and beginning a dialogue with my colleagues on these important issues that, hopefully, will lead to better solutions.

Prepared Statement of Brandon Marshall, Executive Chairman and Co-Founder, Project 375

Thank you, Mr. Chairman, Ranking Member Wyden, and members of the committee. I'm grateful for the opportunity to speak before the U.S. Senate Finance Committee on an issue which not only affects me, but millions of people across America: the impact of stigma in the mental health community, and the critical need to make it easier for people to get assessed and treated and be able to lead a normal, fulfilled life.

My name is Brandon Marshall—father, husband, son, friend, a man of faith, wide receiver in the NFL, and co-founder with my wife Michi Marshall of the nonprofit Project 375. Our mission is to end the stigma surrounding mental illness, fostering open dialogue that encourages people to recognize symptoms and seek help.

As a public figure, my actions have been in the spotlight for years, both on the gridiron and off. I was diagnosed with Borderline Personality Disorder in 2011. Before then, as many people may know, my life was a living hell. Yet I didn't know why. It was hard to control my emotions and manage my life effectively, and the situation was only magnified by the tough-it-up culture of football.

For me, the tipping point came when I became so isolated and depressed that I stopped talking to my wife and family. I descended further and further, but it simply felt like the new normal. What the tabloid headlines said wasn't the true reality of my suffering—the isolation and depression were.

Finally, I was persuaded to visit McLean Hospital near Boston and got evaluated in a supportive environment where I felt people actually understood me. Just getting the diagnosis made me feel 50 percent better. And getting the right treatment plan transformed my life.

Why did it take so long to get help? The biggest factor was the stigma surrounding mental illness. I saw how ashamed others felt. This was what motivated me and my wife to launch Project 375. The journey I went through was difficult. I wanted to help others take that first step, the hardest one to take. By many accounts, I am the first public figure to stand up and publicly admit to the world a diagnosis of BPD. Going public was hard. It's no less hard for others struggling with undiagnosed mental illness.

In football, there's stats—lots of them. People obsess over the stats. My fans can rattle off mine. Here are three:

- I hold the record for most receptions—21—in an NFL game.
- I'm one of only five players in NFL history to have at least 100 receptions in three seasons.
- I hold the NFL record for most receiving touchdowns in a single Pro Bowl game.

In the realm of football, those numbers are impressive. But there are other stats that should make more of an impression on everyone here today. Here are 10 of them:

- 1 in 3 people will experience a psychiatric disease in their lifetime.
- Over 60 million Americans are afflicted by mental illness during any one year.
- The suicide rate has risen over 24 percent since 1999, making mental illness one of the only illnesses that has seen an increase in mortality rates.
- An estimated 17 million youth in the U.S. live with a psychiatric disorder, more than the number of children with cancer, diabetes and AIDS combined.
- Anxiety disorders are the most common mental illness, affecting close to 18 percent of adults in the U.S.
- Among the 20 million American adults who experience a substance use disorder, more than 50 percent have a co-occurring mental illness.
- Nearly 8 percent of Americans will experience PTSD at some point in their lives. People who suffer from PTSD are nine times more likely to experience issues of drug and alcohol abuse and dependence.
- Mental illness is associated with increased occurrence of chronic diseases such as cardiovascular disease, diabetes, obesity, asthma, epilepsy, and cancer.
- According to the American Psychiatric Association, while awareness of mental illness is increasing in the United States, there is a worsening shortage of psychiatrists.
- One silver lining: Many Americans do not understand that common mental illnesses can be successfully treated most of the time, including a 70 to 80 percent success rate for treatment of depression.

The prevalence of mental illness in the United States is reflected across society: from homelessness to incarceration to suicide. Often it goes unreported, or simply unnoticed, until it claims the life of a well-known figure, such as Robin Williams. The stigma surrounding mental health issues is our last great fight on this frontier.

Ask yourself: would you feel ashamed being diagnosed with cancer? No, of course not. With the first symptoms you'd get diagnosed and treated, whether through surgery, radiation or chemotherapy. Would you be afraid you'd be fired from your job if you were diagnosed with HIV/AIDS? We've conquered that frontier—the answer is no. However, many people still wonder: Are you sure you won't be fired if you're diagnosed with Bipolar II or BPD? Would your child be invited to a birthday party or sleepover if he or she is diagnosed with anxiety disorder, OCD, or maybe schizophrenia?

A staggering 75 percent of those who need help do not seek it because of the stigma. Because they fear what others may think, and how it may negatively impact them. Without help and treatment the consequences are dire—unemployment, incarceration, substance abuse, and even death. According to Dr. Scott Rauch of McLean hospital and a board member of Project 375, people are still hiding in corners, avoiding treatment, fearful of being labeled, afraid of losing their jobs.

I founded Project 375 with my wife out of our shared pain—and an understanding that millions of others could be helped by my stepping into the light. Talking about my BPD was liberating, but it was also scary—because of the stigma, I could have lost everything. Every time we release a video, send a tweet or publish a post, we hear from people who were inspired to finally take that step forward, to seek help, and to share their story.

We need to provide health coverage for brain Illnesses in the same way we would any other physical illness or, in other words, treat the brain like we would any other organ in the body, making "Check Up from the Neck Up" part of routine exams, so we normalize treatment of mental health and addiction. We must accept mental illness as a disease, and like any other disease, it needs better research, screening and funding. We need better recognition of new therapeutic treatments that are proven to work. We need more robust education in schools, the enlightened support of news and entertainment media, and the advocacy of high-profile figures, like myself, willing to step forward. None of this happens if we still remain silent about these issues!

As an NFL wide receiver, I've caught hundreds of passes during my career. Today, I'm throwing one, to you. Thank you.

Prepared Statement of Linda Rosenberg, MSW, President and CEO, National Council for Behavioral Health

Thank you to the members of the committee for inviting me to be with you today. On behalf of the National Council for Behavioral Health, I appreciate the opportunity to talk with you about the challenges and opportunities facing our mental health system.

Last week, the Centers for Disease Control and Prevention released data showing a steady growth in suicide rates in the United States each year since 1999, increasing by 25 percent in the last 15 years. Deaths by suicide are rising among adolescents and youth . . . among middle-aged Americans . . . and among older adults.

This news was especially difficult for me because I serve on the Executive Committee of the Action Alliance for Suicide Prevention. Despite growing attention to the issue of suicide prevention, our Nation hasn't been able to move the needle. Shining the spotlight of public attention into the shadows of mental illness is not enough.

There is rising public attention everywhere we look. This week, the *New York Times* featured a story about the Portland Police Department's efforts to improve how they handle crises. As Portland's police chief put it, "we are working in the backdrop of a fractured mental health system that has gotten worse and worse."

Talk of mental health and addictions has reached the presidential campaign trail, where candidates are making the issue a major platform of their campaigns. Governor Kasich, whose brother has been diagnosed with schizoaffective disorder and whose home State of Ohio saw more than 2,700 residents die of a drug overdose in 2014, has called for more services. And on the other side of the aisle, Hillary Clinton has released a comprehensive plan to address treatment and recovery.

Six hundred thousand Americans have taken a Mental Health First Aid course. The public is hungry to learn how to recognize the signs of mental illness, to be able to respond in an emergency, and to know where you can get help. Teachers, first responders, veterans, clergy, construction crews—the demand continues to grow.

So, yes, everyone—from Portland cops, to the candidates for President, to friends and colleagues—is talking about mental health and addictions. But as the numbers show, it is not enough. It's not enough for the more than 41,000 Americans who died by suicide last year. It's not enough for the more than 28,000 who died from an opioid overdose.

It's not enough, but not because of stigma, and not because we don't know what works in preventing these tragic deaths. It's because of how rarely those interventions are available—across settings—to reach people in their moment of need.

Life-saving treatments are too often delivered through Federal, State or local grants. When patients have cancer or heart disease, getting access to chemotherapy or a stent doesn't depend on their local clinic having a grant that targets those conditions. Treatment for mental illness and addiction should be no different.

Today, Congress has the opportunity to change the course of millions of lives. The question before you is not, "where are we now?" but "where do we need to be?" To get there, we need to move from talk to action: from raising awareness to connecting people with help. Here's how we can do it:

- Access: Expand access to a full continuum of services delivered in the context of robust and sustainable community-based delivery systems.
- Science-based care: Invest in evidence-based services, delivered by a skilled workforce that leverages technology and is held accountable for outcomes.
- Integration: Ensure mental and physical health care is integrated, services are coordinated, and high-need, high-cost populations are targeted.

Access

To answer the question of "where do we need to be?" let me begin with the issue of the shortage of psychiatric hospital and residential beds. Currently, the Medicaid Institutes for Mental Disease (IMD) exclusion makes it difficult for inpatient and residential facilities to expand. This has led to proposals to eliminate the IMD exclusion entirely or raise the permitted number of beds.

In some communities there is a need for more beds, and these inpatient facilities represent an important part of the spectrum of care. However, at their core, these services are designed to help people experiencing a sudden and severe deterioration of their health. Inpatient services will never be fully effective in a vacuum. Instead, they must be delivered in the context of a continuum of care. Only community-based services can prevent re-admissions, trauma, and disruptions to home and work. At a time when we are growing Accountable Care Organizations and Medical Homes, beds aren't enough.

That's why the National Council is so proud to support the Excellence in Mental Health Act, which enables and sustains quality community treatment systems, and facilitates the coordination of care across health care settings.

The Excellence Act demonstration established criteria for Certified Community Behavioral Health Clinics (CCBHCs) that provide mental health and substance use services and primary care screening—along with care coordination. When care in a different setting is needed, CCBHCs coordinate with that facility to ensure seamless transition into and out of care. CCBHCs must also collaborate with schools and justice systems to keep individuals out of jail, at work, and in school. In turn, organizations that meet the criteria to be a CCBHC qualify for a Medicaid reimbursement rate that supports expanding services, serving new populations, and engaging patients and families outside the four walls of their clinics.

The comprehensive array of services envisioned under the Excellence Act includes crisis services. There has been talk in policy circles about investing in crisis services, and for good reason: timely access to high-quality crisis care can be the difference between an individual getting the intervention they need and that same individual ending up in the emergency room, jail, or worse.

This is not the first time crisis services have gained prominence in our policy debates—they were also touted in the 1980s as a way to alleviate the burden on overcrowded, understaffed hospitals. Crisis respite centers opened but many, funded by grants, struggled to survive. And, just as with psychiatric hospitals and residential facilities, standing alone, they were not enough.

The integration of crisis care into broader community-based delivery systems is a cornerstone of the Excellence Act, with CCBHCs required to directly delivery 24- hour crisis care (including mobile teams). CCBHCs must also coordinate with law enforcement and criminal justice agencies to ensure they're supporting public safety officers who too often are first responders to a psychiatric crisis.

Importantly, CCBHCs must also coordinate with veterans-serving agencies. As members of our armed forces return from Iraq and Afghanistan, rates of post- traumatic stress disorder and traumatic brain injury are on the rise. Unfortunately, too many veterans cannot access the services they need, in some cases because VA facilities are overburdened or simply inaccessible. CCBHCs are tasked with providing culturally competent care to veterans and members of the armed forces, and are responsible for coordinating that care with other agencies that serve veterans.

The integration of crisis care with community-based care envisioned in the Excellence Act could transform the way people access crisis services in this country—it could quite literally save lives. Unfortunately, it won't be available to all Americans.

Under the Excellence Act demonstration, 24 States are currently planning the comprehensive mental health service reforms that will allow them to certify, pay, and monitor CCBHCs. Yet, the law sets an 8-State limit on those who may ultimately participate—meaning that two-thirds of the planning States will have to stop in their tracks. Every State that wishes to create and sustain quality service systems should be able to do so, and that's why the National Council urges you to allow all 24 States to participate in the demonstration.

Science-Based Care Delivered by a Skilled Workforce with the Support of Technology

To get our Nation's mental health and addiction services to where they need to be, it's not enough to expand access—we must ensure that services are high- quality, evidence-based and delivered in a way that both enables us to measure what's working (or what isn't) and holds us accountable for outcomes.

Unfortunately, the adoption of practices based upon the best available research is limited by a reliance on grants. For example, recent data from the NIMH Recovery After an Initial Schizophrenia Episode (RAISE) study showed the effectiveness of a multi-pronged intervention for individuals experiencing their first episode of psychosis. The intervention included evidence-based practices such as cognitive behavioral therapy along with medication, family psychoeducation, case management, supported education and employment. Despite research here in the United States and around the world, and the allocation of block grant funding, it's not enough. Most communities will be unable to implement the requisite interventions and tens of thousands of young people will be relegated to a life of disability.

Certified Community Behavioral Health Clinics hold the promise of expanding Americans' access to science-based care. CCBHCs are required to offer evidence- based services to meet the specific needs of their communities—and they can be paid a rate inclusive of these activities. Through data tracking and outcome monitoring, clinics will be held accountable not just for delivering these services, but for measuring patients' progress and adjusting course when treatments aren't working as hoped. Clinics that do well will be rewarded with quality bonus payments, another step in our Nation's move toward linking payment with performance, toward much discussed value-based purchasing.

But a key challenge to delivering timely, high-quality services lies in our Nation's shortage of mental health and addiction treatment professionals. The behavioral health workforce needs additional capacity and support to fully meet Americans' need for services. Texas, Iowa, Indiana, Idaho, Nevada, and Wyoming all have fewer than 6 practicing psychiatrists per 100,000 people—in fact, a mere 34 psychiatrists practice in the entire State of Wyoming. Just last week, I spoke with a medical director at a clinic in Texas who has been trying for more than 3 years to recruit a child psychiatrist. His situation isn't unique. Clinics all over the country struggle to recruit and retain staff.

One way Congress can help is by permitting licensed mental health counselors and marriage and family therapists to directly bill Medicare for their services. Technology can also help, playing a crucial role in extending the workforce. Using state- of-the-art streaming video technology, staff can connect with patients to adjust medications, deliver cognitive therapies, and educate and support children and parents. Online treatment platforms such as my Strength help patients manage in their daily life. Mental health and addiction organizations can be helped to adopt electronic health records—a proposal that has received strong bipartisan support—to better track patient outcomes, facilitate the exchange of health information, and coordinate care.

But the fundamental limitation underlying all discussions on the workforce is that most clinics cannot afford skilled staff or the necessary ongoing investments in technology. Those of you on this panel who have ever run a business know this is unsustainable—and it's no way to successfully treat Americans with mental illness and addictions. If we are ever going to alleviate the workforce shortage, we need clinics to be able to afford to hire the right staff and pay them what they deserve. And we need sustainable financing mechanisms that reimburse providers at a rate inclusive of technology costs.

The Excellence Act demonstration offers certified clinics a Medicaid payment rate that bears a rational relationship to the costs they incur. Under the Excellence Act, clinics will be able to hire critical staff—including psychiatrists, midlevel professionals and peers—and leverage new technologies to further extend the reach of those clinicians. They will be to do this because they will receive a sound, predictable and sustainable payment rate that—unlike grant funding—supports the full array of activities of a high-performing clinic and does so in a way that will continue into the future.

Integration

Data show that individuals with serious mental illness have an average age of death at 53, the same as the U.S. life expectancy in 1917. The primary drivers of that early mortality are preventable and/or treatable chronic conditions like heart disease, lung disease, and cancer. Data also tells us that people with chronic physical illnesses often have co-morbid mental illnesses, especially depression and anxiety, that lead to poor health outcomes. Integrated care improves outcomes for both groups.

Earlier this month I had a first-hand experience with integrated care. On a Sunday, I went to an urgent care clinic. Unbeknownst to me, that urgent care clinic was part of an Accountable Care Organization that also included my primary care physician—which I discovered upon showing up at her office on Monday and finding out that they already knew all about the problem that had brought me to urgent care! They had access to my electronic health record and knew what treatment I had received. When my primary care doctor ordered a sonogram, the ACO followed up with a phone call asking if I'd like to use their sonogram provider. That's smart business AND it's good care. The two can, in fact, go together.

Unfortunately, my experience is still all too rare. Far too few health care organizations are equipped to fully coordinate and integrate care in such a way that every patient could reap the benefits I did. But behavioral health is aware of the need to better integrate care, and we are at a tipping point. The Excellence in Mental Health Act, through its creation of CCBHCs, represents a foundational opportunity in the behavioral health safety net to advance the way care is integrated and coordinated.

CCBHCs are required to provide basic primary care screening and monitoring to all their patients, with referrals to and coordination with local primary care providers. In this way, they help reverse the trend of early mortality due to preventable causes among people with serious mental illness; and help primary care providers better address their own patients' ongoing mental health needs.

We know through the SAMHSA Primary Care-Behavioral Health Integration program, which has been funded by Congress since 2009 and has served over 70,000 Americans, that investing in integrated care improves health and reduces costs. For example, after one year in the PBHCI program, results from one grantee site in Travis County, Texas indicated patients had 618 fewer emergency room visits and spent 155 fewer days hospitalized. These outcomes resulted in $1,193,000 saved in a year.

These results were from one clinic operating under a time-limited grant. Just imagine what we'll see when the Excellence Act demonstration's CCBHCs start their operations in January of next year.

Conclusion

The question before you is not, "where are we now?" but "where do we need to be?" Shining the spotlight of public attention into the shadows of mental illness is not enough. We need to move from talk to action and from pockets of excellence to the widespread availability of effective interventions.

The Excellence in Mental Health Act—CCBHCs—is where our mental health system needs to be—financially sustainable continuums of evidence-based treatments supported by and integrated with primary care, 24/7 high-quality crisis services, and a revitalized behavioral health workforce. That's what we can call reform.

Prepared Statement of Doug Thomas, Director, Division of Substance Abuse and Mental Health, State of Utah

Chairman Hatch, Ranking Member Wyden, and members of the committee, my name is Doug Thomas; I am the Director of the Division of Substance Abuse and Mental Health in the State of Utah and I am honored to be here with you today along with these distinguished guests.

Medicaid is the backbone of the public mental health system in Utah and throughout the United States. It provides the infrastructure and economy of scale necessary for States to standardize evidenced based practices to provide high quality care to individuals with serious mental health needs. The various Medicaid waivers and alternative benefit plans available to States allow them needed flexibility to customize plans to fit the unique challenges, needs, and resources of each State. Case Management, Peer Support Services for individuals and families, Psychosocial Rehabilitation and Respite services are great examples of Medicaid reimbursable services that help people stay in their communities despite serious illness and allow people the opportunity to reintegrate in place of being alienated from their families and communities of origin.

In 2009 the Institute of Medicine (IOM) issued a lengthy publication about the prevention and early intervention of mental, emotional and behavioral (MEB) disorders. The report highlights that almost one in five young people have a MEB disorder at any given time and that "among adults in the United States, half of all of these disorders were first diagnosed by age 14 and three-fourths by age 24." First symptoms usually precede a disorder by 2 to 4 years giving us a window of opportunity. Narrowing the gap between the onset of symptoms and evidenced based intervention is critical as the research is showing us that this early intervention preserves executive functioning and allows people, especially young people and people suffering from the first-episode of illness to recover more quickly with less life disruption. This allows them to accomplish and maintain important developmental tasks, such as "establishing healthy interpersonal relationships, succeeding in school, and making their way (into and succeeding) in the workforce." For young people with Medicaid we are able to intervene early with positive outcomes showing that people can and do recover from mental illness. Treating a person's mental illness improves physical health outcomes and reduces overall healthcare costs as well. There have been various Medicaid and other Health systems studies which show that collaborative physical and mental health care lowers costs and improves health outcomes. In Utah 3 years ago with a new State Legislative Appropriation and County matching funds we began to act on the IOM report with what we call Mental Health Early Intervention. This consists of three programs, School Based Behavioral Health, Mobile Crisis Outreach Teams for Youth in four of our five most populous Counties and Family Resource Facilitation with Wrap-Around to Fidelity. Over the last 3 years we have increased services to almost 5,000 more youth, the majority with Medicaid funding. Office Disciplinary Referrals are down,

Literacy scores are up, symptoms of mental illness are being reduced often to the community norm, and families are receiving the supports they need to keep their children safely at home, in their own school, and enhancing their family's natural support system through Peer Support.

Utah recently passed a limited Medicaid expansion designed to target people with the lowest income in the greatest need, parents with dependent children already on Medicaid, people who are chronically homeless, people with mental illness and substance use disorders involved in the criminal justice system and people with mental illness and substance use disorders. We must have Medicaid work with us to find a way to approve a waiver allowing Utah to extend Medicaid coverage to these additional people in need.

People want to be served in the safest, least restrictive environment and providers want to provide these types of services. Sometimes children and adults need care beyond what can be provided appropriately in an outpatient or home like setting. Allowing Medicaid residential services the ability to bill and be paid for room and board would be a great step in the right direction. Room and board is covered during a more costly inpatient hospital stay, but not covered during a more economical residential stay. This disincetivizes local, lower cost, short term residential services in lieu of more costly inpatient hospital care.

With the Patient Protection and Affordable Care Act, The Mental Health Parity and Addiction Equity Act and more integrated care being provided there is a need to modernize the Medicaid Institutes for Mental Diseases (IMD) Exclusion. I applaud the efforts of the Substance Abuse and Mental Health Services Administration, Centers for Medicare and Medicaid Services and the Department of Health and Human Services to modernize rule, including the option of State waivers around the IMD exclusion. It must be done cautiously and systematically to ensure we are not re-institutionalizing people but that we are providing a short-term crisis intervention meant to help people stabilize and rejoin us in our communities where we all work and play and live.

Thank you for the opportunity to testify before you today. If there are any questions I would be happy to respond.

Prepared Statement of Hon. Ron Wyden, a U.S. Senator from Oregon

The Finance Committee is responsible for the programs—Medicare and Medicaid—that spend more on mental health than any others in America. That's why this committee, working in conjunction with others including HELP and Judiciary, must develop a fresh approach for protecting and caring for Americans with mental illness. The focus of that approach should be breaking health care, social service programs, and law enforcement out of their individual silos and bringing them together in a coordinated system that deploys their strengths to help people dealing with mental health issues.

The Wyden family knows a little bit about this subject. My brother struggled with schizophrenia for decades, and he had a lot of health care bills covered by Medicaid. In and out of halfway houses, confrontations with law enforcement officers, problems securing funds for services or treatments—it was certainly something that has confronted millions of families and demonstrates the need for a fresh approach to helping those with mental illnesses.

Instead, because of the lack of appropriate places to go, patients who deal with a lot of the same issues Jeff Wyden did have been boarded in emergency rooms. They've been in fights with police, sometimes deadly. Or they've wound up in prison, where more than half of all inmates suffer from mental health problems, and minorities are vastly overrepresented.

I'll be the first to say that mental health is not an issue that falls neatly under any one Senate committee's jurisdiction. A lot of different members with different areas of expertise will have to pull the same end of the rope to make progress on this front. Senator Stabenow, right on this committee, is a champion of mental health. Senator Murray, the Democratic leader on the HELP Committee is also right at the forefront.

In my view, our efforts on mental health have to be concentrated on three priorities. First, there needs to be a sharp new focus on preventing mental illness. People need better care earlier on to keep illnesses from escalating. And furthermore, there are nearly 2 million low-income, uninsured Americans suffering from mental illness or addiction in States that have not expanded their Medicaid programs. That's 2 million Americans who, without treatment or help, are far more likely to fall into homelessness, far more likely to be incarcerated, far more likely to suffer from addiction, far more likely to commit suicide. The choice to expand Medicaid and give new hope to those 2 million individuals and their families, in my view, should be an easy one to make.

Second, services from health care to social work need to be better coordinated. It doesn't make much sense to tell a person struggling with an illness that they're on their own managing treatments, figuring out what specialists to see, scheduling appointments and handling medications. Even outside the doctor's office there are a lot of areas where people with mental illnesses often need help they're not getting today. Paying the bills. Making it to appointments. Maintaining a home. Taxpayer dollars need to reach deeper into our communities and improve coordination to help people who the system today overlooks.

Third, there needs to be a better link between mental health and law enforcement. In a lot of cases that's going to mean more training on what to do when responding to a person with mental illness. Too many people who should be in proper health care facilities are winding up in jail cells instead. In Portland, the Police Bureau has recently put a lot of work into building a team of specially-trained officers to handle these challenges safely, and it's paying big dividends in the early going. In my view, more agencies around the country ought to follow suit.

The big hurdle in all of this is funding. Each year, mental illness costs the U.S. $450 billion, only a third of which is actually spent on medical care. At roughly $75 billion combined, Medicare and Medicaid make up the biggest slice of the pie. Those are huge numbers, and a lot of the overall total goes to emergency room visits and jail time. In my judgement, if you can shift some of that funding to the three priorities I talked about—preventing mental illness, better coordinating care and services, and linking law enforcement with mental health—you'll see a lot more people successfully managing their mental illnesses and living healthier lives.

This is a tough challenge, and it's going to require a lot of bipartisan teamwork. But I'm optimistic that members will come together to make real progress, and I look forward to today's hearing.

COMMUNICATIONS

American Academy Of PAS (AAPA)

22318 Mill Road, Suite 1300
Alexandria, Virginia 22314
www.aapa.org

On behalf of the more than 108,500 nationally certified PAs (physician assistants) represented by the American Academy of PAs (AAPA), we appreciate the Senate Finance Committee's interest in the state of the American mental healthcare system. While there are numerous policy challenges in this area, the most pressing may be the current shortage of mental healthcare providers. In light of the historical use of PAs to alleviate healthcare provider shortages, the increased number of PAs practicing in psychiatry, and the growing movement towards the integration of primary care and specialty care, AAPA believes that PAs should be—and are well-equipped to be—better utilized in the provision of mental healthcare.

According to the Substance Abuse and Mental Health Services Administration (SAMHSA), an estimated 43.6 million Americans experienced some type of mental health issue in 2014. While the Affordable Care Act (ACA) attempted to make mental healthcare more accessible, many individuals who suffer from mental illnesses continue to go without treatment. For instance, SAMHSA's National Survey on Drug Use and Health found that in 2014, more than 15 million adults reported having a major depressive episode in the previous year. Yet, one third of those individuals did not seek the assistance of a mental healthcare provider. Although a variety of factors likely account for this disparity, the U.S. Department of Health and Human Services recently estimated 90 million people lack access to mental health and addiction medicine providers. Many of these individuals live in rural and medically underserved areas, where there are little or no options for public transportation and the nearest mental healthcare provider may be hours away. It is clear that more must be done to make treatment for mental illnesses more accessible for this population, as well as the public at large.

While early intervention for suspected mental illness is essential to ensuring positive mental and physical health outcomes for all patients, it is particularly important in the populations served by Medicare, Medicaid, and the Children's Health Insurance Program (CHIP), as they are typically less likely to have access to comprehensive and coordinated healthcare. SAMHSA has found that half of adults who have mental illnesses began showing symptoms by age 14. In 2014, more than 11% of youth between ages 12 and 17 had experienced a major depressive episode in the prior year. However, fewer than half of them received treatment or counseling. When combined with the everyday struggles of many families who rely on Medicaid or CHIP, it is easy to see why early intervention in mental healthcare issues within this population is essential.

At the same time, SAMHSA has estimated that 25% of older Americans have reported some kind of mental health problem, and 6.5 million seniors have been diagnosed with depression. As in younger populations, treatment for mental health issues in the Medicare population is necessary to ensure better healthcare outcomes across the board. Yet, an ongoing shortage of mental healthcare providers combined with continued struggles to better coordinate healthcare for all populations has meant that many individuals who are in the highest-need demographics are falling through the cracks. While there are many factors involved in creating a better mental healthcare system, AAPA believes better utilization of PAs in federal healthcare programs is essential to solving the overall access problem.

PA Education and Practice

PAs receive a broad education over approximately 27 months which consists of two parts. The didactic phase includes coursework in anatomy, physiology, biochemistry, pharmacology, physical diagnosis, behavioral sciences, and medical ethics. This is followed by the clinical phase, which includes rotations in medical and surgical disciplines such as family medicine, internal medicine, general surgery, pediatrics, obstetrics and gynecology, emergency medicine, and psychiatry. Due to these demanding rotation requirements, PA students will have completed at last 2,000 hours of supervised clinical practice in various settings and locations by graduation.

The majority of PA programs award a master's degree. PAs must pass the Physician Assistant National Certifying Examination and be licensed by a state in order to practice. The PA profession is the only medical profession that requires a practitioner to periodically take and pass a high-stakes comprehensive exam to remain certified, which PAs must do every 10 years. To maintain their certification, PAs must also complete 100 hours of continuing medical education (CME) every 2 years.

PAs practice and prescribe medication in all 50 states, the District of Columbia, and all U.S. territories with the exception of Puerto Rico. They manage the full scope of patient care, often handling patients with multiple comorbidities. In their normal course of work, PAs conduct physical exams, order and interpret tests, diagnose and treat illnesses, assist in surgery, and counsel on preventative healthcare. The rigorous education and clinical training of PAs enables them to be fully qualified and equipped to manage the treatment of patients who present with both physical and mental illnesses.

PAs and Mental Healthcare

PAs are recognized along with physicians and nurse practitioners under Medicare, ACA, and other federal healthcare programs as one of the three types of primary care providers. Overlap between primary care and mental healthcare has traditionally existed, particularly in settings which provide care for the medically under-served like hospitals, community health centers, rural health clinics, free clinics, and jails and prisons. This is largely due to the fact that many of these facilities' patients suffer from both physical and mental ailments and have little ability to obtain either primary or mental healthcare. In these situations, providers will often work to treat the whole patient. The interface between primary care and mental healthcare is becoming more common due to the growth of alternative payment models within Medicare, as well as efforts to better coordinate patient care at the federal level. As a result, primary care providers in all settings are beginning to offer mental health screenings, arrange "warm handoffs" to a mental health specialist, or work in tandem with a specialist via telemedicine or other means.

Many of the mental healthcare bills currently before Congress acknowledge the interface between primary healthcare and mental healthcare. Today, there are approximately 30,000 PAs practicing as primary care providers who are on the "front lines" of care. This means even if they do not specialize in mental healthcare, a significant number of PAs care for patients who reside in medically underserved areas and present with complex or comorbid conditions affecting both their physical and mental health. According to data collected by AAPA in 2015, 10% of all patients cared for by PAs suffer from depression. An additional 5% suffer from behavioral or other psychiatric conditions other than depression. PAs who practice in primary care are qualified to provide a full spectrum of healthcare services for these patients, including conducting patient histories and examinations, performing psychiatric evaluations and assessments, ordering and interpreting diagnostic tests, establishing and managing treatment plans, prescribing medications, and ordering referrals as appropriate, and they should be fully utilized as members of the care team.

At the same time, it is important to note that a growing number of PAs are receiving additional education to specialize in psychiatry. While Medicare recognizes these PAs as reimbursable mental healthcare providers, they are not always included in legislation as mental health professionals along with psychiatrists, psychologists, clinical social workers, and psychiatric nurse practitioners. PAs in psychiatry work in behavioral health facilities, jails and prisons, and psychiatric units of rural and public hospitals. These PAs are credentialed and privileged affiliate members of the medical staff who provide both initial and ongoing care to patients. Given the current shortage of providers in this field, it is critical that PAs in psychiatry be fully included as part of the mental healthcare team.

Recent Legislative and Administrative Actions

There have been some notable efforts in recent proposals by both Congress and the administration to better integrate PAs into mental healthcare. In March, the Senate Committee on Health, Education, Labor and Pensions (HELP) favorably reported S. 2680, the Mental Health Reform Act of 2016, a comprehensive bill directed at improving access to mental healthcare. AAPA supports this legislation because it acknowledges the role of primary care providers in assisting patients with mental illnesses, aims to increase coordination of care for patients needing primary and mental health care, and includes PAs in psychiatry among the specialty providers listed in the bill.

Additionally, the Health Resources and Services Administration (HRSA) recently acknowledged the role of PAs in mental healthcare and addiction medicine in its FY17 budget request by including them in the definition of "behavioral health workforce." AAPA is pleased by this recognition, and we support HRSA's efforts to further integrate primary care providers like PAs into mental healthcare by encouraging the use of screenings, referrals, and telemedicine to connect patients with mental health specialists when appropriate, all of which have been shown to improve patient outcomes and mitigate gaps in coverage caused by too few providers.

AAPA Legislative Recommendations

As the Committee works on solutions to the mental healthcare access problem, AAPA hopes you will consider the following recommendations:

1) Affirmatively including PAs in mental healthcare legislation as members of the healthcare team. This inclusion is important for all types of healthcare legislation, but it is especially important in mental healthcare given the critical level of provider shortages in this field. Moreover, as the Committee works on continuing to integrate primary care into mental healthcare, PAs should continue to be counted among primary care providers who may assist their patients in receiving mental healthcare when it is appropriate.
2) Including "PAs in psychiatry" as mental healthcare providers. Mental health legislation has historically included a number of specified mental healthcare providers, but left out PAs who specialize in psychiatry. There is a growing number of PAs who receive additional education to specialize in this field, and they work in behavioral healthcare centers and other high-need facilities. These PAs should

be included in any definition of mental healthcare provider as a result of their qualifications and experience. S. 2680, the Mental Health Reform Act, is an example of how PAs can be included as part of the solution to mental healthcare provider shortages.

AAPA looks forward to working with the Committee as you move forward on these important issues.

American Association for Geriatric Psychiatry (AAGP)

The American Association for Geriatric Psychiatry (AAGP) appreciates this opportunity to comment on the status of Mental Health in America. AAGP is a professional membership organization dedicated to promoting the mental health and well being of older Americans and improving the care of those with late-life mental disorders. AAGP's membership consists of geriatric psychiatrists as well as other health professionals who focus on the mental health problems faced by aging adults. Thus AAGP brings a unique perspective to the consideration of unmet mental health needs that plague our public healthcare services. We would like to take this opportunity to highlight the geriatric mental health workforce crisis that has crossed our nation's doorstep.

The 2012 Institute of Medicine (IOM) report "The Mental Health and Substance Use Workforce for Older Adults: In Whose Hands?" clearly highlights that our current and future capacity to manage the complex medical needs of older adults with mental health or substance use conditions is grossly insufficient.

The aging of the baby boomer generation will result in an increase in the proportion of persons over 65 from 12.7 percent currently, to 20 percent in 2030, with the fastest growing segment of the population consisting of people age 85 and older. During the same period, the number of older adults with major psychiatric illnesses will more than double, from an estimated 7 million to 15 million individuals, meeting or exceeding the number of consumers in discrete, younger age groups. In addition, 8 million Americans are estimated to have Alzheimer's disease by 2030, nearly all of who will have neuropsychiatric or behavioral symptoms that will require expertise in geriatric mental health from all clinical disciplines.

Virtually all health care providers need to be fully prepared to manage the common medical and mental health problems of old age. In addition, the number of geriatric health specialists, including mental health providers, needs to be increased to provide evidence-based care for those older adults with the most complex issues and to support and train the rest of the workforce as partners in collaborative care.

Unfortunately, workforce estimates for geriatric mental health do not look promising. By 2030, it is estimated there will be only 1,500 geriatric psychiatrists across the country, compared to the 4,000 to 5,000 needed based on estimates from the National Institute on Aging. Current rates of training geriatricians (~175 fellows per year) lag far behind what is needed (~1,200 fellows per year) to reach the goal of having 30,000 trained and providing care to our elders in 2030. Geriatric training is also rare among other common members of the geriatric mental health care team. For example, only 1% of Nurses, Pharmacists and Physician Assistants; ~2.6% of Advanced Practice Nurses; and ~4% of Social Workers have geriatric certification. Only 3% of Psychologists work primarily in elder care.

The 2012 IOM report recommended Congress appropriate funds that authorize training, scholarship, and loan forgiveness for individuals who work with or are preparing to work with older adults who have mental health or substance use conditions. We strongly encourage the Committee to ensure funding opportunities prioritize mental health training that focuses on the needs of vulnerable groups across the life span, including older adults.

Supporting training for geriatric mental health will improve access to evidence- based, high quality health care for our elders and will ensure recruitment and retention of top professionals into geriatric mental health practice. The well-being and dignity of our elders requires action now to ensure the workforce is prepared.

Submitted by: Christopher Wood
Executive Director
American Association for Geriatric Psychiatry
6728 Old Mclean Village Drive
Mclean, VA 22101, (703) 556–9222

Statement Submitted by John Boronow, MD

I am a practicing psychiatrist who has lived in Maryland for 35 years. I specialize in the treatment of schizophrenia and other "severe and persistent" mental disorders. I worked at Sheppard Pratt back in the days of the IMD exclusion, when there were no Medicaid adults. Later came the waiver, and since then, the State of Maryland has supported Medicaid patients until last autumn. I have treated Medicaid inpatients for nearly 20 years, in addition to the Medicaid outpatients I have always treated since opening my practice. I also am an Associate Clinical Professor of Psychiatry at the University of Maryland and teach residents and medical students daily about public policy toward this patient population.

The IMD exclusion is simply another example of an historical anachronism that has lingered on well beyond its original intended life span. It was created in an era before deinstitutionalization, when asylums and private hospitals ran a parallel existence and when there were virtually no psychiatric inpatient units in general medical hospitals. Medicaid was invented right alongside the Community Mental Health Act in the mid 1960s to transform the delivery of behavioral healthcare. The intent of the IMD exclusion was to prevent state hospitals from gobbling up new Federal dollars to maintain an otherwise dying model of care, and to prevent rich private hospitals from accessing funds for institutions that frankly did not need them.

When Sheppard Pratt first treated our Medicaid adults in the late 1990s, we had already started to build a continuum of care including day hospitals, crisis residential care, and residential rehabilitation programs in suburban apartment complexes.

For us, access to Medicaid enabled us to treat thousands of severely and persistently ill mental patients who were in Maryland emergency rooms. What we brought to the table was expertise: a small 20 bed general psychiatric unit has to treat all comers, and it is impossible to be expert at all things. But a large IMD with great depth is able to do more than just do crisis intervention, and can actually successfully treat complex cases which would otherwise be overwhelming to small programs.

It is time to end the IMD exclusion. Deinstitutionalization is done, and it was done so poorly that in fact we have transinstitutionialized patients from state hospitals to the criminal justice system. We need now to finish the work: to deinstitutionalize the laws (which limit commitment to bricks and mortar facilities instead of to a system of care in the community) and to update the funding rules like the IMD exclusion, which exclude patients from centers of excellence that can actually solve difficult clinical challenges instead of just kicking them down the road in the endless cycle of "revolving door" hospitalizations. IMDs are now part of the solution, they have changed with the times, and the funding should now finally follow suit.

Statement Submitted by Evelyn Burton

Thank you for allowing this opportunity for public input on how the Finance Committee can improve the Mental Health System.

Limited Medicaid funds need to be targeted more to treatment of those with Serious Mental Illness who are at high risk for homelessness, incarceration, victimization, and suicides. This will save both lives and money.

I urge the repeal of the discriminatory Medicaid Institutions for Mental Diseases (IMD) exclusion which denies medically necessary appropriate psychiatric hospital care to adults with severe mental illness. For no other conditions are Medicaid services excluded in certain medical institutions.

If you decide to limit the number of days authorized in an IMD, I urge you to allow at least 30 consecutive days, regardless to the month. The proposed rule of allowing 15 days per month in an IMD is unworkable from a medical prospective. If the intent is to allow 30 days to a patient who enters an IMD on the 15th of the month, why should others who require a 30 day stay and enter an IMD on the first of the month be kicked out after 15 days? Will patients be encouraged to wait in the ER until the 15th of the month or told by their doctor to wait 15 days and increase the risk of criminalization, or suicide? Will the IMD try to discharge them to a general hospital for one day and then readmit them? This type of rule encourages high risk game playing with the lives of the seriously mentally ill.

The IMD exclusion policy of Medicaid is a barrier to hospital treatment and stabilization, and also reduces the incentive for expansion of hospital beds.

I have personally seen individuals, with schizophrenia and bipolar disorder, in many families, that cycle continually between Community Hospital, homelessness, and jail, because they are never adequately stabilized in the very short hospitalizations provided by most general hospitals, Those lucky enough to have private insurance that pays for a longer stay in an IMD have been better stabilized and are less likely to be quickly rehospitalized or incarcerated.

I even know of one family that withdrew their family member from Medicaid so that they could pay privately for a 6 week stay at an IMD, to achieve stabilization and stop the frequent hospitalizations. It was very successful. That individual has not been hospitalized now for over 10 years, thus saving Medicaid millions of dollars. Those on Medicaid should have the same opportunity for stabilization.

The IMD exclusion is a disincentive for expansion of critically needed hospital beds and has contributed to a shortage of hospital beds nationwide. This results in Emergency Room boarding and driving vast numbers of those with serious mental illness into the criminal justice system. In Maryland over 90% of the state hospital beds are now taken by forensic patients, and there is no availability for non-forensic patients. Also those in my County jail may wait for weeks for a hospital bed, denying their right to proper medical treatment.

The IMD Waiver Demonstration Program for hospitals has shown reduced costs with the use of IMDs. It is past time to act on those results, stop discrimination against those with serious mental illness, and save lives.

The IMD exclusion for outpatient residential services is also highly detrimental for those with serious mental illness and needs to be repealed entirely or at a bare minimum, allow for much larger facilities than 16 beds. Some with serious mental illness do NOT recover to the point of being able to live independently or with part time supervision. However they can live in the community with intensive supervision and this is much less costly and more humane than frequent hospitalizations or incarcerations. Allowing Medicaid payment for outpatient residential treatment in facilities over 16 beds would allow for the economic expansion of critically needed residential treatment beds. Larger facilities do not mean that the residents would be "institutionalized." Just like those living in Senior Communities, or Assisted Living Facilities, those in a residential outpatient treatment program can be engaged in community activities.

I also urge repeal of the discriminatory Medicare lifetime limit on psychiatric hospital days. There is no lifetime hospital limit for any other illness. It denies critical treatment to the most vulnerable of our elderly population and contributes to the very high suicide rate in the elderly.

Thank you for your consideration.
Sincerely,
Evelyn Burton, consumer and family advocate.

Clinical Social Work Association (CSWA)

P.O. Box 10
Garrisonville, Virginia 22463
(Office) 703–522–3866
(Fax) 703–522–9441
www.clinicalsocialworkassociation.org

The Clinical Social Work Association (CSWA) would like to thank you for the opportunity to comment on this hearing. CSWA serves as the Voice of Clinical Social Work, representing the 240,000 licensed clinical social workers in the country, the largest single group of independent mental health clinicians.

It is well documented that untreated or undertreated behavioral health problems tend to become more severe, and often exacerbate other medical conditions as well. That coverage for mental health conditions continues to be less broad than what is offered for medical conditions turns logic on its head, ultimately increasing overall health care costs.

When the Paul Wellstone and Pete Domenici Mental Health Parity and Addiction Equity Act of 2008 (MHPAEA) passed, licensed clinical social workers and their patients were hopeful that the ways in which mental health disorders were under-treated and under covered by insurers would be resolved. Sadly, what we have seen instead are numerous coverage restrictions on mental health treatment, imposed by insurers by means of limits on "acceptable" diagnoses and/or treatment methods, frequency of sessions, length of treatment, and patient access to out of-network clinicians.

The lack of precise definitions for parity standards has been a major failure of MHPAEA. This problem can be seen clearly in area of "non-quantitative" treatment limitations, where insurers restrict treatment authorization on the basis of "treatment progress" when in fact there is no absolute way to determine treatment progress except when the patient has fewer hospitalizations, when the patient and clinician agree the patient has less emotional suffering, has *more significant and continuing impact* on improved mental health (Levy, et al., "The Efficacy of Psychotherapy," *Psychodynamic Psychiatry,* 42(3) 377–422, 2014). Additionally, the cross- discipline surveys done by *Consumer Reports* (1995, 2004 and 2008) show that psychotherapy provided by psychologists and licensed clinical social workers have widely positive results in treating depression, anxiety, trauma-based disorders, and even psychotic disorders.

Where in-patient mental health treatment is concerned, we understand that budgetary consequences must be addressed—and decisions based—on a realistic assessment of the costs of providing adequate mental health and physical health care. However, we would be remiss if we failed to point out two glaring gaps in mental health treatment for chronic and severe conditions:

- The limitation to 190 days of inpatient treatment for psychiatric reasons. There is no such limitation on medical conditions, and clearly this violates MHPAEA.
- The lack of *any* coverage for Medicaid beneficiaries who need inpatient mental health care in what are called Institutes for Mental Disease. The IMD restrictions are unfair, and cause harm to those who need inpatient care for mental health conditions.

We ask that the Task Force add these two coverage gaps—limitations which have a devastating effect on individuals coping with chronic mental health conditions (as well as their families and communities)—to the range of issues under consideration.

On a more general level, CSWA would like to note the following concerns:

- As clinicians, we have long been aware of the inadequate coverage of chronic mental health conditions on the inpatient and outpatient level. We are concerned, as well, that the critically important integration of medical/surgical care and mental health/substance use care continues to be elusive.
- Another area of CSWA concern is the general lack of attention to diversity that we believe has been a major factor in the successful delivery of health care and mental health treatment. Cultural competence is not just basic to our clinical social work approach to treatment, but fundamental to any health or mental health treatment. Understanding of the patient's ethnicity, gender, sexual orientation, economic levels, race, age, religion, and other areas of personal identity is essential.
- Finally, Accountable Care Organizations, with their goal of creating delivery systems that would share profit and loss with providers, have great potential for controlling overall healthcare costs in America. However, mental health treatment is, at present, seriously underfunded, and we fear that ACOs will not be viable as health care delivery systems for treatment of chronic mental health conditions

without a significant increase in funding. The fiscal targets that are to be met must be realistic or this form of funding mental health treatment is likely to fail.

There is no question that mental health treatment is cost effective in the long run, often preventing other health problems and/or more severe mental health problems. We applaud the work of the Task Force in reviewing the range of issues hindering parity in mental health and substance use treatment, and look forward to your final report.

Thank you for the opportunity to make these comments.

Healing Minds NOLA

2206 Soniat St.
New Orleans, LA 70115
(504) 274–6091

Statement Submitted for the Record by Janet Hays Dear Chairman Hatch and respected members of the committee,

I am the wife of someone with a serious mental illness (SMI) as well as an advocate for alternatives to incarceration, homelessness and death for mentally ill people in my community.

As the director of Healing Minds NOLA, an organization I began last year, I hear from many residents who struggle with the broken mental healthcare system. The most tragic stories always involve the inability of the caregiver to ensure that their loved ones with serious mental illness are getting—and taking—medications necessary to manage their illness. Funding should be directed to evidence-based programs and services that provide support to that group of people.

- Assisted Outpatient Treatment (AOT) is legal in almost every State in the nation and avoids hospitalization. It's a compassionate and creative approach to getting care to more difficult cases where a person's disease has become more powerful than the person. AOT ensures that a person follows their treatment plan in order that they can make competent decisions for themselves. When a person is medication compliant, it reduces conflicts that can escalate in families and communities and helps to prevent incarceration for unacceptable behavior. By keeping sick people out of corrections institutions, they preserve their civil rights and right to self-determination and stay out of the downward spiral that leads to further deterioration and further costs to society. AOT should be funded and scaled up.

Our son doesn't have a behavior problem, he suffers a brain disease; he should be put into an AOT program, ordered by a judge, not dropped from a useless program because he didn't follow rules he signed in a contract. Many uninformed preach, it's all about stigma. They're wrong, it's all about non-treatment.

Treatment before tragedy is what we need, not yoga and art classes that are wonderful for relaxation and enjoyment but do nothing in the needed medical care for the sickest of the sick in this country right now.

Parents need to be able to take part in their adult child's commitment and care, not even notified their loved one is in a psychiatric hospital until after being released after the 72 hour hold and being homeless because they have rights.

As our son is so ill he has a human right to medical care to be a productive person again, hopefully. What some in power to make changes in this broken system of ours don't realize is that some don't get well, some untreated don't even live.

We need a workable bill to help families in mental illness crisis, not a watered down one like those representing their own personal interests here to keep their federal and state jobs are pushing for. They callously don't want to believe our son has a medical disease and has a right to treatment. H.R. 2646 offers all this to bring on reform.

Thank you for the opportunity, Nancy J. Jones.

Statement Submitted by Marilyn Martin

1) There are three *Federal laws* that need to change, the first two within your purview: (1) the IMD exclusion, which excludes Medicaid patients from psychiatric facilities that have more than 16 beds, such as Sheppard Pratt in Maryland. (2) The lifetime Medicare hospitalization limit is discriminatory. There are no other limitations on physical illnesses. My son's schizophrenia is a neurobiological disease. (3) HIPAA laws that prevent caretaker families like mine from knowing basic information that would be helpful in keeping our loved ones in care. For example, I should have been notified that my son had just fired his clinic provider a couple of weeks prior to his recent assault on my husband. Since I had no HIPAA release (because my son had lost insight to his illness), I was not notified. I later learned that he had even run out of the pills that were no longer working, but they did help him sleep. Lack of sleep is a trigger for psychosis.
2) *Professional Shortages:* We need more neuro-psychiatrists, and we need for them to be better compensated—because treated SMI (neurological brain diseases) can be extremely challenging, and often dangerous. We also need more incentives for clinical licensed social workers to treat the SMI rather than the "worried well." My son was able to find one therapist at his clinic who was effective for a few months before she left the clinic to return to school. She was the only therapist he was

willing to see during the entire 8 years since his first psychosis. These community clinics have high turnover and difficulty in attracting highly qualified professional staff.

3) *Beds.* Maryland needs more beds for psychiatric disorders. This is especially crucial for patients such as my son, who has had to wait for a bed on several occasions.
4) Many disorders and diseases currently referred to as mental illnesses are actually neurological disorders, according to NIH. My 32-year-old son has schizophrenia. Although I believe that early treatment provides better outcomes, I do not believe that the word, "prevention" has meaning for the families of those with serious neurological brain diseases. (I believe in higher funding for brain research would help with that.)
5) My son was recently placed on a new injectable antipsychotic that I believe is effective. His SSDI and SSI payments are so low that he would not be able to afford any increase in paying for them should Medicare reduce reimbursement. He does not need another excuse for opting out of his monthly injections. He's already done that in the past. To save money, perhaps injectables could be administered by a nurse rather than a doctor?
6) Limited funds need to be focused on the more serious brain illnesses. One reason treatment is expensive is that many of our state-level "behavioral health" treatment laws actually *promote* disability. For example, my son recently spiraled into a serious psychosis after decompensating on a medication that had stopped working—he had developed a tolerance to it. Every time a person relapses like this, the likelihood of his returning to his previous level of functioning is lowered because he's lost grey matter. Many states, such as mine, will only allow us to get our loved ones who lack insight back into appropriate treatment when they become "dangerous." *States should be rewarded for having more reasonable commitment standards.* Hence, we had to wait until my son became psychotic and assaulted my spouse. He is now awaiting trial. *States should be rewarded for having an Assisted Outpatient Treatment statute.* This way, those few with a history of decompensating repeatedly could be kept out of the criminal justice system before it is too late. If my son is fortunate enough to receive long-term in-patient care rather than jail time, he should be able to be stabilized enough to learn how to manage his chronic illness, thereby staying appropriately medicated. An additional problem is that my state's "disabilities law center" emphasizes getting out of the hospital within 72 hours rather than focusing on keeping these patients in treatment. Promoting very short stays places limits on stabilizating on new medications. This is counterproductive for a patient with a serious illness like schizophrenia, who would need at least 2–3 weeks to stabilize on a new antipsychotic medication. My son has had at least 16 hospitalizations within the

past 8 years, all very short. Mr. Cornyn seems to have some understanding of the issues we have with noncompliance. Thank you, Mr. Cornyn.

Thank you for your interest in mental health for which we have a good system. I had no trouble finding good trauma therapy for PTSD after my son's recent assault. However, for serious mental illness (brain disorders) there is no reliable system, and family care givers are worn out, stressed out, often fearful, and left out from useful information from providers due to HIPAA. Please take action soon to help us save lives, keep our loved ones out of prisons, or trying to survive as homeless.

Mental Illness Policy Org

Unbiased Information for Policymakers + Media
50 East 129 Street, Ph7, New York, NY 10035
http://mentalillnesspolicy.org

We thank Senator Hatch for his opening statement which identified the single most important core issue:

> As we talk about solutions, we need to note that the distinction between mental health, mental illness, and severe mental illness is crucial, because each group requires different clinical and policy prescriptions. For example, the current system, proportionally speaking, provides far more support for mental health than severe mental illness. We need to review these priorities and find an equitable solution to ensure that all needs are being met.

One-hundred percent of Americans can have their mental health improved. Twenty percent have a mental health diagnosis. These are often mild and remit on own. But only 4% have a serious mental illness like those suffered by the brother of Senator Wyden (schizophrenia) and father of Senator Stabenow (bipolar disorder).[4] Those serious mental illnesses are not preventable or identifiable before the symptoms become manifest which is usually in late teens and twenties. So elementary school age interventions are not likely to bend the curve.

It is seriously mentally ill adults, not children or the worried-well who are most likely to become homeless, arrested, incarcerated, suicidal, and dangerous to themselves or others. Congress should reject pressure to move funds to younger groups, groups without mental illness, and programs that promise "prevention." Congress should keep its eye on

---

[4] Substance Abuse and Mental Health Services Administration (SAMHSA). *"NSDUH 2013 Report:* Substance Use and Mental Health Estimates from the 2013 National Survey on Drug Use and Health: Overview of Findings." Rockville, MD, September 2014. Available at http:// store.samhsa.gov/shin/content/NSDUH14-0904/NSDUH14-0904.pdf.

getting treatment to adults known to have serious mental illness. Congress has tended to balkanize funding. It funds programs for children, seniors, veterans, pregnant women, LGBT, high school students, college students, African Americans, Native Americans, immigrants and other special sub-populations. The mental health industry has convinced funders that bad grades, single parent households, unhappy marriages, underemployment, unemployment, sexual confusion, criminal involvement, and other issues are "risk-factors" and diverted funding for them. For example, there are 5,500 suicides of individuals under age 24 and Congress allocates $55 million to preventing those. But there are 37,500 suicides in those over 24 and Congress only allocates $2 million to them.[5] Under pressure from the mental health industry, Congress is spending where suicide is not, rather than where it is. Creating these multiple priority populations, leaves less for the elephant in the room: getting treatment to adults known to have serious mental illness, what should be the core population. But there are rarely programs targeted to them.

Congress should ensure that both *existing funds and incremental funds* are spent on interventions that meet these three criteria: have independent evidence; improve a meaningful outcome like reducing homelessness, arrest, incarceration, homelessness and hospitalization; and reduce violence in people with serious mental illness.

Programs to Eliminate

Virtually none of the programs funded by SAMHSA meet those three criteria. We have documented SAMHSA's failure at http://mentalillnesspolicy.org/samhsa.html. SAMHSA funds antipsychiatry and pseudo-science. It declares non-evidence based practices to be evidence based, encourages states to use mental health block grant funds Congress appropriated for mental illness on people without mental illness, refuses to focus on the seriously ill, refuses to focus on improving meaningful outcomes, and wastes money. There is little support for SAMHSA other than from those who receive funds from it. Their own employees rated is the 319th worst federal agency and its former top doc just wrote an op-ed explaining that she left SAMHSA largely for the reasons I just explained. Congress should take funds that go to CMHS unit of SAMHSA that don't help the seriously ill move them to programs that do help. Any CMHS programs that are worthy of continuing can be moved to NIMH, IOM, CDC, DOJ and other entities that will use them more appropriately.

PAIMI. PAIMI has moved off its original purpose of preventing abuse of the institutionalized mentally ill to preventing treatment of the seriously ill. There is not a mental health director who has tried to improve services for the seriously ill who has not found a PAIMI advocate on the other side. PAIMI responsibilities can be moved to the CRIPA unit within DOJ which is largely duplicative.

---

[5] Testimony of SAMHSA Acting Director Kana Enomoto at House Appropriation Hearing: Substance Abuse and Mental Health Services Administration Budget, March 2, 2016. Available at https://www.youtube.com/watch?v=Mke5HKRusMI.

Programs to Support

Programs that have independent evidence they improve a meaningful outcome in people with serious mental illness and should be expanded include:

- Assisted Outpatient Treatment (AOT). We no longer have to make a binary choice between the total removal of rights via incarceration and involuntary commitment and unfettered freedom in the community. By allowing judges to order a small group of the most seriously ill *who already have a history of violence, incarceration, or homelessness* to accept mandated and monitored treatment in the community, it reduces homelessness, arrest, incarceration and violence in the 70% range. This is all the more outstanding because AOT is only for the most seriously ill who have not been helped by voluntary services. By replacing expensive inpatient hospitalization and incarceration with less expensive outpatient treatment, it cuts the cost to taxpayers in half. A fact sheet is enclosed.
- Access to hospitals. Eliminate the IMO Exclusion. As a result of the IMO Exclusion, states lock the front door and open the back causing incarceration of the seriously ill. There are 10 times as many mentally ill incarcerated. Because IMO amelioration can be expensive (because CBO does not score offsetting savings) we suggest starting with providing IMD relief to non-forensic state hospital beds. There are very few of those left, so the cost would not be excessive. Congress could also raise the number of beds from 16 to say, 24 which would allow IMO funds to go to the seriously ill without dramatically increasing costs. Another approach would be to allow IMO relief for X number of hospital days. CMMI issued regs that allow 15 days of hospital care per month, but that only affects capitated patients. Congress should mandate it for non-capitated ACA enrollees. A *Washington Post* op-ed is enclosed.
- Group Homes. Some of the most seriously mentally ill do not do well in the independent supported housing currently being promoted. They are now well enough to manage a household and drive-by case management is not enough. They need on-site 24/7 support of the kind that can be found in group homes.
- Clubhouse Model programs. Congress should establish (or direct CMMI to establish) a bundled Medicaid rate for clubhouse programs. Clubhouses, like New York's Fountain House, are unique in that they serve the most seriously ill. However, the unique model, whereby several patients can be served at once does not neatly fit the Medicaid model.

Finally, we urge Congress to give those of us who provide housing and case management services to seriously mentally ill out of love, the same access to information paid providers receive. HIPAA and FERPA prevent the families of people from seriously ill from knowing the diagnosis, treatment, medications and pending appointments. We are therefore powerless to see prescriptions are filled and appointments kept.

As Michael Biasotti, former President of the NYS Chiefs of Police told a House Energy and Commerce Committee, "We have two mental health systems. The traditional mental health system helps those well enough to volunteer for services. Those who are not well enough to volunteer are turned over to criminal justice. The mental health system seems unwilling to accept responsibility for this more symptomatic group." The main task of the Finance Committee should be to reorient services back to the seriously ill. Thank you. Attached are fact sheets on some of these issues.

Sincerely,

D.J. Jaffe Executive Director

How the Federal Government Can Help the Most Seriously Mentally Ill

Focus on the 4% with serious mental illness, not just the 18% with poor mental health.

Background: Some of the most seriously mentally ill (SMI), unlike people with less severe "mental health issues" hallucinate, are delusional, psychotic, and can't think straight (cognitive impairment). Some need periodic hospital care, a small group will never recover, and some as a result of cognitive impairments and anosognosia, are unwilling or unable to stay in treatment even when available and offered to them. Most mentally ill are not violent, but when the seriously mentally ill go untreated, they are at higher risk of violence.

Policy	Which seriously mentally ill does it help?	How it helps
Fund Assisted Outpatient Treatment	AOT helps a very small but important group of the most seriously ill who because of inability or unwillingness to stay in treatment *already* accumulated *multiple* incidents of homelessness, arrest, violence, incarceration, or hospitalization *after* being offered voluntary services that were made available to them. This small group, because of their known history, is the most likely to again become hospitalized, homeless, arrested, incarcerated and possibly violent. Note: AOT is *not* an alternative to community services. AOT is a way to help the seriously ill access community services. http://mentalillnesspolicy.org/national-studies/aotworks.pdf	*Extensive replicated research* shows AOT helps SMI stay in existing community treatment and avoid expensive and rights-depriving inpatient commitment and incarceration. • 74% fewer participants experienced homelessness • 77% fewer experienced psychiatric hospitalization • 83% fewer experienced arrest • 87% fewer experienced incarceration • 81% said AOT helped them get and stay well • Reduces hospitalization incarceration costs 50%.

Policy	Which seriously mentally ill does it help?	How it helps
Repeal Institutes for Mental Disease (IMD) Reform	IMO repeal would help a small group of the most seriously mentally ill who even if there were perfect community services cannot survive safely in the community be- cause medications and other treatments do not work for them or they require the much more intensive support than the higher functioning. The IMO Exclusion prevents reimbursement for this care and is federally sanctioned discrimination against the seriously ill. It affects no other group and should be eliminated. (http:// mentalillnesspolicy. org/imd/imd-nasmhpd.html)	Hospitals reduce incarceration America's mentally ill held in— Prison 2001: 600,000 Mental Hospitals 2001: less than 50,000
Remove "HIPAA Handcuffs"	HIPAA reform would help seriously mentally ill who have families willing to provide housing, case management, and financial support to them. But HIPAA prevents families from being told the diagnosis, what medications and rehabilitation is needed, and therefore cannot see prescriptions are filled and transportation arranged. (http://mentalillnesspolicy.org/ national studies/HIPAA_handcuffs.pdf)	By giving Moms and Dads who provide care out of love the same information that paid providers receive parents can prevent their relatives from becoming too psychotic to keep at home and from becoming a government responsibility.
Eliminate or Reform SAMHSA	*SAMHSA elimination* would help the most seriously ill who need help based on the scientific "medical model" rather than the SAMHSA-invented "recovery model" which requires patients to self-direct their own care, something some of the most seriously ill cannot do. (http://mentalillnesspolicy.org/samhsa. html)	SAMHSA elimination would free states of the SAMHSA-instituted obligation to use Mental Health Block Grants for people without mental illness and curtail SAMHSA funded consumer trade association from lobbying against hospitals and other treatments that help the most seriously ill. It would stop SAMHSA funding antipsychiatry, the certification of programs that do not have independent evidence, etc. This would save taxpayers money while helping SM get care. The few useful programs can be transferred to CDC, NIMH, IOM, etc.
Require PAIMI to focus on abuse and neglect	Persons with serious mental illness who have been subjected to "abuse or neglect." (http://mental illnesspolicy.org/myths/ paimifails2011sam hsaevaluation.html)	PAIMI primarily focuses on "freeing" the non-seriously ill from care, rather than helping the seriously ill access it. Threat of suits prevents states and hospitals from helping the seriously ill. Having PAIMI focus on abuse and neglect would reduce both.

The Washington Post, December 30, 1999

Pretending these issues don't exist is causing massive homelessness and incarceration of the seriously ill. Federal legislation tends to focus on higher functioning, and/or less important issues. Following are specific policies that would help persons with the most serious mental illnesses. Prepared by Mental Illness Policy Org. http://mental illnesspolicy.org, May 14, 2015.

FEDERAL NEGLECT OF THE MENTALLY ILL

D.J. Jaffe and Mary T. Zdanowicz

The recently released Surgeon General's Report on Mental Health is the equivalent of describing the maiden voyage of the Titanic without mentioning the iceberg. While the report criticizes private insurance companies for failing to provide "parity" in their coverage of mental illnesses, it is totally silent on the failure to provide parity in Medicaid, the federal government's insurance program.

For the most severely mentally ill, private insurance is essentially meaningless. Because of their illnesses, most are indigent, and private insurance is a luxury they cannot afford and are not in a position to obtain through employment.

Many of these individuals do have insurance through Medicaid a federal insurance program that covers their care, except for a single exception—inpatient care in psychiatric hospitals. The federal government's Institution for Mental Diseases (IMD) exclusion prohibits Medicaid from reimbursing for most individuals who need care in a psychiatric hospital. If you have a disease in your heart, liver or any other organ and need treatment in a hospital, Medicaid contributes. But if you have a disease in your brain and need care in a psychiatric hospital, Medicaid does not.

As a result of this federally sanctioned discrimination, state psychiatric hospitals are locking the front door and opening the back, making it increasingly difficult for the most severely ill to get inpatient treatment. They are discharging patients sicker and quicker in a headlong dash to make them Medicaid eligible by ending their inpatient residency.

There were about 470,000 individuals receiving inpatient psychiatric care in state hospitals when the Medicaid program started in 1965, compared with fewer than 60,000 today Hospital closures have actually accelerated in recent years. Forty state hospitals shut their doors between 1990 and 1997, nearly three times as many as during the entire period from 1970 to 1990, and many more closings are planned.

Of the 3.5 million Americans with schizophrenia and manic-depression, 40 percent (1.4 million) are not being treated. Medicaid's denial of coverage results in homelessness, incarceration, victimization and even death for many people who are so ill they are unable to care for themselves. By the Justice Department's own statistics, there are currently about 283,800 mentally ill people locked up in the nation's jails and prisons.

All Studies Show Assisted Outpatient Treatment (AOT) Reduces Homelessness

AOT Study/Source	Findings
Substance Abuse and Mental Health-Services Administration (SAMHSA) National Registry of Evidence based Practices and Programs (NREPP) 2015.	"Although numerous AOT programs currently operate across the United States, it is clear that the intervention is vastly under utilized."
Agency for Healthcare Research and Quality (AHRQ) U.S. Department of Health and Human Services Management Strategies To Reduce Psychiatric Re- admissions May 2015.	AOT "programs improve adherence with outpatient treatment and have been shown to lead to significantly fewer emergency commitments, hospital admissions, and hospital days as well as a reduction in arrests and violent behavior."
Department of Justice "Crime solutions: assisted out- patient treatment" http://www.crimesolutions.gov/ 2012.	Assisted outpatient treatment is an effective crime prevention pro-gram.
Bruce Link, Matthew Epperson, Brian Perron, Dorothy Castille, Lawrence Yang. "Arrest outcomes associated with outpatient commitment in New York State." *Psychiatric Services* 62, no. 5 (2011): 504–508.	"For those who received AOT, the odds of any arrest were 2.66 times greater (p<.01) and the odds of arrest for a violent offense 8.61 times greater (p<.05) before AOT than they were in the period during and shortly after AOT. The group never receiving AOT had nearly double the odds (1.91, p<.05) of arrest compared with the AOT group in the period during and shortly after assignment."
Allison Gilbert, Lorna Mower, Richard Van Dorn, Jeffrey Swanson, Christine Wilder, Pamela Clark Robbins, Karli Keator, Henry Steadman, Marvin Swartz. "Reductions in arrest under assisted outpatient treatment in New York," *Psychiatric Services* 61, no. 10 (2010): 996–999.	"The odds of arrest for participants currently receiving AOT were nearly two-thirds lower (OR=.39, p<.01) than for individuals who had not yet initiated AOT or signed a voluntary service agreement."
Marvin Swartz, Christine Wilder, Jeffrey Swanson, Richard Van Dorn, Pamela Clark Robbins, Henry Steadman, Lorna Moser, Allison Gilbert, John Monahan. "Assessing outcomes for consumers in New York's assisted outpatient treatment program." *Psychiatric Services* 61, no. 10 (2010): 976–981.	"The likelihood of psychiatric hospital admission was significantly reduced by approximately 25% during the initial six-month court order . . . and by over one-third during a subsequent six-month renewal of the order. ... Similar significant reductions in days of hospitalization were evident during initial court orders and subsequent renewals. ... Improvements were also evident in receipt of psychotropic medications and intensive case management services. Analysis of data from case manager reports showed similar reductions in hospital admissions and improved engagement improved services."
Jo Phelan, Marilyn Sinkewicz, Dorothy Castille, Steven Huz, Bruce Link. "Effectiveness and outcomes of assisted outpatient treatment in New York State." *Psychiatric Services* 61, no. 2 (2010): 137–143.	Kendra's Law has lowered risk of violent behaviors, reduced thoughts about suicide, and enhanced capacity to function de-spite problems with mental illness. Patients given mandatory outpatient treatment—who were more violent to begin with—

AOT Study/Source	Findings
	were nevertheless four times less likely than members of the control group to perpetrate serious violence after undergoing treatment. Patients who underwent mandatory treatment reported higher social functioning and slightly less stigma, rebutting claims that mandatory outpatient care is a threat to self- esteem.
New York State Office of Mental Health, Kendra's Law: Final Report on the Status of Assisted Outpatient Treatment. Report to Legislature, Albany: New York State, 2005, 60.	Danger and violence reduced • 55% fewer recipients engaged in suicide attempts or physical harm to self • 47% fewer physically harmed others • 46% fewer damaged or destroyed property • 43% fewer threatened physical harm to others • Overall, the average decrease in harmful behaviors was 44% Consumer outcomes improved • 74% fewer participants experienced homelessness • 77% fewer experienced psychiatric hospitalization • 56% reduction in length of hospitalization • 83% fewer experienced arrest • 87% fewer experienced incarceration • 49% fewer abused alcohol • 48% fewer abused drugs Consumer participation and medication compliance improved • The number of individuals exhibiting good adherence to meds increased 51% • The number of individuals exhibiting good service engagement increased 103% Consumer perceptions were positive • 75% reported that AOT helped them gain control over their lives • 81% said AOT helped them get and stay well • 90% said AOT made them more likely to keep appointments and take meds • 87% of participants said they were confident in their case manager's ability • 88% said they and their case manager agreed on what was important to work on

(Continued)

AOT Study/Source	Findings
Jeffrey Swanson, Richard Van Dorn, Marvin Swartz, Pamela Clark Robbins, Henry Steadman, Thomas McGuire, John Monahan. "The cost of assisted outpatient treatment: can it save states money?" *American Journal of Psychiatry* 170 (2013): 1423–1432.	In New York City net costs declined 50% in the first year after assisted outpatient treatment began and an additional 13% in the second year. In non-NYC counties, costs declined 62% in the first year and an additional 27% in the second year. This was in spite of the fact that psychotropic drug costs increased during the first year after initiation of assisted outpatient treatment, by 40% and 44% in the city and five-county samples, respectively. The increased community-based mental health costs were more than offset by the reduction in inpatient and incarceration costs. Cost declines associated with assisted outpatient treatment were about twice as large as those for voluntary services.
Marvin Swartz, Christine Wilder, Jeffrey Swanson, Richard Van Dorn, Pamela Clark Robbins, Henry Steadman, Lorna Moser, Allison Gilbert, John Monahan. "Assessing outcomes for consumers in New York's assisted outpatient treatment program." *Psychiatric Services* 61, no. 10 (2010): 976–981. Marvin Swartz, Jeffrey Swanson, Henry Steadman, Pamela Clark Robbins, John Monahan. "New York State assisted outpatient treatment program evaluation." Duke University School of Medicine, Durham, NC, 2009	"We find that New York State's AOT Program improves a range of important outcomes for its recipients, apparently without feared negative consequences to recipients." • **Racial neutrality:** "We find no evidence that the AOT Program is disproportionately selecting African Americans for court orders, nor is there evidence of a disproportionate effect on other minority populations. Our interviews with key stakeholders across the state corroborate these findings." • **AOT improves the likelihood that providers will serve seriously mentally ill:** "It is also important to recognize that the AOT order exerts a critical effect on service providers stimulating their efforts to prioritize care for AOT recipients." • **AOT improves service engagement:** "After 12 months or more on AOT, service engagement increased such that AOT recipients were judged to be more engaged than voluntary patients. This suggests that after 12 months or more, when combined with intensive services, AOT increases service engagement compared to voluntary treatment alone." • **Consumers Approve:** "Despite being under a court order to participate in treatment, current AOT recipients feel neither more positive nor more negative about their treatment experiences than comparable individuals who are not under AOT."

AOT Study/Source	Findings
Michael Heggarty. "The Nevada County Laura's Law experience." Behavioral Health Department, Nevada County, Nevada County, CA, November 15. 2011	In Nevada County, CA, AOT ("Laura's Law") decreased the number of Psychiatric Hospital Days 46.7%, the number of Incarceration Days 65.1%, the number of Homeless Days 61.9%, and the number of Emergency Interventions 44.1%. Laura's Law implementation saved \$1.81–\$.2.52 for every dollar spent, and receiving services under Laura's Law caused a "reduction in actual hospital costs of \$213,300" and a "reduction in *actual* incarceration costs of \$75,600."
Marvin Southard. "Assisted Outpatient Treatment Program Outcomes Report" Department of Mental Health, Los Angeles County, Los Angeles, CA, February 24, 2011.	In Los Angeles, CA, the AOT pilot program reduced incarceration 78%, hospitalization 86%, hospitalization after discharge from the program 77%, and cut taxpayer costs 40%.
Virginia Hiday, and Teresa Scheid-Cook. "The North Carolina experience with outpatient commitment: a critical appraisal." *International Journal of Law and Psychiatry* 10, no. 3 (1987): 215– 232.	In North Carolina, AOT reduced the percentage of persons refusing medications to 30%, compared to 66% of patients not under AOT.
Mark Munetz, Thomas Grande, Jeffrey Kleist, Gregory Peterson. "The effectiveness of outpatient civil commitment." *Psychiatric Services* 47, no. 11 (1996) 1251–1253.	In Ohio, AOT increased attendance at outpatient psychiatric appointments from 5.7 to 13.0 per year. It increased attendance at day treatment sessions from 23 to 60 per year. "During the first 12 months of outpatient commitment, patients experienced significant reductions in visits to the psychiatric emergency service, hospital admissions, and lengths of stay compared with the 12 months before commitment."
Robert Van Putten, Jose Santiago, Michael Berren "Involuntary outpatient commitment in Arizona: a retrospective study." *Hospital and Community Psychiatry* 39, no. 9 (1988): 953–958.	In Arizona, "71% [of AOT patients] ... voluntarily maintained treatment contacts six months after their orders expired" compared with "almost no patients" who were not court-ordered to outpatient treatment.
Barbara Rohland. "The role of outpatient commitment in the management of persons with schizophrenia.'" Iowa Consortium for Mental Health Services, Training and Research, 1998.	In Iowa "it appears as though outpatient commitment promotes treatment compliance in about 80% of patients. After commitment is terminated, about ¾ of that group remain in treatment on a voluntary basis."
Treatment Advocacy Center. "Success of AOT in New Jersey 'Beyond Wildest Dreams.'" Treatment Advocacy Center. September 2, 2014.	In New Jersey, Kim Veith, director of clinical services at Ocean Mental Health Services, noted the AOT pilot program performed "beyond wildest dreams." AOT reduced hospitalizations, shortened inpatient stays, reduced crime and incarceration, stabilized housing, and reduced homelessness. Of clients who were homeless, 20% are now in supportive housing, 40% are in boarding homes, and 20% are living successfully with family members.

(Continued)

AOT Study/Source	Findings
Virginia Hiday, Marvin Swartz, Jeffrey Swanson, Randy Borum, H. Ryan Wagner. "Impact of outpatient commitment on victimization of people with severe mental illness." *American Journal of Psychiatry* 159, no. 8 (2002): 1403–1411.	"Subjects who were ordered to outpatient commitment were less likely to be criminally victimized than those who were released without outpatient commitment."
Jeffrey Swanson, Marvin Swartz, Richard Van Dorn, John Monahan, Thomas McGuire, Henry Steadman, Pamela Clark Robbins. "Racial disparities in involuntary outpatient commitment: are they real?" *Health Affairs* 28, no. 3 (2009): 816–826.	"We found no evidence of racial bias. Defining the target population as public-system clients with multiple hospitalizations, the rate of application to white and black clients approaches parity."

The Los Angeles County Jail and New York's Riker's Island are currently the two largest "treatment facilities" for the mentally ill in the country. Another 150,000 to 200,000 mentally ill are homeless, and 28 percent get at least some of their meals from garbage cans. More than 10 percent will die from suicide. Others will commit acts of violence against family, friends, and total strangers.

Not only does federal discrimination hurt the mentally ill, it affects the standard of living for everyone else, too. Many parks and public libraries, once enjoyed by all, are now rendered nearly unusable to the general community by the visions of lost, psychotic souls who need inpatient care but are locked out by the discrimination embedded in Medicaid law. Seemingly random acts of violence committed by individuals with a history of mental illness are frequently reported on the evening news. No amount of preaching by the Surgeon General against "stigma" will overcome the acts of a Russell Weston, a Ted Kaczynski or an Andrew Goldstein, all persons with untreated schizophrenia.

The federal government must accept its share of criticism for a policy that discriminates against individuals solely on a diagnosis of mental illness. We must steer clear of the iceberg that sank our state psychiatric hospital system and eliminate the Medicaid IMD exclusion.

D.J. Jaffe is Executive Director of Mental Illness Policy Org. Mary Zdanowicz is (former) Executive Director of the Treatment Advocacy Center.

Some of the Problems at the Substance Abuse and Mental Health Services Administration (SAMHSA)

Summary

Congress directed SAMHSA "to target . . . mental health services to the people most in need" (Conference Committee May 19, 1992) (ADAMHA Reorganization Act 1992).

Priority populations were defined as adults with a serious mental illness and children with a serious emotional disturbance (U.S. Congress n.d.). SAMHSA refuses to focus on the most seriously ill and refuses to focus on the most consequential issues like reducing violence, incarceration, hospitalization, and homelessness.

In a 2015 survey of federal employees, SAMHSA was ranked 317th worst government place to work out of 320 government agencies (Partnership for Public Service 2015). Employees cited ineffective leadership as biggest problem. A 2015 General Accountability Office audit found SAMHSA fails to coordinate the nation's mental health policies, most of its mental health programs don't serve the seriously ill, and most programs that do serve the seriously ill go unevaluated (GAO 2015). Former SAMHSA Administrator Pam Hyde told Congress on a scale of one to ten, "SAMHSA is a ten."

SAMHSA's Strategic Plan Ignores Serious Mental Illness

SAMHSA's 2011–2014 strategic plan directed its mental health resources toward "creating a high-quality, self-directed, satisfying life integrated in the community for *all Americans*" (emphasis added) (SAMHSA 2011). A top SAMHSA official told *Time* magazine: "The behavioral health of the *entire population* is a priority for SAMHSA" (emphasis added) (Sanburn 2013). Of SAMHSA's six 2015–2018 "strategic initiatives" only one mentions serious mental illness and that is limited to preventing it. Serious mental illness cannot be prevented (SAMHSA 2014).[6]

SAMHSA Replaced the Scientific "Medical Model" with a SAMHSA-Invented "Recovery Model"

Instead of medical evidence, SAMHSA relies on popularity contests, convening meetings of "stakeholders" and letting them vote on priorities. SAMHSA stacks their meetings with high-functioning consumers and mental "health" organizations and excludes police, sheriffs, and others concerned about serious mental illness and issues like hospitalization, arrest, violence, homelessness, and incarceration. That's what SAMHSA did when it wanted to replace the proven medical model of treating serious mental illness with a politically correct "Recovery Model."

SAMHSA's Recovery Model includes "10 Guiding Principles of Recovery." The most important is that "self-determination and self-direction are the foundations for recovery." That makes the recovery model dangerous to some as it makes no allowance for the fact that there are individuals with severe mental illness who cannot self-direct their care. "Under the 'recovery model,' John Hinckley was defining his own life goal—the attention of Jodie Foster—when he shot President Reagan" (Torrey and Jaffe 2013).

[6] Of SAMHSA's eight 2011–2014 ''strategic initiatives,'' only one involved getting treatment to adults with serious mental illness, and that was limited to veterans (SAMHSA 2011).

SAMHSA Claims It Knows How to Prevent Serious Mental Illness and Diverts Funds to It

As former NIMH Director Dr. Thomas Insel noted, we can't prevent serious mental illness because "we do not know the cause [and] we lack a biomarker that is 100% accurate for diagnosis" (Insel 2014). But prevention is SAMHSA's number one strategic initiative: "Prevention Works" is part of its motto, and a "National Prevention Week" is held annually (SAMHSA 2011). SAMHSA-funded advocates parade the word "prevention" in front of legislators—along with spreadsheets showing the alleged savings—in order to increase their own funding. SAMHSA often quotes a 1994 Institute of Medicine (IOM) report (IOM 1994). But the report said, "To date, the definitions [of prevention] have been so broad and flexible that almost everything has been labeled prevention at one time or another. *Thus the nation is spending billions of dollars on programs whose effectiveness is not known.*" SAMHSA uses the 2009 update to the 1994 IOM report to justify diverting funds to prevention (IOM 2009). But that report focuses only on youth and specifically excludes "some rare but often severe disorders; for example, schizophrenia and bipolar disorders."

SAMHSA Diverts Millions to Stigma in Spite of Their Own Research Showing It Is Not a Major Barrier to Care

SAMHSA teaches the public and Congress that stigma is an important reason people do not receive care and provides massive funding to this tangential issue. But a 2011 survey by the SAMHSA Center for Behavioral Health Statistics and Quality found stigma (mentioned by 7% of respondents) was low on the list of why people with mental illness do not receive care, far behind cost (50%). Stigma also came behind could handle problem without treatment, did not know where to go for services, lack of time, belief that treatment wouldn't help, anosognosia (did not feel need for treatment), and lack of insurance. SAMHSA does virtually nothing on these other issues, and focuses its resources on stigma.

SAMHSA Knows Peer Support Does Not Improve Meaningful Outcomes in People with Serious Mental Illness But Diverts Funds to It

SAMHSA funds peer supporters, peer travel, peer conferences, peer webinars, and peer support organizations and coerces states to use mental health block grant funds for peer support. (Mental Illness Policy Org. 2013) The Center for Mental Health Services (CMHS) is headed by a peer and focuses on little else. Yet, SAMHSA's own research shows: "The literature [on peer support] that does exist tends to be descriptive and lacks experimental rigor" (SAMHSA–BRSS 2012). SAMHSA "peer-run respite centers" only accept those well enough to volunteer.

SAMHSA Refuses to Certify Programs That Help the Seriously Mentally Ill and Certifies Programs That Don't

SAMHSA encourages states to spend mental health block grants on programs listed in their National Registry of Evidence-based Programs and Practices. NREPP is a sham, little more than an assemblage of privately developed workshops, training sessions, and courses. Little of what's in it are actual treatments, serve the seriously ill, or improve meaningful outcomes. The "evidence" SAMHSA uses to evaluate the programs often comes straight from those who invent, sell, and profit from the listed programs.

- Mental Health First Aid (MHFA) ostensibly teaches people to identify the symptoms of mental illness in others and connect them to help. The three studies SAMHSA relied on to certify it were all done by the owners/vendors of the program (SAMHSA–NREPP 2012). Their research shows only that those who give and receive the training like it; they do not show that it improves outcomes for people with mental illness. There are studies that found no benefit for people with mental illness, but they were not submitted by the vendors to SAMHSA and therefore were ignored by SAMHSA (Mental Illness Policy Org. 2013).
- Four of the five "studies" SAMHSA used to certify Triple-P Positive Parenting, a program that teaches parents of misbehaving children how to be better parents were conducted by the vendor of the program, Prof. Matt Sanders (SAMHSA–NREPP 2014). Numerous independent studies show it doesn't work (Coyne and Kwakkenbos 2013) (Wilson, et al. 2012).
- The two studies used to certify the Wellness Recovery Action Plan (WRAP), which teaches people to develop a wellness plan were conducted at least partially by Mary Ellen Copeland, the vendor of the program. Like MHFA, WRAP is not proven to benefit the seriously mentally ill who receive it (Mental Illness Policy Org. 2013). SAMHSA recently gave Ms. Copeland a large grant.

SAMHSA certifies programs as being "effective" even when they don't improve meaningful outcomes, such as reducing violence, arrest, incarceration, suicide, homelessness, and hospitalization. Many programs SAMHSA certifies as effective only improve soft outcomes, like "satisfaction," "feeling of wellness," "empowerment," "hopefulness," and "resiliency."

SAMHSA refuses to evaluate programs that actually help improve meaningful outcomes in people with serious mental illness including Assertive Community Treatment (ACT) Teams, Intensive Case Managers (ICM), Crisis Intervention Teams (CIT), Assisted Outpatient Treatment (AOT) and Mental Health Courts.

SAMHSA Prevents States from Using Block Grant Money to Help People with Serious Mental Illness

The legislation establishing mental health block grants requires they be used for "adults with serious mental illness" and "children with serious emotional disturbance" and narrowly defines those terms (CMHS 1993). But the SAMHSA instructions and application process ignores that direction and encourages states to use the funds for people without mental illness. (Mental Illness Policy Org. 2013):

> "The focus is about everyone, not just those with an illness or disease, but the whole population" (emphasis added) (SAMHSA 2012, SAMHSA 2014).

SAMHSA Invented a New Mental Illness: Trauma

SAMHSA invented a mental illness it calls "trauma." No reputable psychiatrist considers trauma an illness. Post-traumatic stress disorder (PTSD) is an illness, and even that can run from mild to severe. SAMHSA never exactly defined trauma, but declared "Individual trauma results from an event, series of events, or set of circumstances that is experienced by an individual as physically or emotionally harmful or threatening and that has lasting adverse effects on the individual's functioning and physical, social, emotional, or spiritual well-being" (SAMHSA 2012). These definitions can therefore include anyone who got divorced, found their spouse was cheating, knows someone who died, was in a storm, or had any event they "experienced as . . . emotionally harmful" if it affected their "spiritual well-being."

SAMHSA created a National Center for Trauma Informed Care and has awarded major trauma grants to organizations like the National Association of State Mental Health Program Directors (NASMHPD) (SAMHSA 2006). That is money going to preventing trauma rather than treating serious mental illness.

SAMHSA Funds Antipsychiatry and Antipsychiatrists

SAMHSA is responsible for distributing funds that Congress intended to support programs of "Regional and National Significance" (OMB 2013). Too much of it goes directly to antipsychiatry and other organizations that oppose treatment. It is hard to find an antipsychiatry organization that does not receive financial or PR support from SAMHSA. SAMHSA's *Mental Illness Awareness Week Guide* suggests that schools invite the MindFreedom, the Icarus Project, and the National Coalition for Mental Health Recovery (NCMHR) into classrooms to teach children about mental illness (SAMHSA October 2010). MindFreedom based in Oregon believes "mental illnesses are not brain diseases" (MindFreedom 2008). The Icarus Project believes "these experiences—commonly diagnosed and labeled as psychiatric conditions—are mad gifts needing cultivation and care, rather than diseases or disorders" (Icarus Project 2014). The National Coalition for Mental Health Recovery (NCMHR), the umbrella group for SAMHSA funded peer-run non-profits believes "psychiatric labeling is a pseudoscientific practice of limited value in helping people recover" (NCMHR 2012).

SAMHSA's support of these individuals and organizations has enabled them to prevent states from improving services for the seriously ill by keeping hospitals open, implementing AOT, using ECT, housing seriously mentally ill in congregate settings, hiring professionals in lieu of peers, and has thereby made incarceration of many seriously mentally ill people more likely.

SAMHSA Wastes Money Intended to Help People with Serious Mental Illness

SAMHSA uses its budget to publish and distribute children's books, such as *Play Day in the Park* for 3- and 4-year-olds; *Look What I Can Do!* for 5- and 6-year-olds; coloring books, such as *Wally Bear and Friends;* and my favorite, *The Lion and the Mouse* sing-along (SAMHSA 2011). SAMHSA has scores of free publications covering non-mental illness including "What a Difference a Friend Makes" and publications on oil spill response, hurricane recovery, American Indian and Alaska native culture, peer pressure, social marketing, employment services, and health promotion. But SAMHSA has only a single publication on schizophrenia, and it is out of stock (Torrey and Jaffe 2013). SAMHSA commissioned a $22,500 painting of Native Americans by a Native American artist, "to help raise awareness about the roles of families and the community in mental and substance abuse disorder prevention." It sits in SAMHSA's headquarters.[4] SAMHSA spent $200,000 to put on a party at Paramount Studies in Hollywood (Coburn 2013).

SAMHSA recently led a "National Wellness Week" to encourage "visiting a farmers' market, taking a class on nutritional cooking, 'drinking a veggie or fruit smoothie,' reading poetry, making a collage, taking a walk, joining a song circle, taking a class on how to make sacred drums, . . and join[ing] the Line Dance for wellness . . . because 'dancing is a great stress reliever and also provides social interaction"' (Torrey, The Ridiculous "National Wellness" Week 2014).

SAMHSA Downplays and Minimizes Violence Thereby Stymieing Efforts to Reduce It

Violence is not associated with poor mental health but is associated with serious mental illness *that is allowed to go untreated.* SAMHSA refuses to admit to or address that.

SAMHSA Promotes "Prevention" Knowing Serious Mental Illness Cannot Be Prevented

NIMH had similar problems of mission-creep that were solved when its previous director was replaced by Dr. Thomas Insel. The problem at SAMHSA is not lack of money, it's having too much.

National Alliance to End Homelessness

May 12, 2016

The Honorable Orrin G. Hatch
Chairman
Finance Committee
U.S. Senate
Washington, DC 20510

The Honorable Ron Wyden
Ranking Member
Finance Committee
U.S. Senate
Washington, DC 20510

Chairman Hatch, Ranking Member Wyden, and members of the committee:

On behalf of the National Alliance to End Homelessness, we appreciate the opportunity to submit a statement for the record. The Alliance is a nonprofit, non-partisan organization committed to preventing and ending homelessness in the United States. By improving policy, building capacity, and educating opinion leaders, the Alliance has become a leading voice on this issue.

Evidence indicates that mental illness is a known risk factor for homelessness, and data clearly shows that mental illness disproportionately impacts homeless people. In 2014, almost 20 percent of the adults in the United States experienced any mental illness (AMI), and 4.1 percent had serious mental illness (SMI).[7] In contrast, 18.1 percent of people who experienced homelessness on a single night in 2014 had SMI.[8] Research has shown that integrated treatment which incorporates housing components provides better outcomes than usual care for people who are homeless.[9]

Therefore, we encourage the Committee to ensure that housing supports are included in any legislation as a necessary component of mental health treatment.

The following pending Senate legislation has been endorsed by the Alliance and provides for comprehensive services to meet the needs of people with mental illness who are experiencing homelessness:

---

[7] Center for Behavioral Health Statistics and Quality (2015). Behavioral health trends in the United States: Results from the 2014 National Survey on Drug Use and Health (HHS Publication No. SMA 15–4927, NSDUH Series H–50). Retrieved from http://www.samhsa.gov/ data/.

[8] https://www.hudexchange.info/resource/reportmanagement/published/CoC_PopSub_NatlTe rrDC_2015.pdf.

[9] Hwang, S., Tolomiczenko, G., Kouyoumdjian, F., and Garner, R. Interventions to improve the health of the homeless: a systematic review. *Am. J. Prev. Med.* 2005 Nov; 29(4):311–9.

- S. 2525, Expand Excellence in Mental Health Act: This bill authorizes the expansion of a 2014 demonstration of Certified Community Behavioral Health Centers (CCBHs). CCBHs ensure availability and accessibility of behavioral health services to vulnerable populations including those experiencing homelessness. CCBHs are encouraged to partner with homeless services providers or local continuums of care.
- S. 2680, Mental Health Reform Act of 2016: This bill strengthens mental health and substance abuse care and improve access to treatment. The Act requires state plans for comprehensive community-based health systems that include employment and housing services as well as other supportive services that are essential to ending homelessness. The Act also authorizes the use of funds to provide employment and housing supports.
- S. 524, Comprehensive Addiction and Recovery Act of 2016: This bill encourages housing to be coordinated with medication assisted treatments and behavioral health interventions for the treatment of opioid use disorders.

We hope to continue to work with this Committee to effectively treat mental illness and end homelessness, two national concerns that can be solved.

Sincerely,
Nan Roman
President and CEO

National Alliance on Mental Illness (NAMI)

3803 N. Fairfax Drive, Suite 100, Arlington, VA 22203
703–524–7600
www.nami.org

National Association of Psychiatric Health Systems (NAPHS)

900 17th Street, NW, Suite 420, Washington, DC 20006
202–393–6700
www.naphs.org

April 28, 2016

The Honorable Orrin G. Hatch
Chairman
Senate Finance Committee
219 Dirksen Senate Office Building
Washington, DC 20510–6200

The Honorable Ron Wyden
Ranking Member
Senate Finance Committee
219 Dirksen Senate Office Building
Washington, DC 20510–6200

Dear Chairman Hatch and Ranking Member Wyden,

On behalf of the National Alliance on Mental Illness (NAMI) and the National Association of Psychiatric Health Systems (NAPHS), we want to thank you for convening today's important hearing on "Mental Health in America: Where Are We Now?" We appreciate your focus on this vital issue.

Mental Illnesses are the leading cause of disability and contribute to premature death, yet millions of Americans face discrimination when they need the help the most.

Medicaid is the single largest funding source for people living with mental illnesses, but a little-known provision in the law called the Medicaid Institutions for Mental Disease (IMD) Exclusion prevents adult Medicaid beneficiaries (ages 21–64) from accessing short-term, acute care in psychiatric hospitals.

The IMD Exclusion is discriminatory and for years has disadvantaged Medicaid beneficiaries living with serious mental illness. People are not getting the psychiatric hospital treatment they need, putting families and communities at risk. In the end, this is—pure and simple—a fairness issue. A Medicaid insurance card covers hospital treatment for all other medical conditions, but adults with mental illnesses cannot use their Medicaid insurance card for inpatient psychiatric care in a psychiatric hospital. No other disorder limits hospital choice in the way the IMD Exclusion does.

The Medicaid IMD Exclusion was part of the original Medicaid program in 1965 and was intended to ensure that the states (rather than the federal government) would be primarily responsible for the costs associated with inpatient psychiatric treatments. Long ago, in 1965, the vast majority of inpatient psychiatric care was provided in state mental hospitals and was primarily long-term, custodial care.

Of course, this is no longer the case. Today the vast majority of inpatient psychiatric hospital care is provided in the community in general hospital psychiatric units or freestanding, non-governmental psychiatric hospitals. Inpatient stays today for psychiatric illnesses are measured in days (on average less than 10 days), not in weeks or months.

Over the past two decades, there has been a major decline in the number of inpatient psychiatric beds throughout the country. This has resulted in an increased number of individuals ending up in emergency rooms where they stay for days (and sometimes weeks) before being able to get the crisis inpatient hospital stabilization treatment they so desperately need. A Government Accountability Office (GAO–09– 347) report on hospital emergency departments concluded difficulties in transferring, admitting, or discharging psychiatric patients from emergency departments were factors contributing to emergency department overcrowding.

Community psychiatric hospitals could help relieve these backups if Congress made a targeted, exception to the IMD Exclusion for short-term, acute, psychiatric hospital treatment.

A question that is sometimes asked by policymakers and advocates is whether modifying the IMD Exclusion would lead to more institutionalization. The answer is that this is about people who are in major crisis and need hospitalization to keep them safe. Hospital stays in the community are short and focus on crisis stabilization, helping people continue their recovery in the community.

Some also ask, why not invest in community care instead of hospitals? This is not a question of "either/or." What is needed is a partnership in care. Hospitals are handling the most acute needs of that person (so they don't hurt themselves or others), and then hospitals work with their community partners to handle the next step. This is not dissimilar to someone who has a heart attack, who needs hospitalization to stabilize the situation and then moves onto a rehabilitation facility and then home with continuing supports. What is needed are reforms to the IMD Exclusion that expand access to acute inpatient care and quality measures that ensure connection to outpatient services after a short-term stay in a hospital. In addition, reforms to the IMD Exclusion should also address the disparity that currently excludes non- elderly adults with mental illness from community services funded under state waiver programs.

There are many approaches that have been identified to address the growing crisis of the shortage of inpatient psychiatric beds in this country. And there is growing bipartisan support in both the House and Senate to address the discriminatory and outmoded IMD Exclusion. There are comprehensive mental health reforms bills that have been introduced in the Senate and House, including the Mental Health Reform Act of 2016 introduced by Senators Bill Cassidy (R–LA) and Chris Murphy (D–CT) which includes a targeted, exception to the IMD Exclusion to cover short-term, psychiatric hospital treatment.

Making a change to the IMD Exclusion is the right thing to do and will result in more timely access to life-saving inpatient treatment, reduced emergency backlogs, and a more cost-effective system.

We look forward to continuing to work with the committee to address this unfair and discriminatory policy, so that individuals living with mental illnesses can get the right care at the right time.

Sincerely, Mary Giliberti, JD
Chief Executive Officer
National Alliance on Mental Illness (NAMI)

Mark Covall
President and CEO
National Association of Psychiatric Health Systems (NAPHS)

National Association of Anorexia Nervosa and Associated Disorders (ANAD)

750 E. Diehl Road #127
Naperville, IL 60563
May 9, 2016

Senator Orrin G. Hatch
Chairman
U.S. Senate
Committee on Finance
219 Dirksen Senate Office Building
Washington, DC 20510

Senator Ron Wyden
Ranking Member
U.S. Senate
Committee on Finance
219 Dirksen Senate Office Building
Washington, DC 20510

Dear Chairman Hatch and Ranking Member Wyden:

Thank you for your commitment to improving our nation's mental health care system and for holding a hearing on April 28 to examine the roles that the Medicare and Medicaid programs play in addressing the needs of those with behavioral and mental health issues.

I write today on behalf of the National Association of Anorexia Nervosa and Associated Disorders (ANAD) and the patients we represent. Formed in 1976, ANAD is a non-profit association dedicated to the prevention and alleviation of eating disorders. We focus particularly on anorexia nervosa, bulimia nervosa and binge eating disorder, and we advocate for the development of healthy attitudes, bodies, and behaviors. ANAD promotes eating disorder awareness, prevention and recovery through supporting, educating, and connecting individuals, families and professionals.

Eating disorders are common mental illnesses and can kill. Every 62 minutes at least one person dies as a direct result from an eating disorder.

Anorexia is the third most common chronic illness among adolescents, and it has the highest mortality rate among *all* mental illnesses—between 10 and 20 percent of those who have the illness will die. Further, eating disorders cause medical complications including cardiac arrhythmia, cardiac arrest, brain damage, infertility and osteoporosis, in addition to other mental health conditions such as anxiety and depression.

Appropriate and timely diagnosis and treatment of an eating disorder is absolutely crucial in achieving positive health outcomes for the patient. Eating disorders can be successfully and fully treated but, unfortunately, only about one third of people with an eating disorder ever receive treatment.

Such treatment can often be lengthy—from months to years—but early intervention and proper treatment improve a patient's prognosis and chances of a full recovery. As such, ANAD advocates for the reduction of barriers and obstacles to insurance benefits and discriminatory medical management of those struggling with all eating disorders.

ANAD applauds the steps taken by Congress over the past decade to improve mental health care access and coverage—including mental health parity and related provisions in the Affordable Care Act (ACA). That said, more can and must be done in order to ensure that those suffering from eating disorders are not denied access to the care they need. In particular, steps must be taken to ensure that low-income individuals and families are able to receive coverage for eating disorders treatments under the Medicaid program.

Improvements to Medicaid coverage are imperative to ensuring that all patients have access to the eating disorder treatments that are needed to save their lives. In addition, physicians and counselors in the Medicaid program need the training that is imperative to successfully treating an eating disorder. Skilled clinicians with specific eating disorder expertise are essential for treatment, yet eating disorder specialists are still not available in some communities.

Specifically, ANAD strongly supports the Anna Westin Act (S. 1865), a bipartisan eating disorders bill that was introduced in July 2015 and referred to the Senate Committee on Health, Education, Labor, and Pensions (HELP). The bill is named after Anna Westin, a young Minnesotan who committed suicide as a direct result of her battle with anorexia in February 2000. Since that time, Anna's family has turned their grief into something positive by founding the Anna Westin Foundation and working to ensure that tragedies such as Anna's are prevented in the future.

The Anna Westin Act is a comprehensive eating disorders bill that focuses on both training and treatment measures, and it will help those affected with eating disorders get the treatment they need and deserve. Using current funds from the Department of Health and Human Services (HHS), the bill would help train health professionals, school personnel and the public on how to identify eating disorders and how to help prevent the development of behaviors that may lead to eating disorders. In addition, S. 1865 would clarify the mental health parity law to include residential treatment service coverage—affording the same protections as other illnesses.

The bipartisan Anna Westin Act has 12 cosponsors in the Senate, and its House counterpart (H.R. 2515) has 82 cosponsors. Importantly, key provisions of the bill were incorporated into the comprehensive mental health bill that was approved by the HELP Committee on March 16.

ANAD applauds this bipartisan effort and sincerely hopes that as you work with your HELP Committee colleagues to bring a full scale mental health reform effort to the Senate floor, you will support these provisions that are so important to those suffering from eating disorders, as well as their families and loved ones.

Again, thank you for the opportunity to share our thoughts on the need to improve our nation's mental health care system—particularly from the perspective of treating and preventing eating disorders.

Sincerely,
Laura Zinger
Executive Director

Statement Submitted by Christina Nunez Daw, MPH, PhD

While this hearing's agenda includes information about positive efforts to integrate mental and physical health care delivery, address suicide risk, and meet adolescent mental health needs, it is disappointing that a long-standing barrier to psychiatric and substance addiction treatment is not being discussed—the exclusion of federal Medicaid funding for adult (age 21–64) treatment in IMDs (Institutions for Mental Disease) with over 15 beds. I urge the Committee to support the elimination of the IMD exclusion by ensuring that this provision is restored to S. 2680, the mental health reform bill.

Rather than increasing health care costs, the elimination of the IMD exclusion would *save resources* now spent in hospital emergency rooms, jails, and prisons, and care for homeless mentally ill patients. We are wasting precious resources in these non-treatment settings because our nation is seriously short on inpatient mental health beds and treatment.

Unfortunately, the Congressional Budget Office issued a cost estimate for this provision (eliminating the IMD exclusion) that likely overstates the expenditures needed, while ignoring resulting cost-saving in non-federal expenditures.

- CBO estimated the cost of allowing federal funds for IMDs at $40–$60 billion over 10 years.
- Yet, in the multi-year Medicaid Emergency Psychiatric Demonstration (MEPD), the cost of providing community inpatient mental health treatment for individuals in acute mental illness crisis, averaged $6,724 per admission; the 26 month demonstration covered over 11,500 admissions for just under $78 million (state and federal dollars) in 12 states.[10]
- Even assuming an admission volume of 25 times the number of admissions in the 12-state MEPD demonstration, the total estimated federal expenditure would likely be less than the CBO's estimate.
- Moreover, if we provided treatment instead of jailing mentally ill persons, we would save the $30,000–$50,000 per mentally inmate currently incarcerated.

Hospital emergency room directors have long raised the concerns that the lack of inpatient beds has forced them to board seriously mentally ill persons in crisis, taking up beds in ERs and in wards while delaying admissions of persons with other critical illnesses. Moreover, the IMD exclusion is in clear conflict with mental health parity laws, by discriminating against patients based on type of illness and associated treatment.

The Senate mental health reform bill, S. 2680, lacks this crucial component that was contained in S. 1945 and is still addressed in the current House mental health reform bill. I urge the Finance Committee to restore this provision in S. 2680 and ensure it is preserved in the House-Senate legislative reconciliation process.

Statement Submitted by Patricia Ranney

Urgent need of parity: mental illness = medical illness:

As a concerned parent, grandmother, citizen and constituent, I urge repeal of discriminatory IMD exclusions. Medicaid denies payment to psychiatric hospitals over 16 beds, for patients from 21 to 65 years old . . . but doesn't do same with medical hospitals.

Also repeal lifetime limit of Medicare for treatment of mental illness. . . . Just treat it like other illness without Restrictive CAP.

[10] Data as of November 10, 2015 presented by CMS at the MHA Regional Policy Council.

Absolute critical need for addiction counselors, beds and treatment. . . . Let's show our humanity by treating those in desperate need of mental health services in a hospital, or rehab and not a jail cell or the streets.

Your shared concern is greatly appreciated.

Pat Ranney

THE TREVOR PROJECT

Saving Young Lives
Los Angeles—8704 Santa Monica Blvd., Suite 200, West Hollywood, CA 90069
New York—575 8th Ave., #501, New York, NY 10012
DC—1200 New Hampshire Ave., NW, Suite 300,
Washington, DC 20036
www.thetrevorproject.org

May 12, 2016

The Hon. Orrin G. Hatch, Chairman
The Hon. Ron Wyden, Ranking Member

U.S. Senate
Committee on Finance
219 Dirksen Senate Office Building
Washington, DC 20510

Dear Senators Hatch and Wyden:

The Trevor Project sincerely thanks you for recently holding a hearing entitled "Mental Health in America: Where Are We Now?" and asks that you immediately take steps to pass the Mental Health Reform Act (S. 2680). During the hearing it was very clear that our current mental health system needs a thorough overhaul, and Congress has a great opportunity to enact some of those key reforms by passing the Mental Health Reform Act (MHRA) of 2016. Thankfully, the MHRA has already been passed out of committee and is awaiting a vote on the floor of the Senate. We strongly urge you to request that Senate Majority Leader Mitch McConnell put the bill on the Senate agenda for a full vote as soon as possible. The MHRA is a truly bipartisan bill that addresses many current problems in the nation's mental health system and also reauthorizes vitally important programs such as those created under the Garrett Lee Smith Memorial Act (GLSMA).

The Trevor Project is the leading national, nonprofit organization providing crisis intervention and suicide prevention services to lesbian, gay, bisexual, transgender and questioning (LGBTQ) young people through age 24. We work to save young lives through our accredited free and confidential lifeline, secure instant messaging services which provide live help and intervention, a social networking community for LGBTQ youth, in-school workshops, educational materials, online resources, and advocacy. Trevor is a leader and innovator in suicide prevention, especially as we focus on an important, at-risk population: LGBTQ youth.

When initially passed in 2004, the GLSMA created a suicide prevention grant program to allow states/tribes and colleges to engage in prevention efforts and allocated funding for the national Suicide Prevention Resource Center. Although the inaugural version of the Act expired in 2008, Congress has since continued to reauthorize the measure in recognition of the importance of youth suicide prevention by financially supporting Garrett Lee Smith programs.

The GLSMA currently needs to be reauthorized and is included in the MHRA, providing critical funding for the Suicide Prevention Resource Center ($6 million annually), Youth Suicide and Prevention Strategy Grants to States and Tribes ($30 million annually), and Mental Health and Substance Use Disorder Services and Outreach on campuses ($6.5 million annually). Its funding currently supports suicide prevention programs in all 50 states, as well as the District of Columbia, and the continuation of this funding is necessary to the maintenance of these vital suicide prevention and mental health wellness services in schools and communities nationwide. Through the GLSMA's administration by the Substance Abuse and Mental Health Services Agency, its funding is directed towards providing lifesaving services to individuals at risk of suicide, whether that is through providing mental health counseling; crisis intervention services; running a hotline; conducting a public awareness campaign; or training individuals on how to recognize a person in distress and to appropriately intervene.

Suicide is the second leading cause of death among children ages 10 to 24 in America, as well as the second leading cause of death on college and university campuses.[11] Lesbian, gay, bisexual, transgender, and questioning (LGBTQ) youth are at an exceptionally heightened risk for suicidal behavior: LGB youth are four times more likely, and questioning youth three times more likely, to attempt suicide than their heterosexual peers.[12] Additionally, almost half of young transgender people have seriously considered taking their lives, with approximately 25% having made at least one suicide attempt.[13] LGBTQ youth who experience significant familial rejection are more than 8 times as likely

[11] Centers for Disease Control and Prevention. (2015). *Web-based Injury Statistics Query and Reporting System* [Data file]. Retrieved from www.cdc.gov/ncipc/wisqars.

[12] Kann, L., O'Malley Olsen, E., McManus, T., Kincheen, S., Chyen, D., Harris, W.A., Wechsler, H. (2011). Sexual Identity, Sex of Sexual Contracts, and Health-Risk Behaviors Among Students Grades 9–12—Youth Risk Behavior Surveillance, Selected Sites, United States, 2001–2009, *Morbidity and Mortality Weekly Report* 60(SS07), 1–133.

[13] Grossman, A.H. and D'Augelli, A.R. (2007). Transgender youth and life-threatening behaviors. *Suicide and Life Threatening Behavior* 37(5), 527. Retrieved from http://transformingfamily.org/pdfs/Transgender%20 Youth%20and%20Life%20Threatening%20Behaviors.pdf.

to report at least one suicide attempt than their peers who come from welcoming, accepting family situations.[14]

These statistics are shocking and disheartening, but it is imperative to remember that together we can work to prevent suicide—through awareness and education, as provided by the GLSMA. Reauthorization of the Garrett Lee Smith Memorial Act will preserve the necessary funds for state and tribal organizations, as well as institutions of higher education, in order to allow these programs to continue serving youth in America who are at risk for suicidal ideation, behavior, and/or attempts.

With Congress's upcoming summer recess and its break for campaigning, the bills that are going to pass this legislative session must effectively be passed before the summer break, as we understand it is unlikely for Congress to convene during the lame-duck period. Therefore, we strongly urge you to request that Senate Majority Leader Mitch McConnell put the MHRA on the Senate agenda for a full vote *in the next 2 weeks*. The time has come for mental health reform and the MHRA represents the best opportunity among the last three decades to do just that.

Thank you for your time and consideration of supporting this critical piece of legislation, and for your commitment to improving the mental health of all Americans.

Sincerely,
Abbe Land
Executive Director and CEO

[14] Family Acceptance Project TM. (2009). Family rejection as a predictor of negative health outcomes in white and Latino lesbian, gay, and bisexual young adults. *Pediatrics*. 123(1), 346–52.

In: Focus on Mental Health and Illness
Editor: Isaac Banks
ISBN: 978-1-53615-081-0

Chapter 2

Improving the Federal Response to Challenges in Mental Health Care in America*

U.S. Senate Hearing of the Committee on Health, Education, Labor, and Pensions United States Senate

Opening Statement of Senator Alexander

The CHAIRMAN. The Senate Committee on Health, Education, Labor, and Pensions will please come to order.

Senator Murray and I will have an opening statement. Then we'll introduce our panel of witnesses. Senator Mikulski will introduce the first witness. And then after our witness testimony, senators will each have 5 minutes of questions.

Before we begin today's hearing, I want to briefly mention for the information of committee our progress on two or three items on our agenda. Yesterday, I announced that we plan to hold our first markup on February 9th to consider the first set of bipartisan bills aimed at spurring biomedical innovation for American patients. Senators and staff have been working throughout 2015 on this, on a number of bipartisan pieces of legislation.

The House has completed its work on the 21st Century Cures Act. The president has reiterated his support for a precision medicine initiative and in the State of the Union

* This is an edited, reformatted and augmented version of U.S. Senate Hearing of the Committee on Health, Education, Labor, And Pensions United States Senate One Hundred Fourteenth Congress, Second Session, Publication No. S. HRG. 114–719, dated Wednesday, January 20, 2016.

address for a cancer moonshot. So it's urgent that the Senate finish its work and turn into law these ideas that will help virtually every American.

We've also been working for months together on legislation to help achieve interoperability of electronic health care records for doctors, hospitals, and their patients. We have a lot of agreement on what to do about that, and the committee will be releasing today a bipartisan staff draft of that legislation for public comment.

This February markup will be the first of three committee meetings that have been planned to debate and amend bills as the committee moves forward on the goal of modernizing the FDA and the NIH to get safe, cutting-edge drugs and devices to patients more quickly. The bills that will be considered in February have bipar tisan co-sponsorship by committee members. The same with those that will be considered in April.

In addition, this year, the committee intends to be busy on oversight of the Every Student Succeeds Act. A law that is not implemented properly isn't worth the paper it's written on. So we'll be spending time on making sure the Department of Education implements that the way the Congress wrote it and the way the President signed it.

Of course, we've done a lot of work on reauthorizing Higher Education, which expired at the end of last year. We have a number of bipartisan proposals that will make it easier and simpler for students to attend college and for administrators to manage our 6,000 colleges and universities.

We have a lot that we ought to be able to do this year. One of the most important of those items has to do with the mental health crisis that we're discussing today. I hope—and Senator Murray and I agree on this—that we can move promptly to offer bipartisan recommendations on how to address the mental health crisis. We've already done a lot of work on it. We passed in September the Mental Health Awareness and Improvement Act that Senator Murray and I introduced. The Senate passed that in December.

Senator Cassidy and Senator Murphy have introduced legislation, and Senator Murray and I are working with them. We hope to move promptly to bring a combination of those recommendations to the full committee.

Not everything the Senate may want to do is in our jurisdiction. So we're working with Senator Blunt, who, with Senator Murray, runs the Health Appropriations Subcommittee, on ideas that Senator Blunt has proposed, and we're working with Senator Cornyn on issues that the Judiciary Committee is considering and with the Finance Committee, which will probably have to be involved as well.

What we want to do is to move promptly in this committee to take the things that are within our jurisdiction and have them ready for the floor and work in parallel with the other committees so the leader can bring them to the floor if he chooses to do that.

The reason there is such interest in the mental health crisis today is that about one in five adults had a mental health condition in the past year, according to the Mental Health Services Administration. That's nearly 10 million adults with illnesses such as schizophrenia, bipolar disorder, or depression that interferes with a major life activity.

And 60 percent of adults with mental illness did not receive mental health services in 2014. Only about half of adolescents with a mental health condition received treatment for their condition. Mental health conditions that remain untreated can lead to dropping out of school, substance abuse, incarceration, unemployment, homelessness, and suicide.

Suicide is the 10th leading cause of death in the United States, and 90 percent of those who die by suicide have an underlying mental illness. I hear that from many Tennesseeans. Between 2010 and 2012, nearly 21 percent—that's one out of five adults in Tennessee—reported having a mental illness. Four percent had a serious mental illness. The most recent data shows that our rate of suicide reached its highest level in 5 years a couple of years ago. It was the second leading cause of death.

At our October hearing on mental health, the committee heard from administration witnesses about what the Federal Government is already doing to address mental illness. Today, we look forward to hearing from doctors, nurses, advocates, and administrators who work every day with Americans who struggle with a mental health condition about how the Federal Government can help patients, health care providers, communities, and States to better address these issues. We want people to be able to take advantage of the most innovative research. We heard some about that at our recent hearing, about the RAISE study.

I'm interested to hear how the government can support State efforts to implement evidence-based treatment programs. This will require modernizing our leading Federal agency for mental health. It will require involvement from patients, families, communities, health care providers, health departments, law enforcement, State partners, and many others who are involved. I look forward to hearing from our witnesses about the challenges we face and the solutions that they offer.

Senator Murray.

Opening Statement of Senator Murray

Senator MURRAY. Thank you very much, Chairman Alexander.

Thank you to all of our colleagues who are here today. I am really glad that we have this opportunity today to continue our discussion about ways to improve our mental health care system.

We have a really incredible group of witnesses today joining us to share your expertise and experiences. Thank you all for coming.

As I'm sure all of us do, I hear far too often from families in Washington State about loved ones, friends, and neighbors who are struggling with mental illness and aren't getting the support they need. It is heartbreaking, especially because when someone does get treatment and support, it can truly make a difference.

I recently heard from a woman in Seattle, who I will call Amanda. She was experiencing mental illness so severe that she lived in a dumpster for fear of being abducted by aliens. Case managers were able to get her the appropriate medication she needed. They also connected her with primary care, housing, and supplemental security income benefits. Today, Amanda is enrolled in school and pursuing her degree with hopes of full-time employment. That is quite a change for her.

My constituent, Jack's, story is similarly powerful. Jack is a veteran from King County. He enrolled in outpatient support services after he was hospitalized several times for attempted suicide. He had serious addiction problems and was becoming alienated from his family. But after being connected with support, he was able to find recovery, even while he was being treated for cancer. He now lives independently and is reconnecting with his teenage son.

Amanda's and Jack's stories show that comprehensive, high-quality mental health care can truly give someone their life back. But, unfortunately, a lot of stories don't end that way. In fact, only 63 percent of people with serious mental health illness received treatment in the past year.

I'm going to focus on a few challenges in particular today, ones which I believe our witnesses will have a lot to say about as well. The first is inadequate access to treatment. Far too many communities lack access to mental health professionals. In fact, half of all U.S. counties don't have a single psychiatrist, psychologist, or social worker. That means for many patients and families, it is unclear where to turn for help. So we need to make sure communities have access to trained professionals who can intervene, treat, and support those struggling with mental illness.

And, in addition to strengthening our mental health workforce, we need to make sure that when someone presents in crisis, or simply chooses to seek help, there are providers who can take them in and meet their needs. No patient should be turned away, asked to wait in an emergency room for days, or be left out on the street because there isn't an available bed.

Ms. Blake, I'm sure this is a problem you have seen all too often in the ER. I think we can and must do better on this, and I'm looking forward to hearing all of your thoughts.

Another issue I am really eager to talk about today is the need to truly integrate mental and physical health care. The two stories I shared a minute ago have something especially important in common. Amanda didn't just need psychiatric help. She needed primary care. Jack needed help with addiction and depression, but during the course of his recovery, he also needed treatment for cancer.

The siloes that exist between mental health care and physical health care don't match patients' realities, and that needs to change. The legislation that Senators Murphy and Cassidy have worked on together would take some very important steps to better integrate mental and physical health care.

I am also interested in some innovative steps being taken at the State level. For example, in my State, the University of Washington has a residency program that allows students focused on psychiatry to get experience working in physical health settings.

Dr. Hepburn, I know you are focused on this challenge in your work, and I'm grateful that we'll have your insights today.

And, finally, I want to reiterate something I mentioned at our last hearing. If we are going to confront the challenges I've laid out today and many others within our mental health system, we have to break down the barriers that stigma creates for those suffering from mental illness. That means prioritizing research like Dr. Eaton's, which helps enhance our understanding of and ability to effectively treat mental illnesses. And it means raising awareness so that those struggling don't feel they have to struggle alone.

Today, nearly one in five people in our country experience mental illness in a given year. Far too many of them don't receive treatment when they need it, and part of the reason is that stigma gets in their way.

Mr. Rahim, you've worked for over a decade to raise awareness and promote understanding of mental health in communities across the country. And you've been an inspiration to many people who otherwise might not have had the courage to seek help. So I want to thank you for your work, and I'm eager to hear what you think Congress should do to lend our voices to efforts like yours.

Again, thank you to all of our witnesses who are here today. We have a lot of urgent work ahead of us to make sure that our families and communities have access to the comprehensive, high-quality mental health care they need.

I look forward, Mr. Chairman, to working on a bipartisan effort to strengthen our mental health system and give patients and families the opportunity to lead healthy, fulfilling lives.

Thank you.

The CHAIRMAN. Thank you, Senator Murray.

We welcome our four witnesses, and I thank you for arranging to be here. You all have busy schedules, other things to be doing. We're grateful to you for that.

I'm going to ask Senator Mikulski to introduce one of you since she has a conflict which will require her to leave soon.

Statement of Senator Mikulski

Senator MIKULSKI. Thank you very much, Senator Alexander, and I want to thank you for your continuing progress on holding hearings on the issue of mental health. I know this is the third hearing on the topic, and I want to really salute you and Senator Murray for moving in this direction.

The Subcommittee on Commerce, Justice, Science, and Related Agencies of the Committee on Appropriations is holding a hearing on President Obama's proposals on gun control, and as the vice- chair, I must be at my duty station and will have to excuse myself.

I really wanted to be at this hearing because of the fact that I'm a professionally trained social worker. We've been working on these issues all of my professional life. This is what I live for. This is why I came to the Senate, to listen to good people with great ideas on how we can help our people.

We have two distinguished Marylanders here. One, of course, is Dr. Hepburn, who headed up the State of Maryland's Agency on Health and Mental Health. He is a University of Maryland trained clinician who then went on to try to breathe mental health into a bureaucracy and then bring care to our people in a State that mandates an affordable budget. So we're going to have some great ideas.

Then we have Dr. Eaton here. Dr. William Eaton is a professor of the Department of Mental Health at the famous Johns Hopkins Bloomberg School of Public Health. Dr. Eaton is a professor there, and he chairs the Department of Mental Health. It is the only department-level unit in a school of public health in the world. Usually public health thinks about vaccinations. What Dr. Eaton thinks about is how we can build resilient personalities and do the preventive work.

He will talk to you today about his work, his research, his recommendations. Understanding, I believe, the thrust will be that everybody who has a mental health problem needs individual treatment, but they live in a social world, and we need to look at the social indicators, look at the social epidemiology, and how we can strengthen the anchor institutions of the family and the school.

You're going to learn a lot from him. I've already learned a lot from him, as I do from listening to the folks at Johns Hopkins School of Public Health. I really look forward to where we're going on this issue of mental health, in a nutshell.

When I got out of graduate school, Senator Alexander—I actually went to graduate school on a National Institutes of Health grant— they were training community mental health social workers. President Kennedy led the battle to establish community mental health centers, to get rid of the old snake pit type mental health hospitals.

All the practitioners at the table remember that, and, Mr. Rahim, I'm sure you've heard stories of that, and we welcome you here with your personal courage.

But maybe it's not that we need new institutions. Maybe we have to look at what we thought we were going to do, and we never did it. We never followed through on community mental health centers. Maybe that's the way to go.

We never followed through in the aggressive way to enforce the Wellstone-Domenici Mental Health Parity Act. Maybe that's the way we need to go. And speaking as a social worker, along with the nurses, we know that mental health requires a team approach, and it is both, of course, the psychiatrists, which we need, but it's those of us who are trained in these matters.

I know my colleagues would never think I had a therapeutic personality, but I look forward to working with you in the best way possible to advance the ideas that will come forth and how we can really meet this crisis that's growing and expanding.

Thank you very much, Mr. Chairman.

The CHAIRMAN. Thank you, Senator Mikulski.

We will now hear from our witnesses, and let me present them. Again, Dr. Hepburn has been mentioned. He's the Executive Director of the National Association of State Mental Health Program Directors, which represents mental health service delivery systems in all 50 States. He's been a clinical associate professor of psychiatry at the University of Maryland Medical System for nearly 20 years, and he has cared for patients for more than 20 years.

The second witness is Ms. Penny Blake, a registered nurse working in an emergency department in central Florida. She's been a nurse for 40 years and has worked in an emergency department for 15 years. She chairs the National Advocacy Advisory Council for Emergency Nurses.

Dr. Eaton, who Senator Mikulski mentioned, is a professor at the Bloomberg School of Public Health, an expert in his field who has written hundreds of articles. Much of his work has focused on the co-occurrence of mental health disorders and other chronic health issues, like diabetes and heart disease.

Mr. Hakeem Rahim is the CEO of Live Breathe, an organization focused on mental health advocacy and reducing the stigma associated with mental health. He brings his own invaluable perspective of his own journey of mental illness, which began during his freshman year in college.

We look forward to hearing from the four of you. If you'll each try to summarize your remarks in about 5 minutes, that will leave more time for the senators to have a conversation with you about your testimony.

Why don't we start with Dr. Hepburn.

STATEMENT OF BRIAN M. HEPBURN, MD, EXECUTIVE DIRECTOR, NATIONAL ASSOCIATION OF STATE MENTAL HEALTH PROGRAM DIRECTORS, ALEXANDRIA, VA

Dr. HEPBURN. Thank you very much, Chairman Alexander, Ranking Member Murray, and Senator Mikulski. It's hard to think of Maryland without Senator Mikulski. Thank you.

Thank you for the opportunity today to address this committee on State services regarding mental illness. Thanks go to this committee and its members and other members of the Senate and the House who are working to find ways to support, strengthen, and augment the country's mental health system.

I want to especially thank, in addition to the chair and ranking member, Senators Cassidy and Murphy and also Senator Franken. I also want to congratulate Senator Franken on his second grandchild. That's where it all starts, being a good grandparent.

We appreciate the full Congress passing Senator Cardin's legislation on IMD Demonstration. Also, we appreciate the support from Congress on the First Episode Psychosis Program.

The organization which I represent, the National Association of State Mental Health Program Directors, represents the State executives of the Mental Health Authorities, representing agencies that have $41 billion in public mental health services and deliver services to 7.3 million people. The mission of NASMHPD is to work with the States and partners in order to promote wellness, recovery, and resiliency.

NASMHPD members work to promote prevention and early intervention, integration of behavioral health and physical health, trauma informed approaches, minimized consumer contact with police, develop the workforce, promote supported employment, supportive housing, and decrease homelessness, support the use of data and health information technology.

The State Mental Health Authorities vary widely in terms of how they're organized. However, they share some common functions: planning and coordinating a comprehensive array of mental health services, submitting an annual application to the Block Grant, educating the public, operating and funding inpatient services. This could be with State hospitals, or it could be buying inpatient services in the private sector.

The State Mental Health Authorities work closely with SAMHSA, which has been an excellent partner for us. The acting administrator, Kana Enomoto, is a respected leader in the field. We appreciate having her as a leader and a partner.

SAMHSA has provided strong leadership in promoting the best practices for individuals with severe mental illness. The best example of that is the First Episode Psychosis Program. The First Episode Psychosis Program started with research. The research showed that it was a best practice. NIMH then worked with SAMHSA to promote the First Episode Psychosis Program. Its implementation is now across the country. It's really an excellent way of showing how the Federal Government can work with the States and work with providers in order to promote a best practice.

It's important to note that the role of the State Mental Health Authorities has changed over the last 30 years. Thirty years ago, the States were primarily involved in State hospitals. Seventy-five percent of the budget went to State hospitals. Now, 75 percent of the budget goes to the community.

Thirty years ago, the private sector was not really addressing issues that are in the public sector. Now, it's hard to separate public sector and private sector. When it comes to admissions to State hospitals, now, almost all the admissions are court related. Almost all the civil admissions were previously uninsured individuals going to State hospitals. Now, those uninsured individuals get the same care as insured individuals, and they go to the private sector.

I want to say something about the funding for the State Mental Health Authorities. Basically, the funding for most States is primarily from the States themselves, so that the State budget and Medicaid make up for almost all that's spent in the budget by the State Mental Health Authority. The Block Grant accounts for less than 1 percent of the funding for mental health within the States.

What are some additional actions that Congress and the Administration could take to support the State Mental Health Authorities? One is, as I indicated, the First Episode Psychosis Program, an excellent program. The fact that you've agreed to move it from 5 percent to 10 percent is excellent. What we would ask is for a change in the methodology. The smaller States are not able to move ahead with the First Episode Psychosis Program the way the larger States are because of the Block Grant methodology.

A second is to modify the Medicaid Institution of Mental Disease exclusion so that IMDs can get paid for taking care of individuals with Medicaid who are adults, at least, to start with the private sector. In Maryland, we participated with a demonstration that showed that the average length of stay in the private psychiatric hospitals were 10 days. Cost per episode was about the same as for the acute and general hospital psychiatric units.

We would ask to reauthorize the Medicaid Money Follows the Person. This has been a very important program in terms of helping to keep people——

The CHAIRMAN. Dr. Hepburn, could you wind down your testimony, please?

Dr. HEPBURN. Yes, I'm sorry—to keep people out of institutions, promoting zero suicide, promoting technology, promoting smoking cessation, and supporting mental health and addiction parity. And with that, I will stop.

Thank you very much.

[The prepared statement of Dr. Hepburn follows:]

Prepared Statement of Brian Hepburn, MD

Chairman Alexander, Ranking Member Murray, and members of the Senate HELP Committee, thank you for the opportunity today to address the Senate HELP Committee on State services for individuals with mental illness. And our thanks go to this committee and its members, and other Members of Congress in the Senate and the House, who are working to find ways to support, strengthen, and augment the country's mental health care delivery system through legislation. Thanks especially to the Chair and Ranking Member for their own *Mental Health Awareness and Improvement Act*, Senators Cassidy and Murphy for their *Mental Health Reform Act*, and Senators Franken and Cornyn for their *Comprehensive Justice and Mental Health Act*. We are also appreciative of the full

SMHA mental health services (29 percent of SMHA funds, or $11.9 billion), followed by Medicare (1.7 percent). The MHBG constitutes just 1 percent of SMHA funding. MHBG funding—totaling $450.4 million in fiscal year 2015, varies widely by State under a consumer-based formula; in fiscal year 2015, State MHBG moneys ranged from California's $63.1 million to Wyoming's $535,764.

Among the effective, evidence-based practices identified and promoted by SAMHSA through its National Registry of Evidence-Based Programs and Practices (NREPP) are those intended to address First Episodes of Psychosis (FEP). Recognizing the demonstrated effectiveness of FEP pilots funded by the National Institute for Mental Health (NIMH) since 2008 in reducing incidences of untreated mental illness, Congress for the first time in fiscal year 2014 designated 5 percent of all MHBG moneys—and increased grant funding accordingly—for programs that address first episodes of serious mental illness, including projects based on NIMH's RAISE ("Recovery After an Initial Schizophrenic Episode") FEP model operating in States such as Connecticut, New York, and Maryland. For this fiscal year 2016, Congress has increased the block grant set-aside for FEP initiatives to 10 percent, again increasing block grant funding to cover the expanded set-aside.

States have also become increasingly involved in working with consumer advocates, peer support workers with lived experience, providers, and State insurance divisions to see that insurers comply with the Federal mental health and addiction parity mandates enacted in 2008 and 2010. Full compliance is still a work in progress, but NASMHPD is convinced that continuing education and monitoring of insurers by providers, consumers, and State agencies should eventually ensure that mental health and substance use benefits are subject to no restrictions—quantitative or non-quantitative—greater than those imposed on surgical and medical benefits.

As increased MHBG funding continues to be made available to the States by Congress, the States should be able to effectively grow their FEP services and the other community-based services for which payers and payment are scarce, such as crisis services, wraparound services, supported housing and supported employment, and ACA enrollment outreach. NASMHPD's members are grateful for the assistance provided so far, and we look forward to continuing to work with SAMHSA and Congress in developing a continuum of evidence-based mental health care and services for each community.

What are some additional actions that Congress and the Administration could take to support the State Mental Health Authorities?

- Continue to support the set aside for First Episode Psychosis programs, but consider changing the allocation methodology so that States with smaller consumer populations and thus smaller block grants, like Rhode Island, Alaska, Maine, Vermont, Wyoming, North Dakota, and Delaware, may receive an amount sufficient to fully implement a working FEP program.

- Modify the Medicaid Institution for Mental Disease (IMD) exclusion so that IMDs are able to receive Medicaid funding for adults.
- Reauthorize the Medicaid Money Follows the Person program, due to expire September 30, which States such as Texas are using to help fund behavioral health services for individuals in home- and community-based settings.
- Support the Zero Suicide goal. The National Suicide Prevention Lifeline, with funding from SAMHSA under the Garrett Lee Smith Act, has developed an excellent hotline system across the country, linking callers with needed crisis services.
- Encourage the use of technology for mental health through reimbursement by Medicaid. As stigma has decreased and more persons are seeking mental health services, there is a workforce and access problem. Technology such as telehealth may be able to help with both. Internet services help to reach underserved rural, urban, and frontier areas.
- Support targeted efforts for smoking cessation in persons with mental illness. Persons with mental illness die at a much earlier age than the general population. This is primarily due to smoking.

And, finally, support parity by strengthening monitoring and enforcement mechanisms. Thank you for your attention to and consideration of this testimony.

The CHAIRMAN. Thanks, Dr. Hepburn. Ms. Blake.

STATEMENT OF PENNY BLAKE, RN, CCRN, CEN, STAFF RN EMERGENCY DEPARTMENT, EMERGENCY NURSES ASSOCIATION, NORTH PALM BEACH, FL

Ms. BLAKE. Chairman Alexander, Ranking Member Murray, and members of the committee, thank you for inviting me to testify at this important hearing.

I'm an emergency nurse working full time in the emergency department at Good Samaritan Hospital in West Palm Beach. It's an acute care community hospital. In addition to the work in the emergency department, I'm the chairperson of the Advocacy Advisory Council for the Emergency Nurses Association, which is the largest professional health care organization dedicated to improving emergency care.

As a registered nurse for almost 40 years, my career has been devoted to providing the best possible care to every person who comes into our hospital's emergency department. Increasingly, this involves treating patients who are suffering from mental illnesses.

The emergency department at my hospital has a capacity of 32 actual beds which can be expanded if necessary. It serves a very diverse community that includes extreme poverty and some of the wealthiest neighborhoods in the entire country.

Since the Federal law prohibits hospitals from turning away anyone seeking emergency care, I see practically every kind of urgent medical condition. But on a typical shift, at least 10 percent of our cases involve psychiatric patients.

The reasons for the surge in mental health patients include an increase in drug abuse, veterans returning from Iraq and Afghanistan who suffer from PTSD, and the stresses that are created by a weak economy and joblessness. But in my view, the principal cause is the lack of adequate treatment options and resources in the community. Mental health patients often find they have nowhere to turn for treatment, so they go to the one place, the emergency room, that's guaranteed to be open at all times and willing to care for every patient.

In Florida, a physician or law enforcement officer can invoke a State law that allows for the involuntary hold for up to 72 hours for a person who is deemed to be a threat to themselves or others. After a 72-hour hold is put on the patient, the emergency department physician must clear the patient of any physical illness, and then the patient is placed in a 10 by 10 room until we can find a facility that can accept the patient for evaluation by a psychiatrist, because at my hospital, we do not have any psychiatrists on staff, and we do not have a psychiatric unit.

So all patients requiring inpatient care must be transferred to one of the four psychiatric facilities in Palm Beach County. I cannot think of a single time in the past year that any of our patients has been accepted immediately when that request has been made.

A mentally ill patient typically stays in our ED between 12 and 24 hours before they are transferred to a psychiatric care facility. However, 2, 3, or even 4 days boarding in the emergency department is not unusual. This is also the case in other hospitals in Palm Beach County, and the problem is made worse by the lack of insurance coverage for people who suffer from mental illnesses.

Our experience is consistent with research conducted by the Emergency Nurses Association that found that the average boarding time in the emergency department is 18 hours for psychiatric patients versus only 4 hours for all other types of patients. Inadequate community health services and extended boarding times are detrimental both for emergency departments and the care received by mental health patients.

For hospital EDs, mental health patients are both resource and personnel intensive. Not only do these patients stay in the emergency department much longer than other patients, but they often require close supervision by multiple staff and personalized medical attention. By necessity, it diverts nurses, doctors, and technicians from the treatment of the other patients who come through our doors.

Whenever a patient is placed on a 72-hour hold, we have a certain protocol we must follow in order to ensure that patient's safety. A security guard in our facility is placed at the door. For the patients who are experiencing a mental health crisis, the emergency department is far from the ideal place to receive care. EDs are chaotic, often loud areas in the hospital, and the nurses and physicians are stretched to their limits in caring for the other patients.

Our emergency physicians are understandably reluctant to prescribe psychoactive medications for these patients because it's not their area of expertise. So if a patient needs medication, we usually just give some form of antianxiety agent. They don't begin any kind of therapeutic interventions because there's no one there with professional psychiatric training to help provide it.

Imagine that you are stressed, anxious, possibly suicidal and/or psychotic, perhaps having hallucinations, and you're confined to a small space. All your belongings are taken away from you so you can't hurt yourself. A guard is at your door, and there's constant chaos, noise, and motion. And because of the shortage of inpatient beds or community-based treatment and psychiatric options, this situation continues for many hours or even days.

Mental health care patients would be better served in facilities that have specialized expertise. The most important thing that we feel is needed is that communities must have the health care infrastructure and funding to provide resources needed to keep this population healthy. They need to have parity for insurance and the same kind of coverage that people with physical illnesses have and a high-quality, community-based mental health system which would include acute and longer term care, access to community mental health clinics, inpatient and outpatient treatment, and the availability of 24-hour crisis psychiatric care and services that will allow the patient to be integrated more fully into society.

I want to thank you for allowing me the opportunity to represent and speak for my fellow emergency nurses. We passionately care about providing the best possible care to all of our patients, and we strive for them to have the best outcomes possible for their illnesses. That includes those who are the most vulnerable in our society, the person who is suffering from mental illness.

Thank you.

[The prepared statement of Ms. Blake follows:]

Prepared Statement of Penny Blake, RN, CCRN, CEN

Summary

Chairman Alexander, Ranking Member Murray, members of the committee, thank you for inviting me to testify at this important hearing. My name is Penny Blake and I am an emergency nurse working in the emergency department at Good Samaritan Medical Center in West Palm Beach, FL. I have been a registered nurse for almost 40 years. My entire career has been devoted to providing the best possible care to every person who comes into my hospital's ED. Increasingly, this involves treating patients who are suffering from severe mental illnesses and substance abuse.

Since Federal law prohibits hospitals from turning away anyone seeking emergency care, I see practically every kind of urgent medical condition imaginable. However, at least 10 percent of our cases involve psychiatric patients. This percentage has grown tremendously in the past several decades.

There are multiple reasons for the surge in mental health patients coming to hospital emergency departments. However, in my view, the principal cause is the lack of adequate treatment options and resources in the community. The shortfall in community mental health resources often leads to the boarding of psychiatric patients in the emergency department.

In Florida, a physician or law enforcement officer can invoke the Baker Act, a State law that allows for the involuntary hold for up to 72 hours for a person deemed to be a threat to themselves or others. The typical length of time that a mentally ill patient stays in our ED before being transferred to a Baker Act facility is between 12 and 24 hours. However, 2, 3, or even 4 days boarding is not unusual. This is consistent with research conducted by ENA that found the average boarding time for psychiatric patients is 18 hours versus only 4 hours for all patients in the ED.

Inadequate community mental health services and extended boarding times are detrimental both for emergency departments and the care received by mental health patients. For hospital EDs, mental health patients are both resource- and personnel-intensive. By necessity, this diverts nurses, doctors and technicians from the treatment of other patients.

For patients experiencing a mental health crisis, the emergency department is far from the ideal place to receive care. By their nature, EDs are chaotic, often loud areas of the hospital where nurses and physicians are regularly stretched to their limits taking care of everything from traumatic injuries to heart attacks. In addition, specialists in psychiatric care are not always available to see patients. Mental health patients would be better served in facilities that have the specialized expertise to handle the complex diagnosis and treatment of mental illness.

Our mental health patients and their families deserve better care than we currently give them. Most importantly, communities must have the health care infrastructure and funding to provide the resources needed to keep this population healthy. A high-quality, community-based mental health system would include acute and longer term care, access to community mental health clinics, inpatient and outpatient treatment, the availability of 24-hour crisis psychiatric care and services that would allow for integrating the patient more fully into society.

Thank you for allowing me the opportunity to represent and speak for my fellow emergency nurses. We passionately care about providing the best possible care to ALL of our patients, and strive for them to have the best outcomes possible for their illnesses. This includes those who are among the most vulnerable in our society— the person suffering from a mental illness.

Introduction

Chairman Alexander, Ranking Member Murray, members of the committee, thank you for inviting me to testify at this important hearing. My name is Penny Blake and I am an emergency nurse working full-time in the emergency department at Good Samaritan Medical Center, an acute care community hospital in West Palm Beach, FL.

In addition to my work in the emergency department, I am the Chairperson of the Advocacy Advisory Council for the Emergency Nurses Association (ENA), the largest professional health care organization dedicated to improving emergency nursing care. ENA has 41,000 members throughout the United States and around the world. I am also the Government Affairs Chair for the Florida Emergency Nurses Association and past president of the Palm Beach County chapter of ENA.

The Challenges Confronting Emergency Departments in Caring for the Mentally Ill

I have been a registered nurse for almost 40 years. The majority of that time has been at the bedside in critical care and, for the past 18 years, in the emergency department. My entire career has been devoted to providing the best possible care to every person who comes into my hospital's emergency department. Increasingly, this involves treating patients who are suffering from severe mental illnesses and substance abuse.

The emergency department at Good Samaritan Medical Center has a capacity of 32 actual beds, which can be expanded by utilizing the halls and walls when necessary. It serves a very diverse community that includes extreme poverty and homelessness, as well as some of the wealthiest neighborhoods in the entire country.

Our patient mix varies depending on the time of day or the day of the week. Since Federal law prohibits hospitals from turning away anyone seeking emergency care, I see practically every kind of urgent medical condition imaginable. However, on a typical shift, at least 10 percent of our cases involve psychiatric patients. This percentage has grown tremendously in the past several decades.

There are multiple reasons for the surge in mental health patients coming to hospital emergency departments. These include an increase in drug abuse, the large number of veterans returning from Iraq and Afghanistan who suffer from PTSD, and the stresses created by a weak economy and joblessness.

However, in my view, the principal cause is the lack of adequate treatment options and resources in the community. Mental health patients often find they have nowhere to turn for treatment, so they go to the one place—emergency departments—guaranteed to be open at all times and willing to care for every patient.

In my hospital, the shortfall in community mental health resources often leads to the boarding of psychiatric patients in the emergency department.

In Florida, a physician or law enforcement officer can invoke the Baker Act, which is a State law that allows for the involuntary hold for up to 72 hours for a person who is deemed to be a threat to themselves or others.

At Good Samaritan, after a hold is put on a patient, the ED physician must clear the patient of any physical illness. The patient is then placed in a 10 x 10 room until we can find a facility that can accept the patient for evaluation by a psychiatrist to determine if continued inpatient treatment is warranted.

My hospital does not have psychiatrists on staff, nor do we have a psychiatric unit. Therefore, all patients requiring inpatient care must be transferred to one of the four psychiatric facilities in Palm Beach County. I cannot think of a single time in the past year that any of our patients has been accepted immediately when the request has been made.

The typical length of time that a mentally ill patient stays in our ED before they are transferred to a Baker Act facility is between 12 and 24 hours. However, 2, 3, or even 4 days boarding in the emergency department is not unusual. Based on conversations I have had with colleagues, this is also the case in other hospitals throughout the Palm Beach County area.

Last year, I visited the ED at a hospital in the southern part of the county. They had 14 patients lined up on stretchers in one of their hallway wings, all awaiting placement in inpatient psychiatric facilities. I was told that was a typical day for them. This problem is made worse by the lack of insurance coverage for people who suffer from mental illness.

My personal observations are consistent with research conducted by ENA that found the average boarding time in the emergency department for psychiatric patients is 18 hours versus only 4 hours for all patients in the ED.

Inadequate community mental health services and extended boarding times are detrimental both for emergency departments and the care received by mental health patients.

For hospital EDs, mental health patients are both resource- and personnel-intensive. Not only do these patients stay in the emergency department much longer than other patients, but they often require close supervision by multiple staff and, if available, personalized medical attention. By necessity, this diverts nurses, doctors and technicians from the treatment of other patients.

When a psychiatric patient who is in our emergency department is deemed to require invocation of the Baker Act, we have a certain protocol we must follow to ensure that patient's safety. The patient is assigned to a closed room, their personal belongings are removed, they are given a gown and slipper socks, and a security guard is placed outside their door, within sight of the patient. We do not have designated rooms for psychiatric patients, so we must attempt to modify the room they are in to prevent access to articles that might be used to harm themselves or others.

The nurse who is assigned to that pod of rooms assumes the care for that patient, along with the other four or five patients who are also in that pod. None of the RN's with whom I work has received any in-depth specialized education in the care of the mentally ill. We all may have had some courses during our nursing education, but for many of us, that was a long time ago.

For patients experiencing a mental health crisis, the emergency department is far from the ideal place to receive care. By their nature, EDs are chaotic, often loud areas of the hospital where nurses and physicians are regularly stretched to their limits taking care of everything from traumatic injuries to heart attacks.

In addition, specialists in psychiatric care are not always available to see patients in the emergency department. As I discussed earlier, this is the case in the hospital where I work.

Further, our emergency physicians are understandably reluctant to prescribe psychoactive medications for these patients, as it is not their area of expertise. This usually translates into the patient being medicated with some form of anti-anxiety agent, if needed, and then kept in the room on a stretcher, only being allowed accompanied trips to the bathroom. They receive a blanket, a pillow, a TV with remote control and meals. The assigned nurse assesses their vital signs and functions every 4 hours or more often as indicated. They do not begin therapeutic intervention as there is no one present with professional training to begin a therapeutic dialog.

Imagine being someone who is already stressed, anxious, possibly suicidal and/or psychotic, and perhaps having auditory or visual hallucinations. Then, you are confined to a small space, all your belongings are removed so you cannot hurt yourself, a guard is at your door, the lights are on outside the room all the time, and there is constant chaos, noise and motion. Further, imagine that because of the shortage of inpatient beds or community-based treatment options, this situation continues for many hours or even days.

Although we do everything possible to care for all patients in a professional and compassionate manner, mental health patients would be better served in facilities that have the specialized expertise to handle the complex diagnosis and treatment of mental illness.

In rare cases, the boarding of mental health patients and the subsequent overcrowding can also lead to violence in the ED. Although the vast majority of behavioral health patients are no more violent than other patients, there is no doubt that lack of treatment can exacerbate a stressful situation for these patients.

How To Improve Patient Care

Our mental health patients and their families deserve better care than we currently give them. I did an informal poll of my colleagues across the country on what they believe are the most important needs for the behavioral health patients we see in our EDs. Their views exactly reflected mine.

These patients need access to the most appropriate facility for the problem they are having. In most cases, that facility should not be the local emergency department.

Individuals with psychiatric and substance abuse conditions should receive prioritization, resources, and treatment based upon clinical presentation that is equivalent to that provided for other illnesses and injuries.

Individuals with psychiatric and substance abuse conditions must be provided parity with regard to third-party reimbursement.

Emergency psychiatric services need to utilize a consistent practice model, including standardized procedures and protocols, for patient care regardless of facility, day of the week, or time of day.

Most importantly, communities must have the health care infrastructure and funding to provide the resources needed to keep this population healthy. These resources should include all related services. A high-quality, community-based mental health system would include acute and longer term care, access to community mental health clinics, inpatient and outpatient treatment, the availability of 24-hour crisis psychiatric care and services that would allow for integrating the patient more fully into society.

Any program should also promote collaboration and communication between emergency departments and their respective community agencies to effectively coordinate the care of patients with psychiatric and substance abuse conditions.

Conclusion

Thank you for allowing me the opportunity to represent and speak for my fellow emergency nurses. We passionately care about providing the best possible care to ALL of our patients, and strive for them to have the best outcomes possible for their illnesses. This includes those who are among the most vulnerable in our society— the person suffering from a mental illness.

The CHAIRMAN. Thank you, Ms. Blake.

Dr. Eaton.

Statement of William W. Eaton, Ph.D., Professor, Department of Mental Health, Johns Hopkins Bloomberg School of Public Health, Baltimore, MD

Mr. EATON. Senator Alexander, Senator Murray and members of the committee, I think you are doing great work and I appreciate the opportunity to speak to you.

My orientation is from that of epidemiology, especially social epidemiology. The first point I wanted to make is, we all know somebody who has mental illness of one type or other or alcohol or drug abuse, and we feel strongly about this.

But there has been developed a new metric in the field of epidemiology called Disability Adjusted Life Years. That metric allows us to compare the disease burden of all the diseases, the mental and substance use disorders, as well as cancer, stroke, and all the physical diseases. When we do that comparison on a population basis using epidemiologic data, it clearly shows that mental and substance use disorders are the most important category of disease burden, and depression is the single most important disease itself in terms of disease burden.

The importance of mental disorders has been recognized many times in the past—the surgeon general's report, the New Freedom Commission, and so forth. But now we have a metric which establishes scientifically that mental and substance use disorders are the most important form of disease category.

One of the reasons for this is that the mental disorders begin early in life, and they're slow. You talk to somebody who has just had an onset of depressive disorder about it, and it turns out it will have started 10 years earlier. And the consequences of that depressive disorder will not show up sometimes for another 10 years.

The mental disorders, especially depressive disorder, actually predicts onset of stroke, dementia, heart attack, diabetes. It predicts it more powerfully than the common risk factors that we know. For example, a person with a history of depressive disorder has three or four times the risk of a heart attack. That's a higher risk than somebody with high blood pressure or with a family history of heart disease.

The point is that the fact these mental disorders start early, they take a long time, and the consequences for physical illnesses are very strong. We need more research to figure out why these consequences are occurring, but also this argues, as has been stated, for the integration of primary health care with psychiatric care, because now the primary care doctor is interested in saving the life of his patient, the way he should be, and that means he should screen for depressive disorder and other disorders, probably, and learn how to do it. We should make that technology available.

I want to say that there are a range of prevention programs for mental and substance use disorders. There are many of them, and they have beneficial outcomes, proven years or even decades following the intervention. Most of these prevention programs are social interventions early in the life course prior to the onset of the disorder, so in the school system, for example, or even shortly after birth. Those preventive interventions are one of the unused resources, I guess I would say.

As a tiny aside, I would say there have been breakthroughs in genetics, especially the so-called methylation issue in genetics, which shows that the tendency for a gene to operate or not operate is affected by the environment. So in the future, we'll be studying the way genes and environment work together, and when we study that, we're likely to be oriented toward the social environment. The way the social environment works together with genetic material is the way that mental disorders have their occurrence.

The failure to help people with severe mental disorders is the most glaring problem in our mental health system. And it turns out that severe mental illnesses like schizophrenia and bipolar disorder—I think perhaps you know this, Senator Alexander, but they are associated with a shortened life span by even two decades.

Somebody with schizophrenia will die 20 years earlier. They're not dying from schizophrenia. They're dying because we're not paying attention to the preventive activities that you and I receive, like Valsartan for blood pressure or lipid-lowering drugs. So that's almost a criminal issue that these folks are dying so much earlier, and nobody chooses to be schizophrenic. It happens to them. It seems like we owe them that.

Finally, in building programs related to brain research, I want to mention that the National Institute of Mental Health has lost its focus on public mental health, and also it has abandoned what should be its natural interest in diagnostic categories. These new programs at the National Institute of Mental Health have basically confused a huge range of researchers and puzzled the international community. This also has vitiated the probability of developing research-based prevention programs for mental and substance use disorders.

From my point of view, the action is preventive interventions early in the life course, mostly social.

Thank you for your time.

[The prepared statement of Mr. Eaton follows:]

Prepared Statement of William W. Eaton, PhD

Summary

The Senate Hearing on Mental Health is appropriate because it is now established; using new and accepted measures of the burden of disease, that mental and substance use disorders produce a higher burden of disease in the United States than any other category of disease. For specific disorders, Major Depression is the single largest source of disease burden in the United States, as compared with all other diseases; and alcohol use disorders are the fifth largest source of disease burden.

Mental and substance use disorders occurring early in life predict later occurrence of important diseases such as diabetes, cardiovascular conditions, stroke, and dementia, and severe mental illnesses are associated with a dramatically shortened life span.

There are a range of successful population-based programs for preventing mental and substance use disorders. Most of these involve social interventions early in the life course.

Breakthroughs in genetics, including the study of methylation, when combined with measures of the environment including the vagaries of social life, will offer new opportunities to prevent mental and substance use disorders in the future.

The failure to help people with severe mental disorders of psychotic intensity, such as schizophrenia and bipolar disorder, is the most glaring problem in the mental health system.

The National Institute of Mental Health (NIMH) has lost its focus on public health and abandoned what should be its central focus on accepted diagnostic categories.

The mental health efforts of the Federal Government would benefit by careful consolidation of governmental units such as the NIMH, National Institute on Drug Abuse (NIDA), the National Institute on Alcohol Abuse and Alcoholism (NIAAA), and perhaps some programs of the Substance Abuse and Mental Health Administration (SAMHSA).

* * *

This testimony is designed to give a brief and selective review of important aspects of public health as applied to the mental and substance use disorders. The presenter is William W. Eaton, professor and former chair of the Department of Mental Health, Bloomberg School of Public Health, Johns Hopkins University. The testimony represents the opinions of William Eaton and not the viewpoint of the Johns Hopkins University.

It is an opportune time for the U.S. Senate to be conducting hearings about mental and substance use because of the growing awareness of the importance of this topic. This growing awareness is in part due to the creation, about 20 years ago, of an algebra for estimating the overall burden of diseases, which allows comparison of the burden of diseases such as cancer, which are often fatal, to diseases such as depressive disorder, which is impairing and often long-lasting, but not as likely to be fatal [1]. The new metric—Disability Adjusted Life Years, or DALYs—is accepted around the globe. Combining epidemiologic data on incidence, chronicity, and associated mortality for a given disorder, with clinical information about the disability associated with a disorder, it is possible to estimate the number of Disability Adjusted Life Years experienced by the total world population in a year—that is, entire burden of all occurrences of the specific disorder in the world, with this metric. As well, the total number of DALYs experienced as a result of all diseases in the world can be estimated. The broad category of mental and substance use disorders were responsible for 7.4 percent of the total disease burden experienced in the world in 2010—about the same percentage as the category of malignant neoplasms, and less than the 11.9 percent explained by the category of cardiovascular and circulatory diseases [2]. In the United States and Canada in 2004, where the effect of fatal diseases of infancy and childhood is lessened than in the world as whole, the mental and substance use disorders were by far the largest contributor to the total burden of disease (about 24 percent of the total number of DALYs), compared to any other categories, such as cancer (12 percent of total DALYs) or cardiovascular conditions (14 percent) [3]. For more narrow disease conditions, Unipolar depressive disorders were responsible for 8.4 percent of the DALYS in the United States and Canada, the largest source compared to all other diseases (e.g., ischemic heart disease, responsible for 6.3 percent; cerebrovascular disease accounting for 3.9 percent). The fifth most important cause in the United States and Canada was alcohol use disorders (3.4 percent of all DALYs).

The importance of mental and substance use disorders has been emphasized for many years in prior reports such as the Surgeon General's Report in 1999, [4] the President's New Freedom Commission in 2003, [5] and the Institute of Medicine report in 2006 on Improving the Quality of Health Care for Mental and Substance-Use Conditions [6]. Since the development of the Burden of Disease metric, the importance of mental and substance use disorders has been more firmly established.

The estimates of DALYs for mental and substance use disorders are higher than for other sometimes fatal disorders such as cancer because of the lifetime structure of these disorders: the mental and substance use disorders start much earlier in life, during childhood and adolescence in many cases, and a sizable proportion of the mental and substance use disorders endure for many years [7]. But the estimate may actually be biased low, because of the effect the mental and substance use disorders have in raising risk for important medical conditions such as diabetes, heart disease, stroke, and dementia. For example, a person with a history of depressive disorder has about two or three times the risk for onset of diabetes, or having a heart attack or stroke, as someone who has not had an episode of depressive disorder. This enhanced risk associated with depressive disorder is larger than many other well-known risk factors, such as a family history of the physical condition, or, for heart attack as an example the raised risk associated with high blood pressure or high cholesterol. For each of these medical conditions this enhanced risk resulting from depressive disorder has been replicated in more than five studies [8, 9, 10]. There is also enhanced risk for onset of dementia in those with a history of depressive disorder, replicated more than five times [11]. It has been estimated that persons with severe mental illness like schizophrenia and bipolar disorder have 20 years shorter life span [12] than the general population, probably not caused by their mental illness, but rather because the treatment and prevention of other chronic medical conditions is ignored.

There are three important implications of these findings of mental to physical co-morbidity.

- First, the estimates of disease burden for mental and substance use disorders may be biased low because they don't account for mental disorders as early sources of physical disorders.
- Second, the possibility exists to lower the risk for the physical disorders by successful treatment of the mental disorders. Less than half of those with mental and substance use disorders get into treatment, in part due to the stigma of mental and substance use disorders, in part due to the cost involved, and in part due to the difficulty in finding good options for treatment [13]. This logic reflects on the advantages of improving the system of care for mental and substance use disorders.
- Third, the health care system will benefit by integrating systems of primary health care with systems designed for treatment of mental and substance use disorders.

- An aspect of mental and substance use disorders that is not well-appreciated is that there are many viable techniques for preventing their occurrence. The high prevalence of these disorders, their comorbidity, and the difficulty of treating them successfully argues for population-based prevention programs, which typically are aimed at entire populations ("universal interventions") or populations thought to be at high risk for the disorders ("selective interventions"). Because the disorders start early in life, it is logical to take advantage of prevention programs oriented toward childhood, adolescence and young adulthood. These prevention programs typically involve social activities of some sort, as opposed to medical interventions that occur after onset of disorder. For example:
- The Nurse-Family Partnership Program begins by identifying high-risk births and providing assistance to the mothers in the period after birth [14].
- The Good Behavior Game activates a social awareness in first graders with strong beneficial effects which last into adulthood [15].
- The Teenscreen program facilitates schools to identify and get help for adolescents who may be at risk for suicide [16, 17, 18]
- The Adolescent Depression Awareness Program, [19, 20] which is information about depressive disorder, designed in a format similar to information about other medical illnesses already available in the Health curriculum of many High Schools.

These are examples of successful programs which have been widely adopted, but their application could be expanded, and the results would be a diminution of the later occurrence of mental and substance use disorders. In 1994 the report of the Institute of Medicine Committee on Prevention of Mental Disorders concluded that: "There could be no wiser investment in our country than a commitment to foster the prevention of mental disorders and the promotion of mental health through rigorous research with the highest of methodological standards" [21].

This statement is still true.

There have been many advances in understanding the genetics of mental and substance use disorders in the last few decades, including breakthrough statistical techniques involving large samples of subjects (so-called Genome-Wide Association, or GWA, studies) [22]. Although most mental and substance use disorders have a moderate or strong tendency to be inherited, it is increasingly apparent that the inheritance will almost always be very complicated, involving many genes interacting in myriad ways. In the last decade it has become clear that the DNA can be permanently or temporarily activated, or deactivated, throughout the course of life ('methylation") [23]. The sources of the methylation include exposure to toxins, obstetric events, physical illnesses, and the vagaries of social life. Therefore, it seems likely that the next decade will involve increasing research on the way in which genetic background and the biological and social environment interact to change the future risk for mental disorder. In turn, these developments are likely to inform the design of selective intervention programs.

The most glaring problem of this Nation with regard to mental and substance use disorders is the failure to help people with disorders of psychotic intensity (schizophrenia and bipolar disorder), even though the deinstitutionalization movement in the early 1960s was supposed to free them from the asylums which had been designed originally to protect them. People do not choose to have schizophrenia, and it places an enormous and unfair burden on them. Since schizophrenia persists in the population, generation after generation, even though people with schizophrenia have low fertility, it may be that they are carrying the genetic burden for the rest of us—that is, the large number of genes connected to schizophrenia are healthy and life-preserving for most of the population, producing schizophrenia only when the genes combine, rarely, in a very particular fashion (an extension of the theory of heterozygote advantage [24, 25]). So, we owe them! Contrary to some characterizations, schizophrenia is not progressive in its nature: rather, people adapt to the disease over the life course, just as they might adapt to having diabetes [26]. The social environment in which they live is strongly associated with their success in adaptation. The social environment should be free from stigma, stable, with uncomplicated access to medical care, a structured workday, and the presence of friends and acquaintances. This structure is the aim of many rehabilitation programs, including the well-known clubhouse model, which has shown good success in generating stable employment and lower health costs [27, 28, 29, 30, 31].

The organization of government efforts to reduce the burden of mental disorders has become increasingly complex over the last several decades. In the early 1970s the National Institute of Mental Health (NIMH), part of the National Institutes of Health, was split into three institutes, including the NIMH, the National Institute on Alcohol Abuse and Alcoholism (NIAAA), and the National Institute on Drug Abuse (NIDA). The Substance Abuse and Mental Health Services Administration (SAMHSA) was created in the early 1990s. Many of the programs of these four units of the government overlap. For example, there are many separate surveys that estimate the use of marijuana or alcohol use in young people, some on a yearly basis (Monitoring the Future, funded by the NIDA [32]); National Survey of Drug Use and Health (funded by the SAMHSA),33 the National Epidemiologic Survey of Alcohol and Related Conditions (funded by the NIAAA) [33] and National Comorbidity Survey and its replication [34, 35] (NCS and NCS—R, funded by the NIMH). There are programs on prevention of suicide in the NIMH and the SAMHSA, and programs of research on prevention of mental and substance use disorders in all four units. One logical consolidation is to combine the two units focused on substance use, NIAAA and NIDA, into one National Institute on Substance Abuse ("NISA"). There is extensive comorbidity between drug and alcohol use disorders, [36] and many of the basic mechanisms of addiction are shared by the two groups of disorders, so consolidation would likely strengthen research efforts on both these closely related groups of disorders.

Since the formation of the SAMHSA, the public health aspects of the NIH units, especially that of the NIMH, have been diminished considerably. Even though the preventive interventions described above have a social aspect, the focus of research has been increasingly on the brain, missing the opportunity to design and implement effective new population-based interventions. Another departure from public health at the NIMH is the new disregard for diagnostic categories as a focus of research interest, [37] thereby emasculating the field of psychiatric epidemiology, the basic science of public mental health, because epidemiology requires an identifiable outcome. As well, the study of service systems and treatment research is hampered because there is a need for data on diagnoses as outcomes of preventive and clinical trials, and effectiveness of treatment systems as recorded in medical records. This new focus of the NIMH has puzzled the international community [38].

Many SAMHSA programs have a public health focus on prevention in the population, and on treatment systems. Some of these programs are excellent, but others lack a research base. There is relatively little focus in SAMHSA programs on disorders of psychotic intensity (described above), which, though rare, are the most impairing and most in need of attention. It may seem strange, but there is only one epidemiologist at the NIMH, and only one psychiatrist at the SAMHSA! It might be useful and efficient to combine some programs of the SAMHSA into the two NIH units (NIMH and the new NISA mentioned above), to reduce duplication, on the one hand, and to ensure that they retain a public health focus, on the other hand. This consolidation would generate better ability to take advantage of the new developments in gene by environment interactions described above, because the programs would be more likely to stay abreast of the rapidly developing research advances. It would not be appropriate to simply eliminate the SAMHSA because there are so many programs and services around the United States that depend on SAMHSA for guidance and funding, and there are many productive programs in the SAMHSA.

The consolidation of these programs is a complex task and would require the work of a special commission to design the new units and to schedule the consolidation. The result would be more advances in useful research, more effective treatment systems and prevention programs, and more efficient use of funds.

References

[1] Eaton WW, Alexandre P, Bienvenu OJ, Clarke D, Martins SS, Nestadt G, Zablotsky B. The Burden of Mental Disorders. In: Eaton WW, and the Faculty, Students and Fellows of the Department of Mental Health, ed. *Public Mental Health*. New York: Oxford University Press; 2012:3–30.

[2] Whiteford HA, Degenhardt L, Rehm J, Baxter AJ, Ferrari AJ, Erskine HE, Charlson FJ, Norman RE, Flaxman AD, Johns N, Burstein R, Murray CJ, Vos T. Global burden

of disease attributable to mental and substance use disorders: findings from the Global Burden of Disease Study 2010. *Lancet*. 2013;382(9904):1575– 86.

[3] Organization WH. *The Global Burden of Disease:* 2004 update. Geneva: World Health Organization; 2008. The figures for mental and substance use disorders were estimated by subtracting the DALYs associated with Neurological Diseases (Epilepsy, Parkinson's, Multiple Sclerosis, and Migraine) from the overall category of Neuropsychiatric Diseases, in Appendix Table 2.

[4] Goldman HH, Rye P, Sirovatka P. *Mental Health: a Report of the Surgeon General.* Washington, DC.: Government Printing Office; 1999.

[5] The President's New Freedom Commission on Mental Health. *Achieving the Promise: Transforming Mental Health Care in America.* Rockville, Maryland: Department of Health and Human Services; 2003.

[6] The Institute of Medicine Commission on Crossing the Quality Chasm: Adaptation to Mental Health and Addictive Disorders. *Improving the Quality of Health Care for Mental and Substance-Use Conditions.* Washington, DC.: The National Academies Press; 2006.

[7] Eaton WW, Alexandre PI, Kessler RC, Martins SS, Mortensen PB, Rebok GW, Storr CL, Roth K. The Population Dynamics of Mental Disorders. In: Eaton WW, Faculty SaFotDoMH, eds. *Public Mental Health.* New York: Oxford University Press; 2012:125–150.

[8] Mezuk B, Eaton WW, Albrecht S, Golden S. Depression and Type 2 Diabetes Over The life-span: A Meta-analysis. *Diabetes Care.* 2008;31(12):2383–90.

[9] Rugulies R. Depression as a predictor for coronary heart disease: a review and meta-analysis. *American Journal of Preventive Medicine.* 2002;23(1):51–61.

[10] Ramasubbu R, Patten SB. Effect of depression on stroke morbidity and mortality. *Can. J. Psychiatry.* 2003;48(4):250–257.

[11] Jorm A. History of depression as a risk factor for dementia: an updated review. *Australian and New Zealand Journal of Psychiatry.* 2001;35(6):776–781.

[12] Colton CW, Manderscheid RW. Congruencies in increased mortality rates, years of potential life lost, and causes of death among public mental health clients in eight States. *Prev. Chronic Dis.* 2006;3(2):A42.

[13] Mojtabai R, Eaton WW, Maulik PK. Pathways to Care: Need, Attitudes, Barriers. In: Eaton WW, Faculty S, and Fellows of the Department of Mental Health, Bloomberg School of Public Health, eds. *Public Mental Health.* New York: Oxford University Press; 2012:415–456.

[14] Olds DL, Kitzman H, Hanks C, Cole R, Anson E, Sidora-Arcoleo K, Luckey DW, Henderson CR, Jr., Holmberg J, Tutt RA, Stevenson AJ, Bondy J. Effects of nurse home visiting on maternal and child functioning: age–9 followup of a randomized trial. *Pediatrics.* 2007;120(4):e832–e845.

[15] Kellam SG, Brown CH, Poduska JM, Ialongo NS, Wang W, Toyinbo P, Petras H, Ford C, Windham A, Wilcox HC. Effects of a universal classroom behavior management program in first and second grades on young adult behavioral, psychiatric, and social outcomes. *Drug Alcohol Depend.* 2008;95 Suppl 1:S5–S28.

[16] Husky MM, Kaplan A, McGuire L, Flynn L, Chrostowski C, Olfson M. Identifying adolescents at risk through voluntary school-based mental health screening. *J. Adolesc.* 2011;34(3):505–511.

[17] Husky MM, Miller K, McGuire L, Flynn L, Olfson M. Mental health screening of adolescents in pediatric practice. *J. Behav. Health Serv. Res.* 2011;38(2):159–169.

[18] Husky MM, Sheridan M, McGuire L, Olfson M. Mental health screening and followup care in public high schools. *J. Am. Acad. Child Adolesc. Psychiatry.* 2011;50(9):881–891.

[19] Ruble AE, Leon PJ, Gilley-Hensley L, Hess SG, Swartz KL. Depression knowledge in high school students: effectiveness of the adolescent depression awareness program. *J. Affect. Disord.* 2013;150(3):1025–1030.

[20] Swartz KL, Kastelic EA, Hess SG, Cox TS, Gonzales LC, Mink SP, DePaulo JR, Jr. The effectiveness of a school-based adolescent depression education program. *Health Educ. Behav.* 2010;37(1):11–22.

[21] Mrazek PJ, Haggerty RJ. *Reducing risks for mental disorders.* Washington, DC: National Academy Press; 1994.

[22] Zandi PP, Wilcox C, Dong L, Chon S, Maher B. Genes as a Source of Risk for Mental Disorders. In: Eaton WW, and the Faculty, Students and Fellows of the Department of Mental Health, ed. *Public Mental Health.* New York: Oxford 2012:201–244.

[23] Nestler EJ, Pena CJ, Kundakovic M, Mitchell A, Akbarian S. Epigenetic Basis of Mental Illness. *Neuroscientist.* 2015.

[24] Bihlmeyer NA, Brody JA, Smith AV, Lunetta KL, Nalls M, Smith JA, Tanaka T, Davies G, Yu L, Mirza SS, Teumer A, Coresh J, Pankow JS, Franceschini N, Scaria A, Oshima J, Psaty BM, Gudnason V, Eiriksdottir G, Harris TB, Li H, Karasik D, Kiel DP, Garcia M, Liu Y, Faul JD, Kardia SL, Zhao W, Ferrucci L, Allerhand M, Liewald DC, Redmond P, Starr JM, De Jager PL, Evans DA, Direk N, Ikram MA, Uitterlinden A, Homuth G, Lorbeer R, Grabe HJ, Launer L, Murabito JM, Singleton AB, Weir DR, Bandinelli S, Deary IJ, Bennett DA, Tiemeier H, Kocher T, Lumley T, Arking DE. Genetic diversity is a predictor of mortality in humans. *BMC Genet.* 2014;15:159.

[25] Doi N, Hoshi Y, Itokawa M, Yoshikawa T, Ichikawa T, Arai M, Usui C, Tachikawa H. Paradox of schizophrenia genetics: is a paradigm shift occurring? *Behav. Brain Funct.* 2012;8:28.

[26] Eaton WW, Bilker W, Haro JM, Herrman H, Mortensen PB, Freeman H, Burgess P. Long-Term Course of Hospitalization for Schizophrenia: Part II Change with passage of time. *Schizophrenia Bulletin.* 1992;18:229–241.

[27] Everett A, Lee SY. Community and Public Mental Health Services in the United States: History and Programs. In: Eaton WW, and the Faculty, Students, and Fellows of the Department of Mental Health, ed. *Public Mental Health*. New York: Oxford University Press; 2012:396–414.

[28] Macias C, Jackson R, Schroeder C, Wang Q. What is a clubhouse? Report on the ICCD 1996 survey of USA clubhouses. *Community Ment. Health J.* 1999;35(2):181–190.

[29] Macias C, Rodican CF, Hargreaves WA, Jones DR, Barreira PJ, Wang Q. Supported employment outcomes of a randomized controlled trial of ACT and clubhouse models. *Psychiatr. Serv.* 2006;57(10):1406–1415.

[30] Warner R, Huxley P, Berg T. An evaluation of the impact of clubhouse membership on quality of life and treatment utilization. *Int. J. Soc. Psychiatry.* 1999;45(4):310–320.

[31] Hwang SW, J.; Eaton, W.W. *Analysis of the Association of Clubhouse Membership with Overall Costs of Care for Mental Health Treatment*. Baltimore 2016.

[32] Biondo G, Chilcoat HD. Discrepancies in prevalence estimates in two national surveys for nonmedical use of a specific opioid product versus any prescription pain reliever. *Drug Alcohol Depend.* 2014;134:396–400.

[33] Grucza RA, Abbacchi AM, Przybeck TR, Gfroerer JC. Discrepancies in estimates of prevalence and correlates of substance use and disorders between two national surveys. *Addiction*. 2007;102(4):623–629.

[34] Kessler R, Merikangas K. The national comorbidity survey replication (NCS- R): background and aims. *International Journal of Methods in Psychiatric Research.* 2004;13(2):60–68.

[35] Kessler RC. The national comorbidity survey: Preliminary results and future directions. *International Journal of Methods in Psychiatric Research.* 1995;5:140–151.

[36] Eaton WW, Alexandre P, Kessler RC, Martins SS, Mortensen PB, Rebok GW, Storr CL, Roth K. The Population Dynamics of Mental Disorders. In: Eaton WW, and the Faculty, Students and Fellows of the Department of Mental Health, ed. *Public Mental Health*. New York: Oxford; 2012:125–150.

[37] Insel T, Cuthbert B, Garvey M, Heinssen R, Pine DS, Quinn K, Sanislow C, Wang P. Research domain criteria (RDoC): toward a new classification framework for research on mental disorders. *Am. J. Psychiatry*. 2010;167(7):748–751.

[38] Phillips MR. Will RDoC hasten the decline of America's global leadership role in mental health? *World Psychiatry*. 2014;13(1):40–41.

The CHAIRMAN. Thank you, Dr. Eaton.

Mr. Rahim.

Statement of Hakeem Rahim, EDM, MA, CEO, Live Breathe LLC, Let's Talk Mental Illness, National Alliance on Mental Illness, Hempstead, NY

Mr. RAHIM. Chairman Alexander, Ranking Member Murray, members of the Health, Education, Labor, and Pensions Committee, Senators Cassidy and Murphy, thank you for taking these initial steps to improve the lives of millions impacted by mental illness.

Let me first share my journey with mental illness. It began in 1998 as a freshman at Harvard University. Three weeks into my first semester, I was struck by my first terrifying panic attack. My journey continued when I had my first manic episode and second one in the spring of 2000.

My next 2 weeks were filled with sleepless nights. I showered less frequently and ate sporadically. I had visions of Jesus, heard cars talking, spoke foreign languages. My parents rushed me to a psychiatric hospital, and I was diagnosed with bipolar disorder.

The last 18 years of my life have been defined by mental illness. Yet through support, proper treatment, and persistence, I have recovered and achieved wellness.

There are millions of Americans who are thriving in the face of mental illness: teachers who rise every morning to face their anxiety and their classroom full of students, veterans with lingering and visible scars of PTSD who will still provide for their families. Many are thriving, but many are not. To serve everyone living with mental illness, we must take steps to address stigma, access to medication, and peer support.

In 2012, I began speaking openly about my struggles to thousands of individuals with mental illness, their family members, law enforcement, faith-based communities, teachers, mental health professionals, and students. Since 2013, I have been a NAMI Queens/ Nassau Let's Talk Mental Illness presenter. I have been delivering presentations to students now, and I've spoken to more than 20,000 students across this country.

After one of my middle school presentations, a petite young African American girl walked up to me and started sharing that she was self-harming. When I asked her if she had told anybody, she said, "No, I have not," and then she lowered her shoulders. I told her, "That's OK. Thank you for being brave and telling me." We walked her over to her school counselor, the same school counselor a friend and a family member advised her not to go to.

Because she saw the importance of openly addressing stigma, and that school saw the importance of openly addressing stigma, the young girl's silence and reticence was dissolved. She was able to get the help that she needed.

Awareness and education is central to ending the shame around mental illness. Many parts of S. 1945 address key components that will break down the barriers from seeking treatment.

For many, medication is also an integral part of treatment. Medication has and continues to play a key role in my life. I still take anti-depressants and anti-psychotics every morning. They are central to my recovery and wellness. Finding the right combination of meds was at times a very harsh task for me. But, thankfully, by working with my doctor, I found the right combinations.

The struggle to find the correct medication is an arduous task for many. Finding the right medication can literally be the difference between life and death. Paul, as I will call him, a young man I know, went through 10 different diagnoses, electroconvulsive therapy, and at least 50 different combinations of medication. Twenty years after his first manic episode, however, he is now a mental health advocate. Because he had access to medication, he is now helping others work toward wellness.

We must keep medications protected, accessible, and affordable to people living with mental illness. Doctors and patients must have a choice in finding the right treatment, as the wrong treatment can lead to vicious cycles of hospital visits, substance abuse, exhausted caregivers, and even death.

However, medication alone cannot sustain wellness. Another key component of this bill is peer support. The power of being able to relate to others going through similar experiences cannot be understated. The peer support group I have interfaced with is the quintessential example of the power of the peer.

In an email chain in this particular support group, a member mentioned that he had relapsed into depression. Within an hour, there were responses to his email, one member even saying that, "Hey, I'll come pick you up." They truly understood the power and emotional strength of that support group, and that emotional support can shatter the weighted chains of depression. I'm happy to say that this group member is doing well, and he's really doing well now.

Having language codifying what a peer specialist is and what peer support looks like is essential to standardizing an invaluable component of mental wellness—peer support.

Mr. Chairman, Ranking Member Murray, and members of the HELP Committee, I am testifying as a voice for people living with mental illness. My journey does not, however, represent the full breadth of experience living with mental illness. My presence here today, however, does give a face to millions of Americans who are struggling, striving, and thriving in the face of mental health conditions.

Recovery from mental illness should be an option for all. Bill 1945 is a pronounced step in that direction, and I deeply and respectfully urge this committee to move forward on this strong bipartisan bill. And I would say that millions of people are depending on a transformation of how we address mental illness in America.

Thank you so much.

[The prepared statement of Mr. Rahim follows:]

Prepared Statement of Hakeem Rahim, EDM, MA

I thank each of you for inviting me to testify before this committee. Moreover I am moved to be able to contribute my voice to an issue that has impacted me well over half of my life—mental illness.

In the spring of 2000, as a sophomore at Harvard University, I was hospitalized for 2 weeks in a psychiatric hospital in Queens, NY. While hospitalized, I was diagnosed with bipolar disorder. I took time off from Harvard and subsequently returned and graduated with honors. After receiving my bachelors, I continued on to graduate school at Columbia University where I received a dual masters in psychological counseling. Currently, I am a mental health speaker, educator and advocate.

In 2012, I began speaking openly about my struggle with mental illness. To date, I have spoken to thousands of individuals with mental illness, their family members, law enforcement officials, faith based communities, teachers and mental health professionals. Since 2013, I have worked with NAMI Queens/Nassau as their Let's Talk Mental Illness presenter. In this role, I have spoken to over 20,000 college, high school and middle school students, delivering well over 300 presentations.

My advocacy work has helped bishops and pastors open up to their congregations; helped mothers and fathers better understand their children; and people with mental illness better understand their conditions. I believe the work I am doing is vital, and saving lives.

My journey does not encompass the full range of experiences of those impacted by mental illness. Living with mental illness is highly individualized; even people with the same diagnosis may have completely unique experiences. As a mental health speaker, educator and advocate, I have been fortunate to hear and see a spectrum of these experiences.

I have heard from people struggling to find work and housing because of barriers due to discrimination related to their mental illness; of parents concerned about their loved ones lack of ability to access treatment; and of people with mental illness who have been incarcerated due to their struggles with symptoms and not because of criminal intent.

Wellness should not be determined by favorable life situations, or serendipitous experiences. Rather, recovery from mental illness should be supported by established, effective, and easily accessible resources.

For this reason, Mr. Chairman, I and advocacy groups I am affiliated with, including NAMI, are very excited about this legislation. I support S.1945, drafted by Senators Cassidy and Murphy (members of this committee) and NAMI is a stronger supporter as well.

Mr. Chairman, Ranking Member Murray and members of the HELP Committee, recovery from mental illness should be a real option for all people living with mental illness. This bill is a pronounced step in this direction. I deeply and respectfully urge this committee to move forward with this strong bipartisan bill—millions of Americans are depending on a collective shift in how we treat and allow people to live their best lives in the face of mental illness.

* * *

Chairman Alexander, Ranking Member Murray, and Members of the Health, Education, Labor and Pensions Committee, I thank each of you for inviting me here today to testify before this committee. Moreover I am moved to be able to contribute my voice to an issue that has impacted me for over half of my life—mental illness.

My journey with mental illness began in 1998 during my freshman year at Harvard University. Three weeks into my first semester, I was struck by my first terrifying panic attack. At the time, I could not find words to describe the deep terror I felt, but I knew something was wrong. My journey continued when I had my first manic episode.

During the spring of 1999, I roamed the streets of my Long Island, NY neighborhood possessed with the delusion that I was a prophet and would save the world with my prophecies. Concerned, my parents sent me to Grenada to relax and be with family. However, there I plunged into a deep depression. I returned to Harvard that fall and struggled with anxiety and depression.

In the spring of 2000, I had a second manic episode. My next 2 weeks were filled with sleepless nights. I showered less frequently and ate sporadically. I had visions of Jesus, heard cars talking and 'spoke" foreign languages. This time my parents rushed me to a psychiatric hospital. I was hospitalized for 2 weeks in Queens, NY. My attending psychiatrist diagnosed me with bipolar disorder and explained that I would be on several medications. Upon my release from the hospital I met with a Brooklyn-based psychiatrist who end up working with me for the next 9 years.

After adjusting to heavy medication, I returned to Harvard University to continue my studies in psychology. However, due to cognitive impairment and other complications, I left school. In 2002, I returned, refocused and persevered to graduate from Harvard with honors. After receiving my bachelors, I continued on to graduate school at Columbia University. I received a dual masters in psychological counseling, and after worked for several years as a college academic advisor. All throughout this journey I have contended with the ups and downs of depression, anxiety and complications from medication including weight gain and cognitive slowing. Yet through this struggle and isolation, I have found ways to thrive and use my pain as a vehicle to fuel my work.

In 2012, I began speaking openly about my struggle with mental illness. To date, I have spoken to thousands of individuals with mental illness, their family members, law enforcement officials, faith based communities, teachers and mental health professionals. Since 2013, I have been the NAMI Queens/Nassau Let's Talk Mental Illness presenter. In this role, I delivered over 300 presentations to more than 20,000 college, high school and middle school students.

My advocacy work has helped bishops and pastors open up to their congregations; a mother seek help for her son who was traumatized by police brutality and another seek professional help after her daughter, an Olympian medalist, died by suicide. I have seen a homeless student, beset by anger issues and diagnosed with bipolar disorder, completely transform after opening up to her school social worker. Students have shared their struggles with me and to adults in their lives because of my mental health presentations. I believe this work is vital in saving lives.

My recovery and this work would not be possible if I did not have a firm foundation anchored in good mental health and wellness. My life has been informed but not limited by my mental illness. I have found ways to thrive and attribute my recovery to perseverance, support and access. The combination of these three factors has been essential to my wellness.

My wellness has been sustained in part due to a strong support network. My family has and continues to play an integral role in providing emotional, mental and financial support. Having this essential and consistent foundation has aided my recovery in innumerable ways. Along with a supportive family structure, upon my return to college, I utilized the readily available support structures at Harvard, including psychiatric visits and psychotropic medications.

Medication has played a huge role in my recovery. Daily I still use key antipsychotics and antidepressants that aid in my stability. This journey to find the right combination of medication has been marked with different dosages and combination of drugs, weight gain, cognitive impairment and long bouts of abysmal depression and paralyzing anxiety.

Along with medications, support groups have played a role in my recovery; the power of being able to confide in and relate to others going through similar experiences cannot be understated. Engaging with peers has shown me that even in my darkest times I am not alone. Along with peer support groups, programs like NAMI's In Our Own Voice, have given me platforms to share my story with communities and other people struggling with mental illness. Communities are an essential component for wellness, hence I am currently developing an online platform for these communities to continue to grow and thrive and for the voices of people impacted by mental illness to be heard.

My journey does not encompass the full range of experiences of those impacted by mental illness. Living with mental illness is highly individualized; even people with the same diagnosis may have completely unique experiences. As a mental health speaker, educator and advocate, I have been fortunate to hear and see a spectrum of these experiences.

Through my personal advocacy and work with NAMI, I have heard from many people struggling to find work and housing because of a variety of barriers including discrimination related to their mental illness. I have spoken to hundreds of people in numerous support groups which have included NAMI Family to Family classes and Depression and Bipolar Support Alliance peer support group. During these conversations, parents have spoken about their struggle to support their loved one, whether due to lack of ability to access treatment or because their loved one refuses treatment. People with lived experience have shared that they are unable to access medication because of insurance issues or loved ones with family members who have been incarcerated due to their struggles with symptoms and not because of criminal intent. Some can point to an experience like mine—full recovery. However many have spoken to the other side of this experience.

Wellness should not be determined by favorable life situations, or serendipitous experiences. Rather, recovery from mental illness should be supported by established, effective and easily accessible resources. I have worked hard to sustain my recovery and wellness living with mental illness however; I have had structures that have lent to my recovery while many do not.

For this reason, Mr. Chairman, I and advocacy groups I am affiliated with, including NAMI, are very excited about this legislation designed to reform our public mental health system—a system which should afford wellness for all. S. 1893, the Mental Health Awareness Act, is a good start, but given what I have experienced and have seen through my advocacy work, more is needed; individuals living with mental illness, and families impacted by mental illness need assistance sooner than later.

Both NAMI and I support S. 1945, drafted by Senators Cassidy and Murphy (members of this committee). A few of the important provisions in S. 1945 that I feel would go a long way toward reforming our mental health system and contributing to a better life for people living with serious mental illness and their families are:

Grants to the States to better integrate physical and mental health;

- Establishment of a new Assistant Secretary for Mental Health and Substance Use at HHS;
- Creation of a new Interagency Serious Mental Illness Coordinating Committee and a National Mental Health Policy Laboratory;
- New transparency requirements and stepped up enforcement of the Federal mental health parity law;
- New requirements in the Federal Mental Health Block Grant program for outreach and engagement to the most difficult to serve.

Mr. Chairman, Ranking Member Murray and members of the HELP Committee, I am aware I am testifying as a voice for people living with mental illness. My experience does not represent the full breadth of the experience living with mental illness, however my presence here does give a face to the millions of people in America struggling, striving and thriving with mental health conditions. Recovery from mental illness should be a real option for all. This bill is a pronounced step in this direction. I deeply and respectfully urge this committee to move forward on this strong bipartisan bill—millions of Americans are depending on a collective shift in how we treat and allow people to live their best lives in the face of mental illness.

The CHAIRMAN. Thank you, Mr. Rahim, and thanks to each of you. We'll now have a round of 5-minute questions for senators.

Mr. Rahim, based on your experience, what advice would you have to someone who knows a person who may need help? How do you persuade them that they should seek help, whether they're a family member, a friend, a student, such as the ones you talked about?

Mr. RAHIM. I get that question all the time. I speak at support groups, like NAMI Family to Family group, DBSA, and that's the billion dollar question, because we can't persuade anybody to do anything that they don't want to do.

The CHAIRMAN. What's your approach? What do you do?

Mr. RAHIM. The key thing I say is education. We can't change anyone's behavior, but we can change how we respond to people. The key thing is educating ourselves, and there are a lot of support groups, there are a lot of educational programs out there that family members of people, say, students, can take, and it can change the way they interact with their friends or their loved ones, and thereby helping them understand what the loved one is going through.

When I was in psychosis, nobody could tell me that I was going through psychosis. But my parents were fortunate enough to bring me to the hospital. Because they changed their way of approaching my condition, they were able to get me help.

The CHAIRMAN. Dr. Eaton, what's your experience? How do you persuade people who need help to seek help?

Mr. EATON. I was going to say one thing that's possible in this area is a program in high schools, which would be built into the health curriculum. There's typically a health curriculum about diseases in high schools, and you can build into that curriculum without too much trouble a module on depressive disorder, psychosis, so people are aware of these and think of them as illnesses just like any other illness. That's part of the stigma reduction idea, and they become less resistant.

There are also in high schools screening programs. The Teen Screen Program was implemented in thousands of high schools around the country, in which you screen high school students, oriented a little bit toward depressive disorder. You mentioned suicide as being the 10th most important cause of death, but for teenagers, it's the 3d most important cause of death. So programs in high schools—I guess that's what I'm saying—to make people aware of the issues around mental illness.

The CHAIRMAN. You were critical of the focus of NIH on——

Mr. EATON. NIMH. Mental Health.

The CHAIRMAN. I mean, the institute that deals with mental health.

Mr. EATON. Right, National Institute of Mental Health.

The CHAIRMAN. And our committee and the Congress has increased funding for that, and there's a bipartisan interest in doing more. If you were there, what would your focus be going forward?

Mr. EATON. I'm completely supportive of more funds for mental health, justified by the burden of disease that I mentioned. We no longer can apply for grants with diagnostic categories as the outcome. It's silly. So I would change that orientation.

SAMHSA is a very important agency, and I think to some extent the NIMH has disassociated itself from the public health orientation, partly because SAMHSA is there, but SAMHSA doesn't have the expertise to do the public health research that the NIMH has. So I made a comment—it wasn't here, but in the written comments—I worked at SAMHSA for 2 days a week last year. There was no psychiatrist there, not even one psychiatrist. As I left, one psychiatrist joined the SAMHSA. There was only one epidemiologist at the National Institute of Mental Health. So that's a failure in public mental health.

The CHAIRMAN. Dr. Hepburn, you mentioned 30 years ago in mental health. I was a Governor at that time, and I've noticed that change. I just have a minute here, but what advice would you have for States based on your experience and perspective about what the focus should be as they move ahead with the dollars that they have, both State, Federal, and private?

Dr. HEPBURN. I think that that's a basic question that commissioners have to deal with on a regular basis, trying to take care of as many people as possible, as cost effective as possible. And what that means is moving further upstream toward prevention and early intervention so that you can take care of more people as they start to show symptoms or where they're at risk for symptoms.

One of the problems we had 30 years ago is that we were waiting until people had severe mental illness before we started treating them. Now, with the public health model, we're trying to move further upstream to early intervention. So trying to spread the dollars out—we obviously still have to take care of the people who are severely mentally ill, but trying to get to people earlier, as we are with the First Episode Psychosis, and even earlier, trying to deal with kids and kids' mental health.

The CHAIRMAN. Thank you, Dr. Hepburn.

Senator Murray.

Senator MURRAY. Thank you, Mr. Chairman.

Mr. Rahim, thank you so much for sharing your story with this committee and for all the work you've been doing with people across the country. It's very impressive. Your message that people aren't defined by their mental illness is really a powerful one, and I appreciate that.

Mr. RAHIM. Thank you.

Senator MURRAY. I wanted to ask you as you talk, particularly with young people, what are the most common forms of stigma that you hear about?

Mr. RAHIM. Some of the most common forms are, I don't want my friends to know. I don't want my family members to know. Students want to talk about what they're going through, but it's their parents that don't want to help them get the help. That's the case sometimes.

Senator MURRAY. They fear their parents will——

Mr. RAHIM. Yes. They fear that their parents will—oftentimes, there's maybe a guilt associated around—is my child broken, or is my child sick? And sometimes it's the parents. When the students come to them, when their daughters and sons come to them, they actually want to help, but sometimes the parents are reticent and not getting them the help that they need. But students—yes, a lot of them are open and willing to talk, especially making and putting that conversation out there.

Senator MURRAY. So having somebody else besides your parent to talk to is critically important.

Mr. RAHIM. That's one of the things.

Senator MURRAY. Resources in the community that they feel comfortable accessing. But I often hear from parents, too, that they don't know who to call. My child is telling me they have this issue, but they don't know who to call. What do you tell them?

Mr. RAHIM. Sometimes there is that bridging the gap between what resources are out there and what is actually known. A key component is that education component, is what is out there, what is available, and knowing that it's OK to seek those resources. Your child is not broken. You're not wrong or bad if something happens to your child. It's really providing that bridge, that knowledge gap, that there are resources, and it's OK to use them.

Senator MURRAY. Great. Thank you very much.

Ms. Blake, let me turn to you. The work you do in the emergency department is a critical part of our health care system. We all know that, and I know the patients that come through your door are at the most vulnerable points of their lives. Otherwise, they wouldn't be walking in that door.

So once a patient is stabilized, and we know they need more specialized care—we know that there is an acute shortage of inpatient psychiatric beds. You referred to that. It's certainly a critical issue in my home State. One study ranked my State 48th out of 50 on the availability of psychiatric treatment beds. We're seeing a lot more press and discussion of that in my State right now.

But I wanted to ask you what happens to a patient in the emergency department if there are no psychiatric treatment beds? You mentioned this in your opening statement. But what do you do?

Ms. BLAKE. What we do is essentially keep them there in that room. We give them three meals, and they are stuck there until we can either find a psychiatric facility that's willing to take them or— sometimes if the 72-hour hold has gone over 72 hours, our emergency room physicians have no choice but to allow that patient to go.

Senator MURRAY. So they go back out into the community?

Ms. BLAKE. They go back out into the community. But, generally speaking, what will happen is they will go from our hospital to the next hospital that's closest and try to get in through that way.

Senator MURRAY. If they seek care. Otherwise, they end up without it.

Ms. BLAKE. Exactly.

Senator MURRAY. Dr. Eaton.

Mr. EATON. Could I just mention that I spent time in Victoria, Australia. They have a linked medical records system. So if someone shows up in an emergency room, and they don't have a bed in that hospital, they can—they've been doing this for decades. They can dial up and find the nearest mental hospital bed in the entire province in a few minutes.

Senator MURRAY. And do you not have that access?

Ms. BLAKE. We do not have that access where I am. In preparation for coming for this, I did an informal poll of my colleagues throughout the country. This is not a problem just in Florida or in Washington. This is every single State in the country, and I would say this is the top issue in emergency departments right now across the country—is holding onto these patients. One hospital in the south part of Palm Beach County I visited earlier this year had 14 patients they were holding, waiting for psychiatric beds.

Senator MURRAY. As Mr. Rahim pointed out, people don't know who to ask. Hospitals don't have a place for them to go, and we have a huge hole in our system.

Ms. BLAKE. Exactly, and it's because there is not enough resources out in the community to be able to place these people, No. 1, to get them screened and get them into treatment programs, but, No. 2, the followup from when they are released from that facility, because they're put out back on the streets. And if they don't have any place to go to followup, to get further treatment, their medications, to have someone that they can go to if they're starting to have a problem—so many of these people are homeless.

If they get put back out, they have no place to go. They have no resources. They have no insurance. They have no way to followup with a physician. They have no way to get their medications. So they show up back in our emergency rooms.

Senator MURRAY. A vicious cycle.

Thank you, Mr. Chairman.

The CHAIRMAN. Thank you, Senator Murray.

I have next Senator Collins, Senator Baldwin, Senator Cassidy, and Senator Murphy.

Senator Collins.

STATEMENT OF SENATOR COLLINS

Senator COLLINS. Thank you, Mr. Chairman.

Dr. Hepburn, particularly in rural States like Maine, patients with serious mental illness all too often lack access to the care that they need. And as I look at Federal policies, at times, Federal policies exacerbate the problem of access. We still don't treat mental illness the same way we treat physical illness in this country from the perspective of Federal reimbursement policies and programs, which is pretty stunning in this day and age.

You mentioned that Congress recently passed Senator Cardin's bipartisan bill, which I was pleased to be a co-sponsor of, which extends an important demonstration project that helps address the psychiatric bed shortage that Ms. Blake has talked about and improve access to critical mental health care services and support. Maine is one of the pilot States under that program and has already seen very promising results, because Federal Medicaid matching payments are being allowed for freestanding psychiatric hospitals for certain emergency psychiatric cases.

Similarly, the Cassidy-Murphy bill, which I've co-sponsored, would go further by lifting the IMD exclusion for psychiatric patients with an average length of stay of 20 days or fewer. That should help more people get the assistance that they need. Could you talk a little bit more about this issue and how the restrictions on Medicaid funding to freestanding psychiatric hospitals affect access to care?

Dr. HEPBURN. Yes. Thank you for the question. Access is a major issue. Following up on the previous discussion, there is a culture problem where individuals are expected to go into a psychiatric unit or a psychiatric hospital. If somebody is in the emergency room for another type of problem and there aren't beds for that particular discipline, they put them into another open bed in the hospital. There isn't any reason that individuals with psychiatric problems couldn't go into a medical bed with a sitter, if some hospitals decide to do that. That's one answer.

The second is increased use of technology may be another way to reach the rural areas. The third, as you talked about, the IMD Demonstration, has shown that private psychiatric hospitals have about the same cost per episode as acute general hospital psychiatric units.

Some 30, 40, or 50 years ago, the private psychiatric hospitals kept people for months, sometimes years. That has changed. The average length of time in a cost per episode is about the same. There really is not a good reason from a financial standpoint or from a clinical standpoint to differentiate between private psychiatric hospitals and acute general hospitals with psychiatric units.

Senator COLLINS. I think you raise an excellent point in your last statement. It says the practices of the past are dictating the reimbursements of today despite changed circumstances. And as we've talked to the administrators and psychiatrists, staff, families, and patients at one of the psychiatric hospitals in Maine, which is part of this pilot project, they are seeing exactly what you've said.

They're not keeping people forever. They're not abusing it. But they're allowing people to get the care that they need because it's being reimbursed for those individuals who are in the age span of 19 to 64, I think it is, that now cannot get reimbursement.

Doctor.

Mr. EATON. Just another comment. Emerging technology may be helpful. So what I was talking about—record linkage in Victoria, Australia. That will be coming in the United States. We'll be able to link records more easily, probably.

But also, in Baltimore, 85 percent of people with schizophrenia own a cell phone, so there is a way of contacting these people. And there are technologies being developed. They're not really therapies, but they're locating devices and devices to talk. I think that's in our future, also.

Senator COLLINS. Thank you.

Thank you, Mr. Chairman.

The CHAIRMAN. Thank you, Senator Collins.

Senator Baldwin had to step out to another hearing, so we'll go to Senator Murphy.

STATEMENT OF SENATOR MURPHY

Senator MURPHY. Thank you very much, Mr. Chairman. Thank you to you and Senator Murray for taking this issue so seriously and for putting us on a path to a bipartisan product coming out of this committee and also a path to bring this to the floor this year. I think this is one of our opportunities in 2016 to be able to move something substantive, something bipartisan, something that makes a difference on the floor of the Senate.

I thank all of you for being here today.

I think we've covered this question of capacity well, and I thank Senator Collins for her specific questions related to the IMD exclusion.

But just for a minute, let's think about how this would relate to our lives. If we were to bring our child to the emergency room around dinner time, and we sat there with our child all evening, we sat with our child overnight, and we didn't get appropriate care for our child until noon the next day, we would call for people's heads at that institution. We would be outraged.

That isn't the outlier when it comes to people being admitted to the ER with mental health diagnoses. That's the average, and yet we sort of have accepted it as commonplace.

But there's a reason why that's happening. We've closed down 4,000 mental health inpatient beds since 2007 in this country. In the last 2 years alone, we went from 91 million Americans living in an area that was designated as a mental health shortage jurisdiction for outpatient services to 97 million Americans. So we're going the wrong way in capacity as need is increasing. It's no mystery as to why we're hearing these stories.

But as Senator Murray pointed out, another failing of our system is the lack of coordination, the fact that we have so many people trying to do good things, but they're not talking to each other. And for really complex patients, it's often not clear who's in charge for a child. Is it the school? Is it the mental health clinic? Is it their primary care physician?

Mr. Rahim, your story was so captivating, and you're so courageous to continue to tell it. I wanted to ask you about this question of coordination. I wanted to ask you a question about the barriers that patients face in trying to find a quarterback for their care, the worry that's involved in just trying to figure out which provider is the best place to start, and where do they eventually go to get the care they need.

How can we do a better job of coordinating all of the good things that are happening in the system so that it's easier for patients to navigate?

Mr. RAHIM. I can take a step back and share what happened with me about 17 years ago. My parents were able to bring me directly to a hospital in Queens. I was in there—and you talk about the waiting area being chaotic. I had hallucinations in the waiting area. I thought that I saw Jesus and prophets.

But I was able to get hospitalized that night, and I was able to get medication that night, and I was able to get in the ward that night, and I spent 2 weeks there. So I think that early care, as Dr. Hepburn was talking about, is so critical. But I was able to get that in that moment.

To speak to the larger issue and larger problem, I think that having that care—the immediacy of care is so critical. I know it was critical for me.

Senator MURPHY. Dr. Eaton, I wanted to explore very quickly an issue that you raised, which is this realization that if we don't spend money on mental health, we're going to spend money somewhere else, and that the fact is that a diabetes diagnosis alone doesn't put you in the top 5 percent of spenders in the Medicare and Medicaid system, and, in fact, a depression diagnosis alone doesn't put you in the top 5 percent of spenders. It's the combination of the two.

And as you point out, if you have depression, if you have a mental health diagnosis, you are, frankly, much more likely to acquire another major and expensive physical health disorder. Can you talk a little bit about the connection between a mental health diagnosis and then a very expensive, very burdensome physical health diagnosis and why a little bit of spending on the mental health side prevents you from spending a lot of money on the physical health side?

Mr. EATON. I wish I knew more, actually, but that finding, depressive disorder predicting to diabetes or stroke or heart attack— that's been replicated 10 times. It's unquestionable, and, therefore, the logic is very strong that on the one hand, treating the mental health disorder will almost certainly lower the risk for the physical disorder later on, but also preventing the mental—moving upstream, even farther than First Episode Psychosis. So if we can identify people at risk for psychosis, not in the first episode, or at risk for depressive disorder, that will have these downstream consequences.

And the problem is it's complicated because it takes a long time. We haven't done enough longitudinal studies to actually understand exactly how depressive disorder contributes to risk for stroke. We don't actually know that, and in the United States, we don't have the tendency to do these longitudinal studies, unfortunately.

I don't think I've answered the question well. But I guess I think we need longitudinal research to actually understand how it is that the body and the mind evolves over time from the age of 15, when somebody's at risk for suicide or depressive disorder, until the age of 45, when they have four times the risk of having a heart attack because of that.

Senator MURPHY. Thank you very much, Mr. Chairman.

The CHAIRMAN. Thank you, Senator Murphy.

Senator Cassidy.

STATEMENT OF SENATOR CASSIDY

Senator CASSIDY. Thank you all. Tremendous testimony. Although this is a topic which is in a sense inherently tragic, on the other hand, the fact that Senators Alexander and Murray and you all are here gives us some room for happiness, of optimism in the midst of this. So thank you all.

Dr. Eaton, let me ask—you describe in your testimony, written and spoken, about the lack of coordination between Federal programs. I'm drawing from that that you feel as if there needs to be some change in how these programs coordinate, or else we'll be spending Federal tax dollars in an ineffective way, et cetera. Your thoughts on that?

Mr. EATON. In the written testimony—and this is the part of it that I know. I do epidemiologic research. There is huge redundancy in the epidemiologic research related to mental disorders. The NIAAA conducts its own survey. The NIDA conducts a survey. The SAMHSA conducts a survey. The NIMH—they're all very similar. I use them all—

Senator CASSIDY. In a sense—I don't mean to cut you off. It's just that I have limited time. In a sense, it would be better to have one person saying, "You shall do this and you shall do that," as opposed to everybody deciding on their own that this is where we need to go?

Mr. EATON. I think it would pay to study the coordination of those agencies. But it's a very difficult thing to figure out.

Senator CASSIDY. Now, let me also ask—you brought up something that Representative Tim Murphy brings up in the House consistently on the House of Representatives side, that the SAMHSA really has a paucity of psychiatrists.

Mr. EATON. They didn't have any when I was there.

Senator CASSIDY. It's kind of amazing that the principal agency for addressing psychiatric illness didn't have a psychiatrist. Or maybe it's not amazing.

Mr. EATON. It is amazing.

Senator CASSIDY. It is amazing. I agree. The epidemiology—by the way, I told Dr. Hepburn when I saw your testimony regarding the need to start basing Federal research on some objective criteria as opposed to inertia, using DALYs as one example, it was like be still my heart.

Right now, I think you're talking about the societal cost. But do you include the cost of incarceration in your societal cost?

Mr. EATON. Those DALYs do not include that cost, typically, and that's something that I didn't get into in my testimony. But, really, incarceration—this is a horrible, horrible problem. I think we now think—many of us think of it—that the prison and jail system is the de facto mental health system in the United States.

Senator CASSIDY. My National Sheriffs Association president, who is from Louisiana, or at least past president, Greg Champagne, says he is the most active mental health provider in his parish.

Mr. EATON. Yes. In Cook County, that's true, also. And we don't even have a good survey of mental disorders in prisons.

Senator CASSIDY. Let me stop. We've heard testimony, Dr. Hepburn, that the right drug is so necessary in order to keep somebody in balance. I've learned, though, that when someone enters a jail, their medicines may be stopped or may be on contract. It will be a drug substituted, et cetera.

If we don't have some way to divert folks who are mentally ill out of the jail, it may be they're going into a setting which would make a dad gum ER look calm—super chaotic. But either no medicine or a different medicine because it is a different—is that a fair statement?

Dr. HEPBURN. Yes, that's one of the big concerns about not having a sequential intercept model that helps to keep people out of being arrested and out of jail. To the point that you made, if somebody comes in on medication and that medication isn't continued, then it can have a negative impact on their ability to recover.

Senator CASSIDY. Thank you.

Mr. Rahim, again, great testimony. Tell me, though—the fact that you're speaking about peer groups as if it is something unique—maybe you're just bragging on the one in which you're involved. But I also got a sense from your testimony that the model needs to be expanded, that as good as it is, we actually don't have peer groups proliferating across the country. This happens to be an exception of which you wish to speak. Is that fair?

Mr. RAHIM. I know that there are peer groups in the country, and I think, knowing the power that——

Senator CASSIDY. Now, there are peer groups. Are they all over the place?

Mr. RAHIM. I couldn't say that they're all over the place, but I know there are peer groups. Certain organizations, like Depression and Bipolar Supporter Alliance—they are based on peers and wellness. NAMI does also have peer groups across the country. But I do think that that is a key component. If I knew that somebody— when I was going through the thick of my medication——

Senator CASSIDY. Let me stop you because I'm out of time. So, in a sense, anything that would promulgate or increase the use of peer groups would probably be a good thing.

Mr. RAHIM. One-hundred percent.

Senator CASSIDY. One-hundred percent. Next, my last question. If we could put you in a bottle and sell you, the whole world would be better off. But oftentimes those who are mentally ill will not take their medicine. And the revolving door comes, and they feel well, and they stop taking their medicine, and they're back with Ms. Blake.

What motivated you to take your medicine, and what do you recommend for those who do not take their medicine? What would you recommend to kind of encourage them to stay on that path of recovery?

Mr. RAHIM. Medication does not define who you are. You are defined by your experience and not your mental illness. Defining mental illness is also how you think about yourself and the things that—how you are labeled.

Senator CASSIDY. So the appropriate mind set, No. 1. What else? Mr. RAHIM. No. 1 is appropriate mind set, and No. 2 is in finding the right medication, knowing that you'll have to go through a com bination. There is no one medication that is a panacea for mental illness, and that's why more research is needed. So know that you have a different combination, know that you're not defined by your medication or your mental illness, and having the ability to self- report to your doctor.

Know how the medications are affecting you. Know how they're impacting your treatment as well as your body, and know that you'll have some sort of response and reaction. I think those are key components. One, trial and error. There's going to be different combinations. Two, know that it'll have an impact on your body. Three, self-report. And, four, know that they do not define who you are. Mental illness does not define who you are.

Senator CASSIDY. Thank you.

I yield back. Thank you, Mr. Chairman.

The CHAIRMAN. Thanks, Dr. Cassidy.

Senator Warren.

STATEMENT OF SENATOR WARREN

Senator WARREN. Thank you, Mr. Chairman. Today, for most insurance plans, mental health parity is the law, but it sure doesn't feel that way for people who need help. A 2015 survey conducted by the National Alliance on Mental Illness found that nearly 50 percent of respondents had been denied coverage for mental or behavioral health care, compared with only 14 percent denied for physical health care. And I hear way too many stories from people in Massachusetts about how hard it is to get insurance coverage for the care that they need.

So let me start here. Dr. Hepburn, what do we really know about how many people are being denied services they need, why they're being denied, if they are filing complaints, and if they ever end up getting the care that they need?

Dr. HEPBURN. It's an important issue. Yesterday, I called the Maryland Parity Project because I wanted to get an update. What they indicated was that it's very hard for them to know what the numbers are, because when people look at how difficult it is to submit a request for review, it's so tedious and it's so detailed, it's going to take months to years to make a difference. So I asked for a recommendation, and they said something has to change in the process.

Senator WARREN. Let's talk about that in just a second. Let's start with what you're saying here. We just don't have even good data on this.

Dr. HEPBURN. No.

Senator WARREN. On any of those four questions.

Mr. Rahim, if someone had trouble getting insurance coverage for mental health services, is there one place that anyone in this country could report a problem and get some help?

Mr. RAHIM. That, I'm not sure of, and——

Senator WARREN. I think that's the information we need right there.

Mr. RAHIM. That's what I'm saying. Being that I'm a mental health advocate and I don't know, that's speaks to that.

Senator WARREN. And that's part of the problem we've got. You know, it's hard to fix any problem if we don't have reliable data.

Connecticut created an Office of the Health Advocate to try to help people navigate the insurance system and assist when they were denied coverage. In 2014, that office returned nearly $7 million to consumers. The most frequent cases they deal with every year are denials of mental health coverage.

My colleague from Massachusetts, Representative Joe Kennedy, introduced the Behavioral Health Coverage Transparency Act last month to try to create a patient parity portal to provide consumers around the country a one-stop shop for information about parity and a central place to submit complaints about coverage.

Let me ask you this, Dr. Hepburn. We'll go back to the question about what to do about this. Would a central place for people to go with problems about insurance coverage for mental health problems help consumers and give regulators better information about where to focus their enforcement actions?

Dr. HEPBURN. Absolutely, yes.

Senator WARREN. So this is something that could make a real difference——

Dr. HEPBURN. Yes.

Senator WARREN [continuing]. From what you're saying. Good.

I just want to say as this committee goes forward on mental health legislation, I would like to work with you, Chairman Alexander and Ranking Member Murray, on making sure that consumers have a central place to turn to for help when they are denied coverage and a central place where we will get the information so that we can enforce the law that's currently on the books.

Thank you, Mr. Chairman.

The CHAIRMAN. Thank you, Senator Warren, for the suggestion.

Senator Franken.

STATEMENT OF SENATOR FRANKEN

Senator FRANKEN. Thank you both, the chairman and the ranking member, for these series of hearings.

Dr. Eaton, in your testimony, you talked about the importance of preventing mental illness.

So did you, Dr. Hepburn.

You, Dr. Eaton, highlight programs such as the Nurse Family Partnership Program, which has been effective at identifying high risk births and assisting moms after birth. I really do believe prevention is important. That's why I authored and helped advance the Mental Health in Schools Act, which will increase access to mental health services in school settings.

Dr. Eaton, what percentage of individuals with mental illness experience onset before the age of 18?

Mr. EATON. It depends on which mental disorder you're talking about. But I think probably before 18, for depressive disorder, the full fledged disorder is probably 20 percent. But the beginnings of it are available—50 percent of the people who will have depressive disorder full fledged in their lifetime, let's say before the age of 30 or 35, are already experiencing symptoms at 15. They would be potentially identifiable, depending on if we can get the tools to do that.

For schizophrenia, it'll be similar. Schizophrenia has much more sudden onset right at 18, 20, 25, something like that. But the signs of psychosis and especially the negative symptoms are there at the age of 15 to 20, I think.

Senator FRANKEN. I think this is why if we expand and enhance mental health services in our schools, we will serve ourselves well.

I want to ask about rural suicides, because a study made by the Journal of the American Medical Association shows that rural adolescents commit suicide at approximately twice the rate as teens in urban areas, and this disparity has just increased over time. Between 2004 and 2013, across all demographic groups, suicide rates rose by 7 percent in metropolitan areas, but by 20 percent in rural areas over the same period.

The research shows that these differences are driven by lack of treatment options in rural areas, provider shortages, and stigma. As the co-chair of the Senate Rural Health Caucus, I find this deeply concerning.

Dr. Hepburn, you have previously served on the National Suicide Prevention Lifeline Advisory Board and now represent the State Mental Health Program Directors. Can you explain why suicide rates have been driven up so dramatically in rural areas?

Dr. HEPBURN. I think you answered it, which is basically access issues. One of the things I think is important is to look at how we can advance technology to try and get to the rural areas. At a time when the Internet is reaching people all around the world, there's really not a good excuse for being unable to reach kids and young people in the rural areas.

One of the problems we sometimes get into is the lack of payment for those services that are done through tele-mental health, and I think that's an important issue that needs to be addressed. In this day and age, tele-mental Internet services should be made available in the same way that every other service is available. And by doing that, we can increase access to those kids.

Senator FRANKEN. Which is one of the reasons we need to make sure every area in America has the Internet, because this is something I hear when I go to rural Minnesota. I support programs that provide financial incentives to mental health service providers in rural areas, actually, we just need them in this country. We have a provider shortage. Is that not right? And would that be helpful?

Dr. HEPBURN. Absolutely. We have a workforce shortage. I think I read the other day that the average age for people in behavioral health in terms of providers in the workforce is 58. So we have to use technology as a way of compensating for that.

Senator FRANKEN. Thank you all for the work you're doing. I think we're beginning to understand how important this is in this Congress and in this country, and we've seen some good things happen in this Congress, beginning to happen, and I want to thank the chairman again and the ranking member.

The CHAIRMAN. Thank you, Senator Franken.

Senator Whitehouse.

STATEMENT OF SENATOR WHITEHOUSE

Senator WHITEHOUSE. Thank you, Chairman. Following up a little bit on Senator Warren's questions, it strikes me that one of the victories that we have achieved has been to bring mental health out of the shadows and de-stigmatize it. Not completely, not as much as it should be, but there have been some real victories in that area. And I want to commend my former delegation member, Representative Patrick Kennedy of Rhode Island, on the work that he did on the Mental Health Parity and Addiction Equity Act, which has really helped make that the law of the land as opposed to just a good social change that we've made.

But in addition to the problem of trying to get insurance coverage, is there not also the underlying problem that our infrastructure for mental health treatment was basically built during a heavily stigmatized period when very few people came forward? So it was designed to address a fraction of the real mental health problem.

I don't know what you all see, but in Rhode Island, we have some of the best mental health facilities in the country. Butler Hospital and Bradley Hospital are best-in-show, world class facilities, and yet they are kind of all there is. And you get beyond that, and you get into really difficult situations, and, very often, there has to be a crisis before somebody can get access and get into the mental health care system, not because the insurance company isn't reimbursing it, but because there simply isn't adequate coverage, particularly in children's mental health.

I see that as the case in Rhode Island. You all have a perspective through your organizations nationally. Do you agree that that is a national problem as well?

[No verbal response.]

Senator WHITEHOUSE. All heads are nodding, let the record reflect.

Do you want to say something?

Mr. RAHIM. Yes. Senator Franken, so key about schools. When I've spoken in 12 different schools, we did a study, a 4-week followup. Are students actually going to seek help? Out of 2,000 students I spoke to, 184 actually went to a school social worker, a school psychologist, or a teacher because they said, "You know what? It's OK to talk about what I'm going through." So if they're ready to seek that help, where do they go?

Senator WHITEHOUSE. Where do they go?

Mr. RAHIM. People are ready to talk, especially the young people. But where do you go once you're ready for that help? That's the question.

Senator WHITEHOUSE. Our victory in the stigma area has now created a problem in the infrastructure area, in my opinion.

In the Judiciary Committee, we will be considering a bill that is jurisdictional to the Judiciary Committee, which is the Comprehensive Addiction Recovery Act, which has a great deal of overlay with mental health issues, very often self-medication as a solution, not a good one, but one that people use when they're really facing a mental health problem.

Could I ask as a question for the record if each of you would have a look—I think your organizations are probably already aware of the Comprehensive Addiction Recovery Act. If you wouldn't mind checking to make sure, and if you have an opinion on it, that we have that. The hearing is going to be coming up in the next couple of weeks, and I'd love to make sure we've got your organization's position on the Comprehensive Addiction Recovery Act in our record here that I can take there.

Senator WHITEHOUSE. And then the last question that I have has to do with emergency rooms. Ms. Blake, that's your world. You live in it. I've spent overnights in our emergency room just to witness what takes place in there. There's an enormous amount of mental health response that's delivered in the emergency room.

People come in in the middle of the night. What they really have is a mental health problem. The police have no place else to bring them. They take them to the ER. Now it's your problem, and an ER isn't really well suited for dealing with that.

Could you just comment a little bit more on how big a role that task that you've been given plays in your workload and how much it is diminishing what else you can do? But I'm also interested in the extent to which you feel comfortable that the electronic health records that you pull up when you bring that person in, or when they come in to you, or when they're brought in to you, are accurate and complete as to the mental health history of that individual?

Ms. BLAKE. Yes, I know what you're asking.

Senator WHITEHOUSE. I've got a feeling that some of the protections we've put in place back when this was heavily stigmatized to keep all this information private is actually keeping it from getting into electronic health records, so that in an ER, you aren't aware of the situation.

Ms. BLAKE. Absolutely. I can actually give you an example of that. Not too terribly long ago, we had a 26-year-old gentleman brought to our emergency room. He was a heroin overdose. He was unconscious. We didn't know a lot about him, except that he had used heroin, because he responded to Narcan when we gave him the Narcan.

We stabilized him, and in the process of taking care of him—I was taking care of him—I got a phone call from a gentleman in Virginia who was trying to locate his son who had been sent down to our county for treatment and rehab for substance abuse, who had walked away from his rehab center. It turned out—he gave me the son's name, and it turned out it was the patient I was taking care of.

The problem was I could not tell him because of the HIPAA law that we had his son in our emergency room, No. 1, because the patient was unconscious and unable to give me permission to do so. But it turned out, too, that his son had a mental health care issue as well. He was bipolar, and he had been off of his medications which was contributing to his problem.

Now, had we been able to release that information or pull that information up somehow, then it might have changed the whole way that we treated this patient. But, more importantly, it broke my heart to not be able to tell this man that his son was safe in the emergency room and was going to be able to recover.

I think maybe if we look at some limited circumstances where certain information could be released—and I certainly understand the privacy issue, but it would be very helpful, because in order to access someone's medical records, you first have to get permission from them in order to do so. And someone who might be in a men tal health care crisis may not have the capacity to be considered able to sign permission for it.

Senator WHITEHOUSE. Thank you. My time has expired, but that was a terrific story and a terrific point. Thank you.

The CHAIRMAN. Thank you, Senator Whitehouse.

Senator Murray, do you have any further comments?

Senator MURRAY. Mr. Chairman, I just want to say this has been a really important hearing, and I really want to thank all of our witnesses today. Clearly, we have a lot of work ahead of us.

We talked about making sure communities have access to mental health professionals, integrating the primary care with mental health care, prioritizing research, and breaking down barriers— continuing to break down barriers that stigma creates. That is a full plate, but it is an important one for us to tackle, and I look forward to working with you on moving this agenda forward.

The CHAIRMAN. Thank you, Senator Murray.

Ms. Blake, thank you for that story, and Senator Whitehouse for bringing that up. Touching HIPAA is like touching an electric wire. But maybe that's what we're paid to do sometimes. So as we look at our mental health legislation, we should consider that story and that circumstance, and given the way we work on this committee, perhaps we can help with that.

If you have a specific suggestion for the kind of exemption that that should be, we'd like to have it. Maybe your organizations have that kind of——

Ms. BLAKE. As chair of the Advocacy Advisory Council, that's definitely something we can put on our agenda to discuss and see what people——

The CHAIRMAN. We're moving pretty fast here.

Ms. BLAKE. We have a meeting today.

The CHAIRMAN. Good.

Senator WHITEHOUSE. They're faster than us.

[Laughter.]

The CHAIRMAN. What Senator Murray and I hope to do is to move promptly through this committee those issues that are within our jurisdiction and do it at the same time that we're working with the Finance-Judiciary Committees and with Senator Murray and Senator Blunt's Appropriations Subcommittee so that we'll be ready to deal with this issue. We have some very good work being done.

I thank you for the testimony today from all four of you.

The hearing record will remain open for 10 days. Members may submit additional information within that time.

The next hearing of this committee will explore issues related to generic drug user fee agreements, and it will be on Thursday, January 28th.

Thank you for being here today. The committee will stand adjourned.

[Additional material follows.]

ADDITIONAL MATERIAL

Prepared Statement of Senator Casey

Thank you, Chairman Alexander and Ranking Member Murray, for continuing with this series of hearings on mental health and substance abuse. I know everyone on this committee is well aware of the fierce urgency of this subject matter. Although the vast majority of individuals with mental illness are not violent, recent years have given rise to tragedies that highlight the need for our Nation to better address this issue. The testimony at the first hearing on mental health, and the second hearing focusing on opioid abuse, has been enlightening, and will help me and the other members of this committee as we decide the best way to move forward on mental health and substance abuse issues.

Mental health is one of the country's most pressing health care needs. Nearly one in five adults experiences a mental illness in a given year. Left untreated, these conditions can destroy lives and tear apart families. The Affordable Care Act built on the landmark mental health parity law by including mental health and substance abuse services as an essential health benefit, and by expanding access to private health insurance and Medicaid. We must work to build upon this progress by strengthening the behavioral healthcare workforce; finding new ways to integrate behavioral health and primary care; providing resources for crisis situations; and strengthening vulnerable communities. We must make good on the promise of insurance parity for mental health and substance abuse services, and work to ensure that cutting edge medical research into mental health and substance abuse receives adequate support and sustained funding.

Today's hearing will provide insight into how we can improve Federal mental health policies. I appreciate the opportunity to hear from the witnesses, who will discuss the challenges faced by State governments, health care professionals, mental health researchers and those that suffer from mental health conditions. I look forward to working with the Administration, as well as my colleagues on the committee, as we use today's testimony to build upon and improve Federal mental health policy.

Prepared Statement of Senator Baldwin

Thank you, Chairman and Ranking Member, for holding this important hearing. My home State of Wisconsin is experiencing a uniquely severe shortage of mental health providers that is drastically reducing access to needed care. Over half of our counties have been designated as mental health professional shortage areas, and estimates show that we would need over 200 psychiatrists to start addressing this shortage.

This has particularly devastating consequences for the tens of thousands of Wisconsin children who are living with untreated mental health issues, forcing parents to wait for months to get their child into care, cross the border for care in another State, or forgo care altogether.

Wisconsin health and community leaders are collaborating on innovative programs to address these issues, but our kids are still in crisis.

Response by Brian Hepburn, M.D.[1] to Questions of Senator Isakson, Senator Murray, Senator Casey, Senator Whitehouse, and Senator Baldwin

Senator Isakson

Question. How does SAMHSA interact with other HHS agencies, Federal departments, and State agencies concerning the development and implementation of mental health policies? What improvements, if any, do you think could be made in this area?

Answer. SAMHSA has a long history of working with the State Mental Health Agencies (SMHAs) and Substance Abuse Agencies in developing programs through grants, sharing evidence-based practices, and seeking input regarding concerns about the upcoming implementation of new Federal programs. SAMHSA meets quarterly with advisory committees for all divisions at the SAMHSA headquarters, and also meets with those advisory committees in aggregate. Acting SAMHSA Administrator Kana Enomoto and Center for Mental Health Services Director Paolo del Vecchio have both long held close working relationships with the SMHAs, relationships founded on trust and a mutual understanding of the essentials of providing services to individuals with serious mental illness and children and youths with serious emotional distress.

A recent illustration of that close working relationship is how SAMHSA and the National Institute for Mental Health worked closely with SMHAs in the implementation of the 10 percent Mental Health Block Grant set-aside for treatment of First Episodes of Psychosis. Soon after enactment of the set-aside, SAMHSA reached out to the SMHAs to solicit input on how the program might best be implemented and then issued guidance to lead the way. Over the last 2 years, technical assistance has provided in the field and by phone to assist States in adopting the most effective, evidence-based approaches to achieve the set-aside's goals.

SAMHSA has specifically provided leadership to our field by:

[1] Stuart Gordon, NASMHPD's Director of Policy, worked with Dr. Hepburn and many individual State mental health directors, in drafting the attached responses to questions that we received from HELP Committee members.

- involving persons experiencing mental illness in shared decisionmaking with their treating providers;
- promoting the importance of peer services (especially at a time when we are facing workforce shortages);
- promoting not just the medical model but also the importance of supportive housing and supportive employment in helping persons avoid disability;
- promoting integration of physical health care and behavioral health; and
- promoting telehealth and the use of health information technology to reach more people.

SAMHSA has been working very closely with officials in the Federal Medicaid program over the past few years on such items as developing quality measures that can be used across programs, and implementation of Section 223 of the Excellence in Mental Health Act conditions for participation. The two agencies have also been increasingly finding projects on which they can collaborate such as the recent CMCS Informational Bulletin on funding early intervention programs under Medicaid authorities. SAMHSA provides input into the National Quality Forum (NQF) Measures Application Partnership which develops recommendations to CMS on quality measures for the Medicaid and Medicare programs.

Senator Murray

Question. In your testimony you discussed the need for adequately funded crisis response services. I'm particularly concerned about the availability of crisis response services in areas with low population density that struggle to maintain services because of the low volume of calls. How can the Federal Government support State and local service providers to ensure that, when patients are in a time of crisis, they always have someone to call?

Answer. Recently the NASMHPD did a survey on how States fund crisis services. Some States pay for crisis services entirely with State general funds. Other States use a mixture of State general funds, block grant funds, local funds and Medicaid.

The percentage of the funds in the exact mixture for the individual States varies greatly. The rural communities are most vulnerable to not having adequate funding because they have a low volume of service utilization and therefore recover less reimbursement on a fee-for-service basis. They are also vulnerable because they have difficulty recruiting mental health professionals, such as psychiatrists. The poorer rural areas are also more vulnerable because there are no local funds which could help support their efforts.

The Federal Government could be helpful in resolving the problem in the rural areas by:

- providing funding to educate the public in how to assist friends and loved ones who are experiencing psychological distress. This would include being able to identify when an individual is in distress, supporting the individual and knowing where to find services for the individual. The goal is to provide the needed intervention as early as possible and avoid escalation into a crisis;
- providing adequate funding of the Suicide Lifeline Network to ensure individuals in crisis in every community will have someone immediately available who is trained in crisis response and knowledgeable about the resources available in the immediate surrounding community;
- providing greater funding for Crisis Intervention Team training of law enforcement personnel and first responders to help ensure that situations do not escalate;
- providing flexibility in Medicaid rules so that services provided remotely could be reimbursed, residential crisis services could be covered, residential crisis services would not be subject to the IMD exclusion, and peer services could be compensated.
- providing educational loan repayments for mental health professionals working in rural crisis programs;
- providing incentives to mental health professional training programs for training those professionals in tele-mental health; and
- providing incentives to develop social media applications directed toward persons in distress/crisis.

Senator Casey

Question 1. As a member of the Committee on Finance as well as the Health, Education, Labor, and Pensions Committee, I frequently hear about the mental health needs of children in the child welfare system, and the challenges current and former foster children have in accessing the mental health services they need. Does the National Association of State Mental Health Program Directors have any recommendations or best practices for State Mental Health Agencies for ensuring that the mental health needs of current and former foster youth are properly met?

Answer 1. As an example, Indiana is utilizing a Children's Mental Health Initiative to provide services to children who have become involved with the Department of Child Services due to their behavioral health concerns but do not have the funding for services. Also in Indiana, there is the Older Youth Initiative that provides youth with mental health services and supports as they approach turning 18 in the foster care system to assist in the transition to adulthood and self-sufficiency.

The Iowa Department of Human Services (DHS) has developed a practice guide, Children in Child Welfare: Mental and Behavioral Health Practice Bulletin, which acknowledges up front that most children who enter the child welfare system have experienced trauma. Thus, mental health screening by licensed mental health providers is one of the first steps taken after a child's entry into the State welfare program. DHS data show that 88 percent of 359 children reviewed between August 2007 and October 2007 had their mental health needs assessed and met.

For a broader look, the Children's Bureau, in collaboration with the Georgetown University Center for Child and Human Development and through the National Technical Assistance Center for Children's Mental Health, has released a series of papers, Integrating Safety, Permanency and Well-Being in Child Welfare, describing how a more fully integrated and developmentally specific approach in Child Welfare can improve both child and system level outcomes. The overview, Integrating Safety, Permanency and Well-Being: A view from the Field (Wilson), provides a look at the evolution of the child welfare system from the 1970s forward. The first paper, A comprehensive Framework for Nurturing the Well-Being of Children and Adolescents (Biglan), provides a framework for considering the domains and indicators of well- being. The second paper, Screening, Assessing, Monitoring Outcomes and Using Evidence-based Practices to Improve Well-Being of Children in Foster Care (Conradi, Landsverk, Wotring), describes a process for delivering trauma screening, functional and clinical assessment, evidence based interventions and the use of progress monitoring in order to better achieve well-being outcomes. The third and final paper, *A Case Example of the Administration on Children and, Youth and Families' Well-Being Framework: KIPP* (Akin, Bryson, McDonald, and Wilson) presents a case study of the Kansas Intensive Permanency Project and describes how it has implemented many of the core aspects of a well-being framework.

We also recommend a 2006 report co-authored by the Georgetown University Center's National Children's Technical Assistance Center, NASMHPD's Children Youth and Families Division, and the National Association of Public Child Welfare Administrators entitled Financing Behavioral Health Services and Supports for Children, Youth and Families in the Child Welfare System. That study surveyed 24 States on their interagency financing strategies and found that 89 percent of child welfare agencies and 83 percent of mental health agencies were involved in those strategies. Medicaid was next at 65 percent, and juvenile justice at 61 percent. The vast majority of the responding States (79 percent) developed partnerships among the involved agencies to implement the funding strategies, and most of them (61 percent) formalized these partnerships.

As an aside, NASMHPD's membership is unanimous in supporting the Administration's initiative to reduce the inappropriate prescribing of psychotropic pharmaceutical agents to kids in the foster care system [estimated at more than $3 billion a year]. That money can be better and more effectively used to enhance Medicaid financing for therapeutic foster care services and other intensive psycho-social interventions targeting the 50,000 children with the most serious emotional disturbances.

Question 2. In what ways do State Mental Health Agencies commonly work with their State child welfare agencies? Is there anything that the Federal Government can do to encourage or promote collaboration between State Mental Health Agencies and the child welfare agencies in their States?

Answer 2. SAMHSA's Children Mental Services Program seeks to establish "systems of care" at the State level to encourage collaboration on a multi-agency basis. As noted above, State child welfare agencies such as Iowa's recognizes that a child in the system has been more than likely to have experienced some level of trauma, and thus includes a mental health screening performed by licensed mental health and substance use treatment providers in the initial physical screening. Other agencies refer youngsters with the most serious behavioral health conditions to specialized services provided by NASMHPD member agencies.

A number of legislative modifications to the Children's Mental Health Services program should be considered including (i) lengthening the average grant cycle under the program (e.g., adding at least 2 years to promote the sustainability of collaborations), (ii) authorizing the Administration's fiscal year 2017 CMHI 10-percent set-aside proposal for funding prodromal approaches to preventing the onset of serious mental illness and the first episode of psychosis, and (iii) using the Children's Mental Health Services Program to promote demonstrations of approaches such as that used in Iowa—a standard mental health/substance use screening and treatment planning protocol for all kids entering the foster care system nationwide.

The Federal Government should also consider providing guidance and funding for collaborations toward the mental health needs of children and families in need. The Indiana Division of Mental Health and Addiction (DMHA) and the Indiana Department of Child Services have collaborated to provide intensive home and community- based wraparound services for youth and families without funding known as Children's Mental Health Initiative.

Senator Whitehouse

Question 1. Along with a bipartisan group of senators including Senators Portman, Klobuchar, and Ayotte, I introduced a bill earlier this year called the Comprehensive Addiction and Recovery Act (S.524). The bill authorizes a series of grants to States and other eligible entities to promote an integrated approach including prevention, treatment, law enforcement tools, and recovery support to the substance abuse epidemic we are facing across the Nation. Among other things, the bill tries to increase screening for, and treatment of, co-occurring mental health and substance use disorders in the juvenile and criminal justice systems and elsewhere.

Do you support the objectives set forth in S.524? How would enactment of S.524 improve your organizations ability to help address the opioid abuse epidemic?

Answer 1. Yes, like our friends at the National Association of State Alcohol and Drug Abuse Directors (NASADAD), NASMHPD strongly supports S.524, but would like to see all grants and programs proposed within the bill fully funded.

Question 2. What additional tools might you like to see at your disposal to address the overlap between substance abuse and mental health issues?

Answer 2. Perhaps language that clarifies that when grant moneys are utilized to treat an individual with a substance use disorder who also has a co-occurring mental illness or emotional disorder that may be impacting or be impacted by the severity or nature of the co-occurring disorder, grant moneys under CARA may be utilized to treat that co-occurring mental illness or emotional disorder without a violation of any SAMHSA program prohibition against the intermingling of program funds.

In a similar vein, in the late 1990s, SAMHSA initiated a dual diagnosis program/ line-item for individuals with both mental health and substance use disorders. It never received much Federal funding, but efforts to revive the initiative in that form or some similar form other would be well-advised.

Senator Baldwin

Question 1. Three Wisconsin health systems in the Fox Valley area have partnered to create a program, called Catalpa, to help improve timely access to mental health care for pediatric patients. This program provides crisis care for children and their families within 24 hours and then regular, followup care, led by a multidisciplinary team in the partnership network. At its main center, wait times have dropped from 54 days to about 5 days.

Answer 1. Dr. Hepburn and Ms. Blake, this is just one example of a program working to address the mental health services crisis facing our children. What steps would you recommend the Federal Government take to help solve our mental health provider shortage and improve access for children throughout the country?

NASMHPD is very supportive of the model that Wisconsin is now using. However, one of the difficulties has been getting funding for programs such as this. They are often funded by State general fund dollars which has slowed their expansion. Federal funding would be very helpful.

NASMHPD strongly supports President Obama's fiscal year 2017 budget recommendation that a 10 percent set-aside be created in the Children's Mental Health Services budget line to fund outreach to and treatment of at-risk troubled children before they reach a level of serious mental illness or serious emotional distress, and certainly before they experience their First Episode Psychosis. Such a program would utilize peers, teachers, counselors, and family members to help identify troubled youths in the schools and in the community and then invite them and their families in for family based cognitive behavioral therapy sessions led by licensed providers. This type of program addressing behavioral health needs further upstream should reduce the need for crisis-focused programs later in childhood development.

Question 2. Mental health is too often thought of as a separate part of the care continuum, resulting in a fragmented mental health care delivery system. To begin integrating mental health into primary care, our Medical College and Children's Hospital of Wisconsin are participating in a State pilot program that offers primary care providers daily consultation services with child psychiatrists. Dr. Hepburn, how can we encourage more of our health systems and local support networks to work together to prioritize mental health and integrate these services into our larger delivery system?

Answer 2. Again, NASMHPD is very supportive of the model that Wisconsin is using. The model has been used successfully in Massachusetts and in Maryland and we would like to see it spread throughout the country. However, as with the first model you mention, the difficulty has been getting funding for programs such as this. They are often funded by State general fund dollars which has slowed their expansion. Federal funding initiatives and also allowing these consultations to be paid for by Medicaid would be very helpful.

An alternative approach might be to utilize telemedicine to help pediatricians consult with the 7,000 to 8,000 licensed child psychiatrists nationwide.

The model that seems to NASMHPD to have the greatest promise for integrating primary care and behavioral health care for persons of all ages is the Health Homes Demonstration Model for persons with chronic conditions enacted under Section 2703 of the Affordable Care Act. This works particularly well because the statute includes, among the conditions considered to be chronic and thus covered under the demonstration, persistent mental health conditions and substance use disorders. The Health Homes Demonstration requires participation of a team of health care professionals that includes physicians and other professionals such as a nurse care coordinator, nutritionist, social worker, behavioral health professional, or any professionals deemed appropriate by the State.

The home health services provided include comprehensive care management, care coordination and health promotion, transitional care and followup, patient and family support, community and social support, and use of health information technology. While most health homes have a primary care provider as the designated lead provider, there is no legal reason why a health homes model for pediatrics could not have a pediatrician as a designated lead provider and, in fact, pediatricians are identified in the list of providers that can so serve.

In contrast to the mostly hospital-based accountable care organizations, the health home team can be free-standing, virtual, or based at a hospital, community health center, community mental health center, rural clinic, clinical group practice, academic health center, or any entity deemed appropriate by the Secretary. Also in contrast to the ACO model, behavioral health providers have been active participants in the Health Home Demonstration project.

RESPONSE BY PENNY BLAKE, RN, CCRN, CEN TO QUESTIONS OF SENATOR ALEXANDER, SENATOR CASEY, SENATOR WHITEHOUSE, AND SENATOR BALDWIN

Senator Alexander

Question. During your testimony, you told a story regarding the disclosure of protected health information under the Health Information Portability and Accountability Act. In that case, you said that you were unable to disclose information to a family member of a patient when that patient was unable to give consent. However, HIPAA does allow disclosure under these types of situations according to the HIPAA Privacy Rule at 45 Code of Federal Regulations 164.510. What should the Federal Government be doing to clarify situations where disclosure of protected health information is permissible under HIPAA? Are there specific parts of HIPAA that you feel are too restrictive or unclear?

Answer. Thank you for highlighting this key issue. Before I begin, please let me recap the specifics of the circumstance, given the relevance to your question.

During the hearing, I noted that a 26-year-old gentleman presented at our emergency room in Florida, unconscious with a heroin overdose, which we ascertained because he responded to Narcan, a narcotics rescue agent. After the patient was stabilized, I received a phone call from a man in Virginia trying to locate his son, who had been previously admitted in the area for addiction treatment but had walked away from the facility and was, thus, missing. The caller mentioned his name, but due to HIPAA restrictions, I was not able to tell the man that his son was in our care due to the HIPAA law.

In my response, I want to highlight two key issues—(1) lack of clarity within HIPAA and our State privacy laws regarding the unique protections associated with substance abuse and mental health records, and (2) how interoperable health care records could have assisted us in treating the patient I described.

But, first, let me turn to the HIPAA clarity issue. While it is correct that 45 CFR § 164.510 does specify permitted disclosures to a "family member, other relative, or a close personal friend of an individual" in the case of an emergency, such disclosures are limited only to "information directly relevant to such person's involvement with the individual's care" [45 CFR § 164.510(b)]1 The regulation further clarifies [45 CFR § 164.510(b)(3)]2 that such involvement may include 'pick(ing) up filled prescriptions, medical supplies, X-rays, or other similar forms of protected health information." At the time that I talked to the parent, the patient was already stable. Therefore, the disclosure would not have been to assist with the patient's care but to provide ease to a family member. As such, it is not clear that such a disclosure is permitted by HIPAA.

The Emergency Nurses Association Code of Ethics, approved in February 2015, was developed as a guide for carrying out emergency nursing responsibilities in a manner consistent with quality of care and the ethical responsibilities of the profession. Regarding an individual's right to privacy and confidentiality, this framework states that 'information pertinent to the care and welfare of a patient may be divulged to those directly involved in the care of the patient."2

This matter is further complicated by the Florida statute requirements, which are stricter than the Federal HIPAA requirements. Specifically, the Florida statute states that "[p]atient records maintained by licensed Florida facilities, including hospitals, are confidential and may not be disclosed without patient consent unless disclosure occurs to specified persons or in specified circumstances (e.g., to physicians for treatment purposes, in response to a court subpoena, etc.)." FL ST § 395.3025. Therefore, without the patient's consent, I am unable to disclose such records due to Florida law. As a result, even if one were to further clarify HIPAA, which is considered a Federal floor and not a ceiling, States (like Florida) can continue to enact more stringent privacy requirements.

In direct answer to your question, I have highlighted the key issues with respect to the HIPAA requirements—namely, the requirement that the information disclosed to family members be limited to that which is "directly relevant to such person's involvement with the individual's care." This requirement, coupled with more stringent State privacy laws, is intended to make disclosure of personal health information difficult. But, as my example highlights, sometimes, it does not serve all those involved.

However, in the story I relayed, the patient was brought to the emergency department with suspected heroin overdose. Given the unique protections associated with substance abuse and mental health records under Federal and State law, it became unclear whether or not the ability to disclose personal health information without the patient's consent was still allowable.

When I recapped the story before, I only alluded to another key component: Had we been able to electronically obtain the patient's medical records at the time that he entered the emergency room, it could have changed the way we treated him. I understand that the HELP Committee is working to promote interoperability, and I hope that you will continue to do so.

ENA urges Congress to clarify situations where disclosure of protected health information is permissible including requiring the U.S. Department of Health and Human Services (HHS) and State departments of health to clarify situations in which disclosures without consent are permitted, particularly when mental health or substance abuse are the cause for an individual's presentation to the emergency department.

In addition, we urge Congress to require HHS to mandate that certified EHR technology include fields for mental health and substance abuse diagnoses.

It would also be helpful if HHS encouraged local and regional health information exchanges (HIEs) to include mental health or substance abuse diagnoses as required data elements, as this information can be critical in emergency situations for treatment purposes. While it is our understanding that HHS cannot mandate this, it could incentivize this activity by making it a requirement of any grant funding for HIEs.

CFR References

(1) (b) Standard: uses and disclosures for involvement in the individual's care and notification purposes—(1) Permitted uses and disclosures. (i) A covered entity may, in accordance with paragraphs (b)(2) or (3) of this section, disclose to a family member, other relative, or a close personal friend of the individual, or any other person identified by the individual, the protected health information directly relevant to such person's involvement with the individual's care or payment related to the individual's health care.

(2) (b)(3) Limited uses and disclosures when the individual is not present. If the individual is not present, or the opportunity to agree or object to the use or disclosure cannot practicably be provided because of the individual's incapacity or an emergency circumstance, the covered entity may, in the exercise of professional judgment, determine whether the disclosure is in the best interests of the individual and, if so, disclose only the protected health information that is directly relevant to the person's involvement with the individual's health care. A covered entity may use professional judgment and its experience with common practice to make reasonable inferences of the individual's best interest in allowing a person to act on behalf of the individual to pick up filled prescriptions, medical supplies, X-rays, or other similar forms of protected health information.

(3) 5. The emergency nurse respects the individual's right to privacy and confidentiality. The emergency nurse protects and safeguards the privacy of their patients, thus preventing uninvited intrusion into the patient's private life, medical history, and current condition. Information pertinent to the care and welfare of a patient may be divulged to those directly involved in the care of the patient. The HIPAA Privacy Rule protects the privacy of patient's health information and, even in the event of public scrutiny, emergency nurses are mandated to preserve the individual's right to privacy and confidentiality. Patient information utilized for peer review, third-party payments, quality improvement initiatives, or risk management processes may be disclosed based on an institution's policies, protocols, or legal mandates.

Senator Casey

Question 1. In your testimony, you discuss the process that Good Samaritan Medical Center, and similar hospitals, follow when patients present with a mental illness. Is this process different for a child or young adult who is admitted with a men tal health problem? Do these patients have unique needs compared to those of adults with mental illnesses, and, if so, should the Federal Government provide any additional support or enact any policy changes to help health care providers address those needs?

Answer 1. At my hospital, the process for handling children and young adults as compared to other mental health patients is the same. Since our hospital does not have a psychiatric unit, we would transfer a mental health patient to one of the two hospitals in our area that admits patients suffering from an acute mental health issue. In such a situation, the patient is first medically cleared by an emergency physician in my hospital. The patient must then be accepted by the emergency physician of the receiving hospital and is transferred by ambulance or law enforcement vehicle to that hospital's emergency department until a bed became available in their psychiatric unit.

Question 2. In your experience, what kind of training do nurses and other health care professionals receive regarding the patient privacy requirements placed on them by HIPAA? Do you feel that access to increased training would be helpful?

Answer 2. In our facility, we must complete a class annually regarding the HIPAA law. The class is taken online in a computerized format. Access to more in depth training would be helpful to nurses and other health care providers. However, based on discussions with colleagues across the United States, I believe the larger problem is the lack of clarity in the HIPAA language.

Additionally, States may have further restrictions on health care information, making the situation more complex for providers. Finally, hospitals protect mental health records even more stringently. As a result, health care providers tend to err on the side of caution when asked to divulge information.

Senator Whitehouse

Question 1. Along with a bipartisan group of senators including Senators Portman, Klobuchar, and Ayotte, I introduced a bill earlier this year called the Comprehensive Addiction and Recovery Act (S.524). The bill authorizes a series of grants to States and other eligible entities to promote an integrated approach—including prevention, treatment, law enforcement tools, and recovery support—to the substance abuse epidemic we are facing across the Nation. Among other things, the bill tries to increase screening for, and treatment of, co-occurring mental health and substance use disorders in the juvenile and criminal justice systems and elsewhere.

Do you support the objectives set forth in S.524? How would enactment of S.524 improve your organization's ability to help address the opioid abuse epidemic?

Answer 1. The Emergency Nurses Association (ENA) strongly supports the Comprehensive Addiction and Recovery Act. Enactment of S.524 would improve the ability if ENA's 41,000 members to address the opioid abuse epidemic in several ways. I will focus on three important provisions contained in the legislation.

First, making naloxone available for use in the first few minutes of an opioid overdose by laypersons, law enforcement officers and other first responders makes a tremendous difference in the outcome for a person who has overdosed. I am proud to say that I helped to get legislation passed in Florida last year making naloxone available in these circumstances. As a result, patients are now much more likely to receive naloxone in the field from first responders. Later, when they arrive in the emergency department, we monitor the patients as the naloxone wears off and, in most cases, we are able to discharge them within several hours. In the past, when patients were much less likely to have access to naloxone as soon as they experienced a heroin overdose, many suffered brain damage caused by lack of oxygen because they had stopped breathing. We would place these patients on respirators in ICU for days just to keep them alive. Tragically, even some who survived an overdose would continue to suffer from long-term cognitive issues.

Second, the bill authorizing the Centers for Substance Abuse and Treatment to award grants to States, units of local government or nonprofit organizations located in geographic areas that have a high rate of heroin or other opioid abuse to expand treat activities, including medication assisted treatment programs, for the treatment of addiction in the geographical areas affected. This provision will be of great benefit to hospitals. Many of the patients we encounter have no place to go for the treatment of their addiction, especially if they do not have financial resources for private programs. Providing programs in the community that can help them safely withdraw from opioids and then manage their ongoing care would not only prevent them from needing emergency care, but it would save communities the costs associated with emergency medical services or police responding to cases of heroin and opioid overdoses.

Finally, the bill's National Youth Recovery Initiative authorizes the Director of Office of National Drug Control Policy to make grants to high schools and colleges to provide support to their students who are recovering from substance use disorders. This section of the legislation would assist both in the prevention of overdoses and achieving long-term recovery. This would lessen the burden on hospital emergency departments, which are not an optimal place to treat patients with substance abuse and often related mental health issues.

Question 2. What additional tools might you like to see at your disposal to address the overlap between substance abuse and mental health issues?

Answer 2. There are several tools that would help to address the overlap between substance abuse and mental health issues. One important change would be to enhance community-based treatment resources for both mental health and substance abuse patients. This will allow emergency departments to direct patients and their families to treatment options in the local community immediately upon discharge.

The time after discharge is when patients are most vulnerable and most likely to seek treatment for their addiction. Sending them directly to a treatment facility or outpatient program greatly increases their chances of recovery from their addiction. I have several friends and acquaintances who are recovered heroin addicts. They all say that they were fortunate to have family that cared enough to get them into treatment at a time they were in crisis.

Also, there is unfortunately still a prejudice by some in the health care field toward addicts. Therefore, it is important to educate health care providers, as well as the public, that addiction is a medical condition that often has a mental health component, and that both must be addressed as part of a successful treatment protocol.

Senator Baldwin

Question. Three Wisconsin health systems in the Fox Valley area have partnered to create a program, called Catalpa, to help improve timely access to mental health care for pediatric patients. This program provides crisis care for children and their families within 24 hours and then regular, followup care, led by a multidisciplinary team in the partnership network. At its main center, wait times have dropped from 54 days to about 5 days.

Dr. Hepburn and Ms. Blake, this is just one example of a program working to address the mental health services crisis facing our children. What steps would you recommend the Federal Government take to help solve our mental health provider shortage and improve access for children throughout the country?

Answer. From your description, Catalpa appears to have all of the components for a successful program. Access to emergency and crisis intervention immediately with referrals and followup resources are the key to a successful community based program. Regarding the mental health provider shortage, I would suggest examining the incentives the Federal Government has provided to address the ongoing shortage of registered nurses. These include the Title VIII Nursing Workforce Development programs that make scholarships and loans available to nurses and nursing students through a variety of grants. Similar programs and incentives could be made available for those embarking on a career in mental health and psychiatry.

In addition, the expanded use of technology should be considered. We have a shortage of neurologists in my area, so we use telemedicine to evaluate patients for possible interventions for stroke symptoms and it works well. Telepsychiatry is in use in some hospitals across the United States.

Also, policymakers should expand the role of nurse practitioners to allow them, with proper education and certification, to evaluate patients with mental health issues for the need for inpatient treatment. Frequently, in my area, we are told that the delay in having a patient transferred to a psychiatric facility is due to the psychiatrist not being available to review their records and evaluate them for intake. Allowing advanced practice registered nurses to review and evaluate patients would save both time and money.

Response by William W. Eaton, PhD to Question of Senator Whitehouse

Question. Along with a bipartisan group of senators including Senators Portman, Klobuchar, and Ayotte, I introduced a bill earlier this year called the Comprehensive Addiction and Recovery Act (S.524). The bill authorizes a series of grants to States and other eligible entities to promote an integrated approach—including prevention, treatment, law enforcement tools, and recovery support—to the substance abuse epidemic we are facing across the Nation. Among other things, the bill tries to increase screening for, and treatment of, co-occurring mental health and substance use disorders in the juvenile and criminal justice systems and elsewhere.

Do you support the objectives set forth in S. 524? How would enactment of S. 524 improve your organization's ability to help address the opioid abuse epidemic?

What additional tools might you like to see at your disposal to address the overlap between substance abuse and mental health issues?

Answer. I support the objectives set forth in S.524. Thanks for the opportunity to comment.

[Whereupon, at 11:31 a.m., the hearing was adjourned.]

In: Focus on Mental Health and Illness
Editor: Isaac Banks

ISBN: 978-1-53615-081-0

Chapter 3

PREVALENCE OF MENTAL ILLNESS IN THE UNITED STATES: DATA SOURCES AND ESTIMATES (UPDATED)*

Erin Bagalman and Ada S. Cornell

SUMMARY

Determining how many people have a mental illness can be difficult, and prevalence estimates vary. While numerous surveys include questions related to mental illness, few provide prevalence estimates of *diagnosable mental illness* (e.g., major depressive disorder as opposed to feeling depressed, or generalized anxiety disorder as opposed to feeling anxious), and fewer still provide *national* prevalence estimates of diagnosable mental illness. This chapter briefly describes the methodology and results of three large surveys (funded in whole or in part by the U.S. Department of Health and Human Services) that provide *national prevalence estimates of diagnosable mental illness*: the National Comorbidity Survey Replication (NCS-R), the National Comorbidity Survey Replication Adolescent Supplement (NCS-A), and the National Survey on Drug Use and Health (NSDUH). The NCS-R and the NCS-A have the advantage of identifying specific mental illnesses, but they are more than a decade old. The NSDUH does not identify specific mental illnesses, but it has the advantage of being conducted annually.

Between February 2001 and April 2003, NCS-R staff interviewed more than 9,000 adults aged 18 or older. Analyses of NCS-R data have yielded different prevalence estimates. One analysis of NCS-R data estimated that 26.2% of adults had a mental illness within a 12-month period (hereinafter called 12-month prevalence). Another analysis of NCS-R data estimated the 12-month prevalence of mental illness to be 32.4%

* This is an edited, reformatted and augmented version of Congressional Research Service, Publication No. R43047, dated January 19, 2018.

among adults. A third analysis of NCS-R data estimated the 12-month prevalence of mental illness *excluding substance use disorders* to be 24.8% among adults. The 12-month prevalence of *serious* mental illness was estimated to be 5.8% among adults, based on NCS-R data.

Between February 2001 and January 2004, NCS-A staff interviewed more than 10,000 adolescents aged 13 to 17. Using NCS-A data, researchers estimated the 12-month prevalence of mental illness to be 40.3% among adolescents. Some have suggested that the current approach to diagnosing mental illness identifies people who should not be considered mentally ill. The 12- month prevalence of *serious* mental illness was estimated to be 8.0% among adolescents, based on NCS-A data.

The NSDUH is an annual survey of approximately 68,000 adults and adolescents aged 12 years or older in the United States. According to the 2016 NSDUH, the estimated 12-month prevalence of mental illness *excluding substance use disorders* was 18.3% among adults aged 18 or older. The estimated 12-month prevalence of *serious* mental illness (excluding substance use disorders) was 4.2% among adults. Although the NSDUH collects information related to mental illness (e.g., symptoms of depression) from adolescents aged 12 to 17, it does not produce estimates of mental illness for that population.

The prevalence estimates discussed in this chapter may raise questions for Congress. Should federal mental health policy focus on adults or adolescents with *any* mental illness (including some whose mental illnesses may be mild and even transient) or on those with *serious* mental illness? Should substance use disorders be addressed through the same policies as other mental illnesses? Members of Congress may approach mental health policy differently depending in part on how they answer such questions.

INTRODUCTION

Congress has demonstrated an interest in mental health and mental illness,[1] and knowing how many people have a mental illness may be helpful in addressing related policy issues. Determining how many people have a mental illness can be difficult, and prevalence[2] estimates vary. While numerous surveys include questions related to mental illness, few provide prevalence estimates of *diagnosable mental illness*, and fewer still provide *national* prevalence estimates of diagnosable mental illness.[3]

---

[1] See, for example, U.S. Congress, Senate Committee on Health, Education, Labor, & Pensions, *Improving the Federal Response to Challenges in Mental Health Care in America*, 114th Cong., 2nd sess., January 20, 2016, https://www.help.senate.gov/hearings/improving-the-federal-response-to-challenges-in-mental-health-care-in-america; and U.S. Congress, House Committee on Energy and Commerce, Subcommittee on Oversight and Investigations, *Federal Efforts on Mental Health : Why Greater HHS Leadership is Needed,* 114th Cong., 1st sess., February 11, 2015, http://purl.fdlp.gov/GPO/gpo62010.

[2] Prevalence is the share of a population affected by a given condition during a specified period of time. The term "12-month prevalence" refers to the share of study participants with symptoms that could be identified as mental illness in the 12 months before the interview. Another way to express prevalence is "lifetime prevalence," which is based on the share of study participants that had *ever* had a mental illness as of the time of the interview. This report focuses on 12-month prevalence because it more closely reflects the number of people with mental illness at a given time, which might translate into need for services at a given time.

[3] See U.S. Department of Health and Human Services (HHS), Centers for Disease Control and Prevention (CDC), "Mental Illness Surveillance in the United States," *Morbidity and Mortality Weekly Report*, vol. 60, Supplement (September 2, 2011), http://www.cdc. gov/mmwr/preview/mmwrhtml/su6003a1.htm; and HHS, Substance Abuse and Mental Health Services Administration (SAMHSA), Center for Behavioral Health Statistics and

This chapter briefly describes the methodology and selected findings of three large federally funded surveys that provide *national prevalence estimates of diagnosable mental illness*: the National Comorbidity Survey Replication (NCS-R), the National Comorbidity Survey Replication Adolescent Supplement (NCS-A), and the National Survey on Drug Use and Health (NSDUH). This chapter presents prevalence estimates of *any* mental illness and *serious* mental illness[4] based on each survey and ends with a brief discussion of how these prevalence estimates might inform policy discussions.

One data source may be preferred over another in specific situations. For example, the NCS-R and the NCS-A are more than a decade old, so the NSDUH (which is conducted annually) may be preferred for more recent prevalence estimates. On the other hand, the NCS-R and the NCS-A provide prevalence estimates for specific disorders,[5] which the NSDUH does not provide.[6]

ESTIMATING PREVALENCE OF MENTAL ILLNESS

In clinical practice, mental health professionals diagnose mental illnesses based on criteria in the American Psychiatric Association's *Diagnostic and Statistical Manual of Mental Disorders* (DSM)[7] and exercise clinical judgment in doing so.[8] Large surveys, however, may not allow for lengthy interviews and use of clinical judgment. Considerations in generating national prevalence estimates of diagnosable mental illness[9]

Quality (CBHSQ), *Comparison of NSDUH Mental Health Data and Methods with Other Data Sources*, March 2012, http://www.samhsa.gov/data/NSDUH/2k12Findings/CBHSQDataReviewC2Mental Health2012.pdf.

[4] Severity of mental illness is generally defined by the number of symptoms (i.e., whether the individual has just enough symptoms to meet diagnostic criteria or has excess symptoms) and/or the degree of functional impairment (e.g., whether an individual with mental illness is unable to work as a consequence of the illness). Each survey discussed in this report uses its own definition of serious mental illness.

[5] Estimates of specific disorders are not presented in this report; they are available in the cited documents. The National Institute of Mental Health also compiles prevalence estimates for selected disorders; see the left navigation bar at "What is prevalence?" http://www.nimh.nih.gov/health/statistics/prevalence/ index.shtml. However, these estimates may come from various studies with different methodologies, and are not necessarily comparable to one another.

[6] The NSDUH provides more detailed information about substance use disorders, but not other mental illness.

[7] American Psychiatric Association, *Diagnostic and Statistical Manual of Mental Disorders, Fifth Edition (DSM-5)*, (Washington, DC: American Psychiatric Association, 2013). Some of the interviews designed for research are based on the fourth edition, text revision (DSM-IV-TR), published in 2000, or the fourth edition prior to the text revision (DSMIV), published in 1994.

[8] A diagnosis of mental illness may be based on what an individual reports about himself or herself; what other people report about the individual (if, for example, a family member is available); and what the mental health professional observes about the individual. People may not be forthcoming with information about certain behaviors (e.g., drug use) or symptoms (e.g., hallucinations); this is a challenge in both clinical settings and research settings.

[9] This report uses the term "diagnosable" as distinct from "diagnosed" in acknowledgement of the potential for surveys to identify people suffering from mental illnesses that have not been diagnosed by a mental health professional. Also important is the distinction between symptoms of mental illness (e.g., feelings of depression or anxiety) and a combination of symptoms meeting DSM criteria for a diagnosis of mental illness (e.g., major depressive disorder or generalized anxiety disorder). While all DSM disorders may be considered mental illnesses, surveys generally do not assess all of them. In this report, some of the prevalence estimates include substance use disorders and others do not.

through large surveys include (1) what survey instrument (i.e., set of questions) is used, (2) who administers it, and (3) how generalizable the findings are. Each of these considerations is discussed briefly below.

Table 1. Examples of Survey Instruments Assessing Mental Illness

Instrument	What It Assesses	Who Administers It	How Long It Takes	Examples of Surveys Using It
Structured Clinical Interview for DSM Disorders (SCID)[a]	Diagnoses	Trained mental health professionals	Approximately 30-60 minutes	NSDUH (for a subsample of respondents)
World Mental Health Survey Initiative version of the Composite International Diagnostic Interview (WMH-CIDI)[b]	Diagnoses, functioning, treatment, risk factors, socio-demographic characteristics, and more	Trained lay interviewers	Approximately 2 hours, but modular so that some sections can be excluded	NCS-R; NCS-A uses a modified Composite International Diagnostic Interview (CIDI)
World Health Organization Disability Assessment Schedule (WHODAS)[c]	Difficulties (due to health conditions) in the areas of cognition, mobility, self-care, getting along, life activities, and participation	Either self-administered or administered by an interviewer (no training required)	Different versions are available; the longest (36 items) takes approximately 15–20 minutes	NSDUH uses a modified version
Kessler-6 Psychological Distress Scale (K6)[d]	Frequency and severity of feeling nervous, hopeless, restless/fidgety, sad/depressed, and worthless	Either self-administered or administered by an interviewer (no training required)	No more than 2 minutes	NSDUH uses a modified version

Note: A survey instrument is a tool for systematically collecting information from survey respondents; each instrument listed in this table is a set of questions that may be asked as part of a larger questionnaire.

[a] DSM = Diagnostic and Statistical Manual of Mental Disorders. Information about the SCID in this table is drawn from U.S. Department of Health and Human Services (HHS), Centers for Disease Control and Prevention (CDC), "Mental Illness Surveillance in the United States," *Morbidity and Mortality Weekly Report*, vol. 60, Supplement (September 2, 2011).

[b] Information about the WMH-CIDI in this table is drawn from Ronald C. Kessler and T. Bedirhan Üstün, "The World Mental Health (WMH) Survey Initiative Version of the World Health Organization (WHO) Composite International Diagnostic Interview (CIDI)," *International Journal of Methods in Psychiatric Research*, vol. 13, no. 2 (2004), pp. 93-121.

[c] Information about the WHODAS in this table is drawn from World Health Organization, Classifications, Classification of Functioning, Disability and Health (ICF), http://www.who.int/classifications/icf/whodasii/en/.

[d] Ronald C. Kessler et al., "Screening for Serious Mental Illness in the General Population with the K6 Screening Scale: Results from the WHO World Mental Health (WMH) Survey Initiative," *International Journal of Methods in Psychiatric Research*, vol. 19 (Supplement 1) (2010), pp. 4-22.

When designing surveys, researchers must weigh the value of detailed information against the time required to collect that information. Longer survey instruments may be better able to identify mental illness accurately by asking all or most of the questions necessary to assess DSM diagnostic criteria. Shorter survey instruments, while more practical to include in a survey, may not identify mental illness as accurately as longer instruments. *Table 1* provides examples of survey instruments assessing mental illness.

Survey instruments may be administered in different ways, which may affect both the accuracy of their assessment of mental illness and the feasibility of their inclusion in large surveys. Some, such as the Structured Clinical Interview for DSM Disorders (described in *Table 1*), require trained mental health professionals. Others require trained interviewers who need not be mental health professionals. Still others may be self-administered or administered by interviewers without extensive training.

The prevalence estimates described in this chapter are weighted to reflect the general U.S. population as closely as possible.[10] This is accomplished by assigning a weight to each survey respondent based on information that is available for both the survey respondents and the general U.S. population (e.g., age and gender, among others). Weighting can correct for known differences between the survey respondents and the general U.S. population (e.g., if people in a certain age range are overrepresented in the survey). Weighting cannot, however, correct for subpopulations that are excluded from the survey altogether (e.g., the homeless). Prevalence estimates are not generalizable to excluded subpopulations.[11]

NATIONAL COMORBIDITY SURVEY REPLICATION

The National Comorbidity Survey Replication (NCS-R) replicated the original National Comorbidity Survey (conducted between 1990 and 1992), which was the first survey to use fully structured research diagnostic interviews to assess a wide range of DSM disorders among a national sample of adults in the United States.[10] The NCS-R was funded primarily by the National Institute of Mental Health within the National Institutes of Health (NIH) of the Department of Health and Human Services (HHS), with supplemental support from the National Institute on Drug Abuse (also within NIH), the Substance Abuse and Mental Health Services Administration (of HHS), the Robert Wood Johnson Foundation, and the John W. Alden Trust.[11] Between February 2001 and April 2003, NCS-R staff conducted in-person interviews with more than 9,000 adults aged 18 or older, drawing the sample from households in the contiguous United States. The sample did not include the

[10] The weighting was done by the researchers whose published results CRS cites in this report, not by CRS.

[11] The weighting was done by the researchers whose published results CRS cites in this report, not by CRS.

[10] Harvard Medical School, Department of Health Care Policy, *National Comorbidity Survey*, http://www.hcp.med.harvard.edu/ncs/.

[11] Ronald C. Kessler et al., "Prevalence, Severity, and Comorbidity of Twelve-month DSM-IV Disorders in the National Comorbidity Survey Replication (NCS-R)," *Archives of General Psychiatry*, vol. 62, no. 6 (June 2005), pp. 617-627. Hereinafter, Kessler et al., NCS-R Prevalence (2005).

homeless, individuals in institutions, or non-English speakers; these exclusions limit the generalizability of findings based on the NCS-R.[12]

Prevalence of Any Mental Illness Among Adults

The NCS-R determined the presence of any mental illness based on the World Health Organization's World Mental Health Survey Initiative version of the Composite International Diagnostic Interview (WMH-CIDI), which assessed 19 specific DSM diagnoses.[13] Analyses of NCS-R data have yielded different prevalence estimates. One analysis of NCS-R data estimated that 26.2% of adults had a mental illness within a 12-month period (hereinafter called 12-month prevalence).[14] Another analysis of NCS-R data estimated the 12-month prevalence of mental illness to be 32.4% among adults; the difference may be attributable to the use of more recent information about the U.S. population in weighting the NCS-R data.[15] Both of these estimates include substance use disorders as mental illness; an analysis of NCS-R data estimated the 12- month prevalence of mental illness *excluding substance use disorders* to be 24.8% among adults.[16]

Prevalence of Serious Mental Illness Among Adults

Additional analyses of NSC-R data were conducted to determine the 12-month prevalence of mental illness at three levels of severity: serious,[17] moderate,[18] or mild.[19] Among the 26.2% of adults identified with a mental disorder in the analysis, serious

---

[12] Kessler et al., NCS-R Prevalence (2005).

[13] The DSM includes more than 19 diagnoses. While all of them may be considered mental illnesses, some are often excluded from definitions of mental illness (e.g., learning disorders).

[14] Kessler et al., NCS-R Prevalence (2005).

[15] Harvard Medical School, Department of Health Care Policy, *National Comorbidity Survey*, "NSC-R Twelve-Month Prevalence Estimates" link at http://www.hcp.med.harvard.edu/ ncs/. This later analysis was based on updated data as of July 19, 2007, and "reflect[s] the latest diagnostic, demographic and raw variable information."

[16] Benjamin G. Druss et al. "Impairment in Role Functioning in Mental and Chronic Medical Disorders in the United States: Results from the National Comorbidity Survey Replication." *Molecular Psychiatry*, vol. 14, no. 7 (July 2009), pp. 728-737.

[17] Kessler et al., NCS-R Prevalence (2005). Any of the following qualified a case of mental illness as serious: "a 12-month suicide attempt with serious lethality intent; work disability or substantial limitation due to a mental or substance disorder; positive screen results for non-affective psychosis; bipolar I or II disorder; substance dependence with serious role impairment (as defined by disorder-specific impairment questions); an impulse control disorder with repeated serious violence; or any disorder that resulted in 30 or more days out of role in the year" (p. 618).

[18] Kessler et al., NCS-R Prevalence (2005). Among cases of mental illness not defined as serious, any of the following qualified a case as moderate: "suicide gesture, plan, or ideation; substance dependence without serious role impairment; at least moderate work limitation due to a mental or substance disorder; or any disorder with at least moderate role impairment in 2 or more domains of the Sheehan Disability Scale [which] assessed disability in work role performance, household maintenance, social life, and intimate relationships" (p. 618).

[19] Kessler et al., NCS-R Prevalence (2005). All cases of mental illness that were not defined as serious or moderate were considered mild (p. 618).

disorders (22.3% *among adults with a disorder*) were less common than moderate disorders (37.3%) or mild disorders (40.4%). The estimated 12-month prevalence of serious mental illness among *all* adults was 5.8%.[20]

NATIONAL COMORBIDITY SURVEY REPLICATION ADOLESCENT SUPPLEMENT

The National Comorbidity Survey Replication Adolescent Supplement (NCS-A) was the first survey to use fully structured research diagnostic interviews to assess a wide range of DSM disorders among a national sample of adolescents in the United States. Like the NCS-R, the NCSA was funded primarily by the National Institute of Mental Health, with supplemental support from the National Institute on Drug Abuse, the Substance Abuse and Mental Health Services Administration, the Robert Wood Johnson Foundation, and the John W. Alden Trust.[21] Between February 2001 and January 2004, NCS-A staff interviewed more than 10,000 adolescents aged 13 to 17, drawing the sample from both schools and households in the coterminous United States. Adolescent participants were interviewed in person, and one parent of each participating adolescent was asked to complete a self-administered questionnaire about the adolescent's developmental history and mental health. The sample did not include the homeless, individuals in institutions, or non-English speakers; these exclusions limit the generalizability of findings based on the NCS-A.[22]

Prevalence of Any Mental Illness Among Adolescents

The NCS-A determined the presence of any mental illness based on a modified Composite International Diagnostic Interview (CIDI), which assessed 15 specific DSM diagnoses. Using NCS-A data, researchers estimated the 12-month prevalence of mental illness to be 40.3% among adolescents.[23] Some have suggested that the current version of the DSM identifies people who should not be considered mentally ill.[24]

---

[20] Kessler et al., NCS-R Prevalence (2005).

[21] Ronald C. Kessler et al., "Prevalence, Persistence, and Sociodemographic Correlates of DSM-IV Disorders in the National Comorbidity Survey Replication Adolescent Supplement," *Archives of General Psychiatry*, vol. 69, no. 4 (April 2012). Hereinafter, Kessler et al., NCS-A Prevalence (2012).

[22] Ronald C. Kessler et al., "Severity of 12-Month DSM-IV Disorders in the National Comorbidity Survey Replication Adolescent Supplement," *Archives of General Psychiatry*, vol. 69, no. 4 (April 2012). Hereinafter, Kessler et al., NCS-A Severity (2012).

[23] Kessler et al., NCS-A Prevalence (2012).

[24] Kessler et al., NCS-A Severity (2012).

Prevalence of Serious Mental Illness Among Adolescents

Additional analyses of NCS-A data were conducted to determine the presence of serious mental illness (called serious emotional disturbance in NCS-A), which was defined as at least one diagnosis accompanied by an estimated score of 50 or less on the Children's Global Assessment Scale (CGAS), indicating either severe functional impairment in one area of living or moderate functional impairment in most areas of living. The CGAS score was not measured directly as part of the NCS-A. Instead the NCS-A used a sophisticated approach that involved (1) selection of a subsample of 347 adolescent-parent pairs from the main study; (2) follow-up telephone interviews conducted by mental health professionals who assigned CGAS scores; (3) development of a statistical model linking CGAS scores to responses to questions in the main study; and (4) application of the statistical model to the full sample to impute CGAS scores based on responses to questions in the main study.[25]

Using the imputed CGAS scores, researchers assessed serious mental illness among 6,483 adolescent NCS-A participants with complete data (including parent questionnaires). This analysis yielded a 12-month prevalence of any mental illness (42.6%) that was slightly higher than the previous estimate and found most cases to be mild (58.2% *among adolescents with a disorder*) or moderate (22.9%), rather than serious (18.8%). The estimated 12-month prevalence of serious mental illness among *all* adolescents was 8.0%. Some people have suggested that most adolescents with mental disorders do not need treatment because their disorders are mild and will resolve on their own; however, some research has shown that mild disorders during adolescence may predict serious disorders during adulthood.[26]

NATIONAL SURVEY ON DRUG USE AND HEALTH

The National Survey on Drug Use and Health (NSDUH) focuses primarily on the use of illegal drugs, alcohol, and tobacco and also includes several modules that focus on mental health issues.[27] The NSDUH is funded by the Substance Abuse and Mental Health Services Administration (SAMHSA). Each year, the NSDUH surveys approximately

---

[25] Kessler et al., NCS-A Prevalence (2012); Kessler et al., NCS-A Severity (2012); and Ronald C. Kessler et al., "The National Comorbidity Survey Adolescent Supplement (NCSA): III. Concordance of DSM-IV/CIDI Diagnoses with Clinical Reassessments," *Journal of the American Academy of Child and Adolescent Psychiatry*, vol. 48, no. 4 (April 2009), pp. 386-399.

[26] Kessler et al., NCS-A Severity (2012).

[27] U.S. Department of Health and Human Services (HHS), Substance Abuse and Mental Health Services Administration (SAMHSA), Center for Behavioral Health Statistics and Quality (CBHSQ), *2016 National Survey on Drug Use and Health: Methodological summary and definitions*, Rockville, MD, September 2017, https://www.samhsa.gov/data/sites/default/files/NSDUH-MethodSummDefs-2016/NSDUH-MethodSummDefs2016.htm. Hereinafter, *2016 NSDUH: Methodological Summary.*

68,000 noninstitutionalized civilians aged 12 years or older in the United States, divided roughly between 51,000 adults (aged 18 or older) and 17,000 adolescents (aged 12 to 17).[28] The NSDUH is conducted in both English and Spanish. Participants are interviewed in their homes using a combination of personal interviewing and audio computer-assisted self-interviewing, which offers more privacy in order to encourage honest reporting of sensitive topics such as illicit drug use. The sample does not include homeless persons not living in a shelter, individuals in institutions, those who speak a language other than English or Spanish, or military personnel on active duty; these exclusions limit the generalizability of findings based on the NSDUH.[29]

NSDUH-based prevalence estimates of any mental illness and serious mental illness among adults aged 18 or older are described below. Although the NSDUH collects information related to mental illness (e.g., symptoms of depression) from adolescents aged 12 to 17, it does not produce *prevalence estimates of mental illness* for that population.

Prevalence of Any Mental Illness Among Adults

The NSDUH determines the presence of any mental illness based on a combination of relatively short modules of questions (including modified versions of the K6 and WHODAS described in *Table 1*) in the main survey and information from an additional follow-up interview conducted with a subsample of adults from the main survey.[30] Unlike the NCS-R and the NCS-A, the core component of NSDUH does not include questions designed to identify specific DSM diagnoses. Instead, the NSDUH uses an approach similar to the one used by NCS-A to impute the CGAS, involving (1) selection of a subsample of adults from the main study; (2) follow-up telephone interviews conducted by mental health professionals who conduct the Structured Clinical Interview for DSM Disorders (SCID); (3) development of a statistical model linking the SCID based diagnosis of mental illness to responses to questions in the main study; and (4) application of the statistical model to the full sample to impute the presence of mental illness based on responses to questions in the main study.[31] According to the 2016 NSDUH, the estimated 12- month prevalence of mental illness *excluding substance use disorders* is 18.3% of adults (aged 18 or older).[32]

---

[28] In 2016, 67,942 respondents completed a NSDUH interview, including 50,833 adults and 17,109 adolescents. (*2016 NSDUH: Methodological Summary*).

[29] *2016 NSDUH: Methodological Summary*. The NSDUH has been ongoing since 1971; prior to 2002, it was called the National Household Survey on Drug Abuse.

[30] 2016 NSDUH: Methodological Summary.

[31] This approach, called the Mental Health Surveillance Study, began with the 2008 NSDUH. The statistical model was changed in 2012; the 2012 model continued to be used in subsequent years, including 2016.

[32] HHS, SAMHSA, CBHSQ, Results from the 2016 National Survey on Drug Use and Health: Mental Health Detailed Tables, Rockville, MD, 2017, Table 8.1B, https://www.samhsa.gov/ data/sites/default/files/NSDUH-DetTabs-2016/NSDUH-DetTabs-2016.htm. Hereinafter, 2016 NSDUH: Mental Health Tables.

Prevalence of Serious Mental Illness Among Adults

The NSDUH identifies adults (aged 18 or older) as having a serious mental illness if (1) they have a mental illness (excluding substance use disorders and developmental disorders) and (2) the illness substantially interferes with or limits at least one major life activity. The same approach used to impute any mental illness is applied to impute serious mental illness. According to the 2016 NSDUH, the estimated 12-month prevalence of serious mental illness *excluding substance use disorders* is 4.2% among adults (aged 18 or older).[33]

CONCLUDING COMMENTS

Knowing how many people are likely to be affected by policies related to mental illness may help policymakers identify specific problems as well as their scope; however, the national prevalence estimates discussed in this chapter may raise as many questions as they answer. For example, given the difference in prevalence estimates between *any* mental illness and *serious* mental illness among adolescents, might policymakers choose to focus on a large group of adolescents that includes many whose mental illnesses may be mild and even transient, or might they choose to focus more narrowly on adolescents with serious mental illness? As clinical practice is moving toward more integrated care,[34] should substance use disorders be included in the definition of mental illness (as in the NCS-R and the NCS-A) and addressed through the same policies, or should they be identified separately (as in the NSDUH) and addressed through different policies? How might policymakers address mental illness among populations that are excluded from the prevalence estimates (e.g., the homeless)? With regard to the NCS-R and the NCS-A, there is an overarching question of whether prevalence estimates based on surveys conducted more than a decade ago remain relevant to current policy discussions. Policymakers may come to different conclusions about the best policy approach depending in part on how they answer such questions.

---

[33] 2016 NSDUH: Mental Health Tables, Table 8.4B.

[34] Like clinical practice, financing is moving toward including substance use disorders with the rest of mental illness. The Mental Health Parity Act of 1996 (MHPA, P.L. 104-204) did not apply to coverage of substance use disorders. The more recent Paul Wellstone and Pete Domenici Mental Health Parity and Addiction Equity Act of 2008 (MHPAEA, P.L. 110-343) applies to both substance use disorders and the rest of mental illness.

In: Focus on Mental Health and Illness
Editor: Isaac Banks
ISBN: 978-1-53615-081-0

Chapter 4

JUSTICE AND MENTAL HEALTH COLLABORATION PROGRAM: FACT SHEET*

Nathan James

People with mental illness comprise a significant proportion of the population involved with the criminal justice system. The Bureau of Justice Statistics reports that at midyear 2005, over half of state prison and local jail inmates had a mental health problem.[1] Mental health courts were developed to respond to the large number of people in the criminal justice systems with mental illness.[2]

The federal government provides funding to support mental health courts across the country through the Justice and Mental Health Collaboration program. The purpose of the program is to increase public safety by facilitating collaboration among the criminal justice, juvenile justice, mental health treatment, and substance abuse systems to increase access to treatment for offenders with mental illness.[3] Authorized funding for this program expired at the end of FY2014, although, Congress has continued to appropriate funding for the program.

---

* This is an edited, reformatted and augmented version of Congressional Research Service, Publication No. R43556, dated February 2, 2016.

[1] Lauren E. Glaze and Doris J. James, *Mental Health Problems of Prison and Jail Inmates*, U.S. Department of Justice, Office of Justice Programs, Bureau of Justice Statistics, Washington, September 6, 2006, p. 3. These are the most recent data available.

[2] The Council of State Governments Justice Center, *Mental Health Courts: A Primer for Policymakers and Practitioners*, p. 2.

[3] U.S. Department of Justice, Office of Justice Programs, Bureau of Justice Assistance, *Justice and Mental Health Collaboration Program (JMHCP)*, https://www.bja.gov/ProgramDetails. aspx?Program_ID=66.

What Are Mental Health Courts?

A working definition of "mental health court"

A mental health court is a specialized court docket for certain defendants with mental illnesses. This court substitutes a problem-solving model for traditional criminal court processing. Participants are identified through mental health screening and assessments and voluntarily participate in a judicially supervised treatment plan developed jointly by a team of court staff and mental health professionals. Incentives reward adherence to the treatment plan or other court conditions. Nonadherence may be sanctioned, and success or graduation is defined according to predetermined criteria.[4]

Despite the expansion of mental health court programs across the country, there is not yet an accepted criteria for what constitutes a "mental health court."[5] The Council of State Governments (Council) reports that the degree of diversity among programs has made agreement on a core definition difficult.[6] Mental health courts vary widely on several aspects including target population, charge accepted (e.g., misdemeanor versus felony), plea arrangement, intensity of supervision, program duration, and type of treatment available. The Council worked with leaders in the field to distill the common characteristics of mental health courts into a working definition.

The Justice and Mental Health Collaboration Program

Grants under the Justice and Mental Health Collaboration program have been awarded since FY2006. They can be used by state, local, and tribal governments to provide mental health and other treatment services for mentally ill adults or juvenile offenders that are overseen collaboratively by a criminal or juvenile justice agency or a mental health court and a mental health agency. Specifically, grants under the program can be used to create or expand

- mental health courts or other court-based programs for preliminarily qualified offenders;[7]

[4] The Council of State Governments Justice Center, *Mental Health Courts: A Primer for Policymakers and Practitioners*, p. 4.

[5] Ibid.

[6] Ibid.

[7] "Preliminarily qualified offenders" means an adult or a juvenile accused of a non-violent offense who (1) previously or currently has been diagnosed by a qualified mental health professional as having a mental illness or co-occurring mental illness and substance abuse disorder or manifests obvious signs of mental illness or co-occurring mental illness and substance abuse disorders during arrest, confinement, or before any court, and (2) has faced, is facing, or could face criminal charges for a misdemeanor or non-violent offense and is deemed

- programs that offer specialized training to criminal and juvenile justice and mental health professionals on how to identify the symptoms of people who might benefit from participating in a mental health courts program;
- programs that support cooperative efforts between criminal and juvenile justice agencies and mental health agencies to provide mental health services and, where appropriate, substance abuse treatment, to individuals with a need for such treatment when they are involved with the criminal justice system; and
- programs that support state and local cooperation with respect to mentally ill offenders.[8]

The Attorney General can also award grants under the program to state, local, and tribal governments for

- programs that offer law enforcement or campus security personnel training in procedures to identify and respond to incidents in which individuals with mental illnesses are involved;
- development of specialized receiving centers to assess individuals in the custody of law enforcement personnel for suicide risk and mental health and substance abuse treatment needs;
- computerized information systems to improve the response to mentally ill offenders; and
- establishment and expansion of cooperative efforts to promote public safety through the use of effective intervention with mentally ill offenders.[9]

AUTHORIZATIONS AND APPROPRIATIONS

The Justice and Mental Health Collaboration program was first authorized by the Mentally Ill Offender Treatment and Crime Reduction Act of 2004 (P.L. 108-414).[10] The act authorized $50 million for FY2005 and such sums as necessary each fiscal year for FY2006-FY2009. The program was reauthorized by the Mentally Ill Offender Treatment and Crime Reduction Reauthorization and Improvement Act of 2008 (P.L. 110-416). The act reauthorized appropriations for the program at $50 million each fiscal year for FY2009-FY2014.

---

eligible by a diversion process, designated pretrial screening process, or by a magistrate or judge, on the ground that the commission of the offense is the product of the person's mental illness. 42 U.S.C. §3797aa(a)(9).

[8] 42 U.S.C. §3797aa(b)(2).

[9] 42 U.S.C. §3797aa(h).

[10] The authorizing legislation for the program is codified at 42 U.S.C. §3797aa.

Congress has appropriated funding for the program since FY2006. Since FY2006, Congress has appropriated an average of $8 million per fiscal year for the program.

Table 1. Authorizations and Appropriations for the Justice and Mental Health Collaboration Program (Authorizations and appropriations in thousands of dollars)

Fiscal Year	Authorization	Appropriation
2005	$50,000	—
2006	SSAN	4,936
2007	SSAN	4,936
2008	SSAN	6,500
2009	50,000	10,000
2010	50,000	12,000
2011	50,000	9,940
2012	50,000	9,000
2013	50,000	8,369
2014	50,000	8,250
2015	—	8,500
2016	—	10,000

Source: The FY2005-FY2011 appropriations were taken from the congressional budget submissions for the Office of Justice Programs for FY2006-FY2012. The FY2012 appropriation was taken from H.Rept. 112-284. The FY2013 appropriation was provided by the Department of Justice. The FY2014 appropriation was taken from the explanatory statement to accompany P.L. 113-76, printed in the January 15, 2014, Congressional Record (pp. H507- H532). The FY2015 appropriation was taken from the joint explanatory statement to accompany P.L. 113-235, printed in the December 12, 2014, Congressional Record (pp. H9342-H9363). The FY2016 appropriation was taken from the joint explanatory statement to accompany P.L. 114-113, printed in the December 17, 2015, Congressional Record (pp. H9732-H9759). Authorized amounts were taken from P.L. 108-414 and P.L. 110-416.

Notes: "SSAN" means "such sums as necessary." Appropriations acts have cited two authorizations for the appropriation amounts presented in Table 1. The first is the mental health courts program authorized by the America's Law Enforcement and Mental Health Project (P.L. 106-515), the second is the program authorized by the Mentally Ill Offender Treatment and Crime Reduction Act of 2004 (P.L. 108-414).

In: Focus on Mental Health and Illness
Editor: Isaac Banks
ISBN: 978-1-53615-081-0

Chapter 5

FEDERAL LAW ENFORCEMENT: DHS AND DOJ ARE WORKING TO ENHANCE RESPONSES TO INCIDENTS INVOLVING INDIVIDUALS WITH MENTAL ILLNESS*

United States Government Accountability Office

ABBREVIATIONS

ATF	Bureau of Alcohol, Tobacco, Firearms and Explosives
BJA	Bureau of Justice Assistance
BOP	Federal Bureau of Prisons
CBP	U.S. Customs and Border Protection
CIT	Crisis Intervention Team
CRCL	Office for Civil Rights and Civil Liberties
CSG JC	Council of State Governments Justice Center
DEA	U.S. Drug Enforcement Administration
DHS	Department of Homeland Security
DOJ	Department of Justice
DSM-IV	Diagnostic and Statistical Manual of Mental Disorders, 4th edition
FBI	Federal Bureau of Investigation

* This is an edited, reformatted and augmented version of the United States Government Accountability Office Report to Congressional Committees, Publication No. GAO-18-229, dated February 2018.

FLETC	Federal Law Enforcement Training Centers
FPS	Federal Protective Service
IACP	International Association of Chiefs of Police
ICE	U.S. Immigration and Customs Enforcement
ODAG	Office of the Deputy Attorney General
PERF	Police Executive Research Forum
Section 504	Section 504 of the Rehabilitation Act of 1973, as amended
TSA	Transportation Security Administration
USMS	U.S. Marshals Service

WHY GAO DID THIS STUDY

Law enforcement encounters with individuals with mental illness may require special training and skills and can sometimes involve volatile situations, risking tragic injuries or even death.

The 21st Century Cures Act includes a provision for GAO to review the practices that federal first responders, tactical units, and corrections officers (for the purposes of this study, "law enforcement officers and agents") are trained to use in responding to incidents involving individuals with mental illness. This chapter addresses

- challenges that federal law enforcement officers and agents face;
- applicable training, policies, and guidance; and (3) existing leading practices, relevant tools, and efforts to leverage information.

GAO selected the five DHS and five DOJ law enforcement components (e.g., Secret Service, Federal Bureau of Investigation) that represent the largest concentration of law enforcement officers within the two departments. GAO reviewed the training, policies, and guidance in place, as well as efforts to enhance them, and discussed these matters with knowledgeable officials. In addition, GAO held discussion groups with a nongeneralizable sample of law enforcement officers and agents, selected through component contacts, to discuss their perspectives. GAO also reviewed studies on law enforcement responses to individuals with mental illness to help identify leading practices and tools and interviewed stakeholders, selected through a structured process, to obtain their perspectives.

WHAT GAO FOUND

Law enforcement officers and agents from the Departments of Homeland Security (DHS) and Justice (DOJ) cited a number of challenges in our discussion groups related to their response to incidents involving individuals with a mental illness.

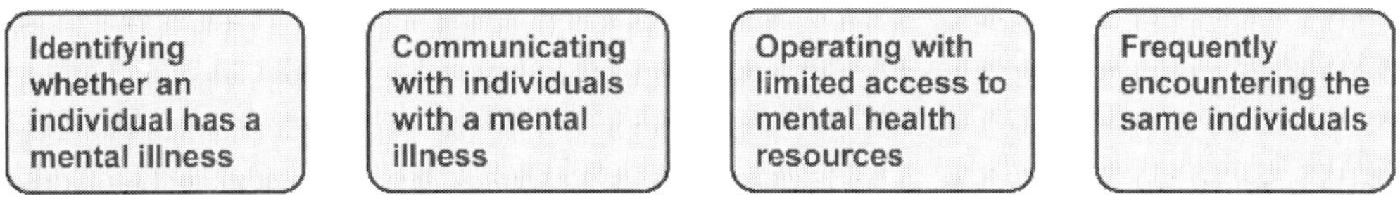

Source: GAO summary of discussion group comments. | GAO-18-229.

Challenges Identified in Law Enforcement Officer and Agent Discussion Groups

All of the federal law enforcement components in GAO's review either offer, receive, or are developing some form of training to their law enforcement officers and agents that addresses responding to incidents involving individuals with a mental illness. Further, all components have relevant policies or guidance in place, and all are undertaking efforts to enhance their practices in accordance with departmental guidance. Since DHS and DOJ components have varying missions and operational needs and interact with the public in different capacities, the nature and scope of training, as well as the number and duration of courses offered in response to individuals with mental illness varies; however, they generally include elements focusing on de-escalation and communication. In addition, DHS and DOJ both have efforts underway to have components review their training and policies under departmental guidance and plan to begin implementing any changes by 2018.

Stakeholders cited leading practices and tools for effective law enforcement responses, and DHS and DOJ components have generally leveraged information from other knowledgeable parties. For example, the Crisis Intervention Team approach involves training selected law enforcement officers on mental health topics and dispatching those officers on mental-health related calls. While models like this are typically used by state and local law enforcement agencies, their benefits could be considered in other settings such as federal law enforcement. DHS and DOJ officials are also using collaborative mechanisms within their departments, such as conference calls and working groups with officials that have helped them leverage information from knowledgeable parties. In addition, DOJ's Bureau of Justice Assistance (BJA), which supports programs and initiatives in the areas of law enforcement, among other activities, has developed and makes publicly available resources such as its Police-Mental Health Collaboration Toolkit. BJA also is working to stand up a national training and technical assistance center to improve law enforcement responses to people with mental illness. While aimed at state, local, and tribal law enforcement, a BJA official also acknowledged that the center could serve as an additional resource for federal law enforcement agencies to consult as they review relevant trainings, policies, and guidance on this topic.

February 8, 2018

Congressional Committees:

According to the International Association of Chiefs of Police (IACP), law enforcement officers nationwide are increasingly called upon to respond to and intervene on behalf of people affected by mental illness.[1] Based on estimates from the Substance Abuse and Mental Health Services Administration—an agency within the Department of Health and Human Services—44.7 million adults in the United States had a mental illness in 2016.[2] Since law enforcement officers can encounter individuals affected by mental illness in the course of their duties, the nature of their interaction has become an issue of national concern. In particular, research has demonstrated that such encounters:

- may require special training and skills to address;
- may depend on the availability of community and mental health resources for a positive outcome;
- are often time-consuming and difficult for law enforcement officers to resolve;
- typically involve repeat contacts with individuals who have unmet mental health needs; and
- can involve volatile situations, risking tragic injuries or even death.

Such concerns and potential safety issues underscore the importance of developing tailored approaches, training, and policies to help guide police departments and law enforcement officials.

To date, most efforts to promote such training or policies have been focused on state and local law enforcement agencies, such as police departments. While federal law

---

[1] IACP, *Improving Police Response to Persons Affected by Mental Illness*, Report from the March 2016 IACP Symposium, Alexandria, Virginia (2016). IACP is a professional association for law enforcement that aims to advance the law enforcement profession through advocacy, outreach, education and programs. For the purpose of our review, we used the definition of mental illness that the National Alliance on Mental Illness developed, which is: "a condition that affects a person's thinking, feeling or mood. Such conditions may affect someone's ability to relate to others and function each day." The National Alliance on Mental Illness is an association of local affiliates, state organizations and volunteers who work to raise awareness and provide support and education on various issues related to mental illness.

[2] Substance Abuse and Mental Health Services Administration (2017). *Key substance use and mental health indicators in the United States: Results from the 2016 National Survey on Drug Use and Health* (HHS Publication No. SMA 17-5044, NSDUH Series H-52). Rockville, MD: Center for Behavioral Health Statistics and Quality, Substance Abuse and Mental Health Services Administration. Retrieved from https://www.samhsa.gov/data/. In that report, adults with a mental illness were defined as having any mental, behavioral, or emotional disorder in the past year that met criteria from the American Psychiatric Association's Diagnostic and Statistical Manual of Mental Disorders, 4th edition (DSM-IV), excluding developmental disorders and substance use disorders.

enforcement agencies typically do not serve as first responders to emergency calls, they do interact with the public in the course of their duties and can encounter individuals with mental illness. At the federal level, the Department of Homeland Security (DHS) and Department of Justice (DOJ) are responsible for enforcing many laws regarding the safety and security of the United States, and these two departments house the majority of federal law enforcement officers nationwide.[3]

The 21st Century Cures Act[4] includes a provision for us to review, among other things, practices that federal first responders, tactical units, and corrections officers are trained to use in responding to incidents involving individuals with mental illness.[5] This chapter addresses the following key questions: (1) What challenges, if any, do federal law enforcement officers and agents at selected DHS and DOJ components face when responding to incidents involving individuals with mental illness? (2) What type of training, policies, and guidance, if any, are in place at selected DHS and DOJ components to prepare federal law enforcement officers and agents for responding to incidents involving individuals with mental illness? (3) What leading practices or tools have relevant stakeholders cited for effective responses to incidents involving individuals with mental illness, and how have DHS and DOJ components leveraged information from other knowledgeable parties?

We focused our review on the training, policies, and guidance put forth by the DHS and DOJ components listed in table 1 below because they comprise nearly all of the federal law enforcement officers in these departments.

To identify the challenges that federal law enforcement officers and agents at our selected DOJ and DHS components face when responding to incidents involving individuals with mental illness, we held discussion groups with six to eleven agents or officers within each selected component to ask about their experiences. We worked with officials at each component to identify officers and agents with varied tenures and experiences. We then summarized the information collected from the discussion groups and identified common themes across the selected components. We worked closely with the departments to organize these discussion groups; however, these officers' and agents' perspectives cannot be generalized to their entire components or to all federal law enforcement components. Nevertheless, their views provided valuable insights into the challenges they face on the job.

---

[3] Specifically, DHS's mission includes preventing terrorism and enhancing security; managing and securing the nations' borders; administering and enforcing immigration laws; and securing cyberspace. DOJ's mission includes enforcing the law and defending the interests of the United States according to the law, ensuring public safety against threats foreign and domestic, providing federal leadership in preventing and controlling crime, and ensuring fair and impartial administration of justice for all Americans.

[4] Pub. L. No. 114-255, div. B., tit. XIV, subtit. B, § 14026, 130 Stat. 1033, 1310-11 (2016). The provision for our study is contained in Division B—the Helping Families in Mental Health Crisis Reform Act of 2016.

[5] For the purposes of our review, we focused on federal law enforcement officers, tactical units, and correctional officers, referring to all under the general term "law enforcement officers" from here forward. We use the terminology "officers and/or agents" to reflect the varying job titles and responsibilities that individuals within these components have. We did not include contractors in the scope of our review.

Table 1. Department of Homeland Security and Department of Justice Federal Law Enforcement Components Selected for GAO's Review and Their Missions

Component	Mission
Department of Homeland Security	
Federal Law Enforcement Training Centers (FLETC)[a]	Provides career-long training to law enforcement professionals to help them fulfill their responsibilities safely and proficiently. Under a collaborative training model, FLETC's federal partner organizations deliver training unique to their missions, while FLETC provides training in areas common to all law enforcement officers, such as firearms, driving, tactics, investigations, and legal training.
Federal Protective Service (FPS)	Provides integrated security and law enforcement services, such as conducting facility security assessments; responding to crimes and other incidents to protect life and property; and detecting, investigating, and mitigating threats to more than 9,500 federal facilities nationwide.
Transportation Security Administration (TSA)	Protects the nation's transportation systems to ensure freedom of movement for people and commerce. TSA does this by, among other things, deploying Federal Air Marshals on U.S. aircraft worldwide. Our review focuses on TSA's Federal Air Marshals, who are to detect, deter, and defeat criminal and terrorist activity targeting transportation systems.
U.S. Customs and Border Protection (CBP)	Protects the borders of the United States from dangerous people and materials, while facilitating lawful international travel and trade.
U.S. Immigration and Customs Enforcement (ICE)	Protects the United States from cross-border crime and illegal immigration that threaten national security and public safety. ICE executes this mission through enforcement of federal statutes and focuses on immigration enforcement, preventing terrorism, and combating the illegal movement of people and goods. Our review focuses on ICE's Homeland Security Investigations office, which investigates cross-border criminal activity, and ICE's Enforcement and Removal Operations unit, which identifies and apprehends removable aliens, detains them when necessary, and removes illegal aliens from the United States.
U.S. Secret Service	Provides physical protection to the nation's highest elected leaders and visiting foreign dignitaries, as well as for facilities and major events, and safeguards the payment and financial systems of the United States from a wide range of financial and computer-based crimes.
Department of Justice	
Bureau of Alcohol, Tobacco, Firearms and Explosives (ATF)	Investigates and seeks to prevent federal offenses involving the unlawful use, manufacture, and possession of firearms and explosives, acts of arson and bombings, and illegal trafficking of alcohol and tobacco products.

Component	Mission
Federal Bureau of Prisons (BOP)	Confines offenders in the controlled environments of prisons and community-based facilities that are safe, humane, cost-efficient, and appropriately secure, and that provide work and other self improvement opportunities to assist offenders in becoming law-abiding citizens. As part of its duties, BOP is responsible for delivering medically necessary health care to inmates in accordance with proven standards of care, including medical, dental and mental health.
Federal Bureau of Investigation (FBI)	Protects the nation from terrorism, espionage, cyber-attacks, and major criminal threats through intelligence-gathering and law enforcement responsibilities. Our review focuses on the FBI's Special Agents, who are primarily responsible for executing this mission, as well as FBI Police Officers, who provide security at FBI facilities.
U.S. Drug Enforcement Administration (DEA)	Enforces the controlled substances laws and regulations of the United States and brings to the criminal and civil justice system of the United States, or any other competent jurisdiction, those organizations and principal members of organizations involved in the growing, manufacture, or distribution of controlled substances appearing in or destined for illicit traffic in the United States.
U.S. Marshals Service (USMS)	Provides federal judicial security, apprehends fugitives and non-compliant sex offenders, secures and transports federal prisoners from arrest to incarceration, executes federal court orders, seizes and manages assets acquired through illegal means, and assures the safety of endangered government witnesses and their families.

Source: GAO summary of information from components. | GAO-18-229.

Note: According to data the departments provided to us, as of the end of fiscal year 2016, the DHS components above—excluding FLETC—employed 42,823 of 43,222 law enforcement officers within DHS, and the DOJ components above employed 43,502 of 43,639 law enforcement officers within DOJ.

[a] FLETC information is presented in this table as the component provides various types of training to a number of federal law enforcement agencies. However, we do not consider it an operational law enforcement component for our subsequent discussions of training in place across DHS components.

To identify the training, policies, and guidance in place, we reviewed documents from each of our selected law enforcement components, when available, and conducted interviews with officials at the selected components responsible for the development or delivery of training or policies. We also reviewed fiscal year 2018 budget justifications for each of our selected components to identify changes in staffing levels or training plans that may be related to officers' and agents' response to incidents involving individuals with mental illness. In addition, since section 504 of the Rehabilitation Act of 1973, as amended (section 504) prohibits discrimination on the basis of disability, which includes mental illness, in federally funded and federally conducted programs and activities,[6] we took steps

[6] 29 U.S.C. § 794. A person with a disability includes anyone who has a physical or mental impairment that substantially limits one or more major life activities, has a record of such impairment, or is regarded as having such an impairment. The definition of disability for purposes of § 504 of the Rehabilitation Act is derived from the Americans with Disabilities Act. 29 U.S.C. § 705(9); 42 U.S.C. § 12102.

to understand the section's applicability to federal law enforcement operations.[7] Specifically, we reviewed departmental guidance related to section 504 and reviewed the selected components' documentation of efforts to review their training, policies, and procedures in accordance with that guidance. We also interviewed department and component officials familiar with the review efforts.

To identify leading practices stakeholders cited for effective law enforcement responses to incidents involving individuals with mental illness, we used a multi-stage process. We first conducted a search of databases and organizational websites to identify published work related to law enforcement responses to individuals with mental illness that had been published on or after January 1, 2007. We then narrowed our search and reviewed only literature review articles, meta-analyses, and summary papers published by academics, think tanks and advocacy groups, or government agencies to identify any potential leading practices.[8] Through our review, we identified two potentially leading practices in the field of law enforcement responses to incidents involving individuals with mental illness. Next, we identified potential stakeholders through a search of literature review articles, meta-analyses, and organizational websites related to law enforcement responses to incidents involving individuals with mental illness. Through our review of these documents and websites, we selected six stakeholders in the field of law enforcement-mental health to solicit their opinions on leading practices. These stakeholders consisted of four organizations and two independent researchers who have either published research or implemented programs, among other criteria, related to law enforcement responses to incidents involving individuals with mental illness. Specifically, we asked stakeholders to validate that the two practices that we had initially identified were in fact leading practices, and to provide any additional leading practices.[9]

To determine if DOJ and DHS components leverage information from other knowledgeable parties, we conducted interviews with or gathered written information from agency officials from the selected components who are responsible for training and policy development. Further details about our scope and methodology can be found in Appendix I. We conducted this performance audit from February 2017 through February 2018 in accordance with generally accepted government auditing standards. Those standards

[7] Regulations and guidance issued by both DOJ and DHS provide that section 504 generally applies to all programs and activities of each department. For example, DOJ guidance states that DOJ's obligations under section 504 and implementing regulations "apply to all members of the public with disabilities whom the Department serves or encounters as part of the Department's traditional law enforcement programs and activities." However, according to this same guidance, "[e]xigencies, dangers, and safety considerations, however, play a significant role in determining whether and to what extent an accommodation [for a member of the public with a disability] is reasonable."

[8] By using the term "leading practices," we refer to practices that are generally effective when officers or agents apply them when responding to incidents involving individuals with mental illness even if robust evaluations of such practices' effectiveness have not been conducted or have shown mixed results.

[9] For the purposes of our report, stakeholders are either academic or independent researchers or advocacy groups who are known to have substantial knowledge or expertise in the area of law enforcement responses to incidents involving individuals with mental illness.

require that we plan and perform an audit to obtain sufficient, appropriate evidence to provide a reasonable basis for our findings and conclusions based on our audit objectives. We believe that the evidence obtained provides a reasonable basis for our findings and conclusions based on our audit objectives.

BACKGROUND

Law Enforcement Interaction with Individuals with Mental Illness

Since the 1960s, the percentage of individuals with mental illness being treated in a hospitalized setting has decreased dramatically in an effort to move care away from institutional settings into a wider range of community-based treatment. This process, known as "deinstitutionalization," has been driven in part by limited funding available for mental health services, changes in treatment philosophy, and medical advancements. According to a 2015 Federal Bureau of Investigation (FBI) publication, one result from this shift is that local police departments have had to meet the growing needs of individuals suffering mental health emergencies (e.g., a schizophrenic episode), and are often the first source of assistance in helping to arrange treatment for these individuals.[10]

Similarly, the IACP reports that police officers often have to "manage situations that result from a history of mental health policy and legislative decisions made by federal and state governments."[11] According to the IACP, law enforcement officers—generally local police—may then find themselves serving in a role similar to that of a social worker in attempting to locate treatment services for such individuals. The IACP also reports that such increasing interactions may result in individuals with mental illness being arrested and placed in jail, rather than receiving treatment from mental health facilities. This can result in a cycle of arrest, imprisonment, and recidivism for such individuals.[12] In addition, interactions between law enforcement officers and individuals with mental illness have the potential to escalate into violence. In recent years, a number of professional organizations and advocacy groups such as IACP, the Police Executive Research Forum (PERF), the National Alliance on Mental Illness, and Council of State Governments Justice Center (CSG JC) have researched and advocated for different approaches that may reduce the likelihood of violent encounters or help officers connect the individuals they encounter with proper

---

[10] Wilcox, Nicolas, M.S., "The Importance of Mental Health Training in Law Enforcement", FBI Law Enforcement Bulletin, July 8, 2015.

[11] IACP, *Improving Police Response to Persons Affected by Mental Illness*, Report from the March 2016 IACP Symposium, Alexandria, Virginia (2016).

[12] We have related work reviewing the incarceration of offenders with mental illness and strategies for reducing recidivism among such offenders that will be issued in early 2018. 21st Century Cures Act, Pub. L. No. 114-255, § 14016, 130 Stat. at 1306-07.

treatment services.[13] In addition, DOJ's Bureau of Justice Assistance (BJA), within its Office of Justice Programs, has created a compendium of existing information and research in the field of state and local law enforcement responses to individuals with mental illness.[14]

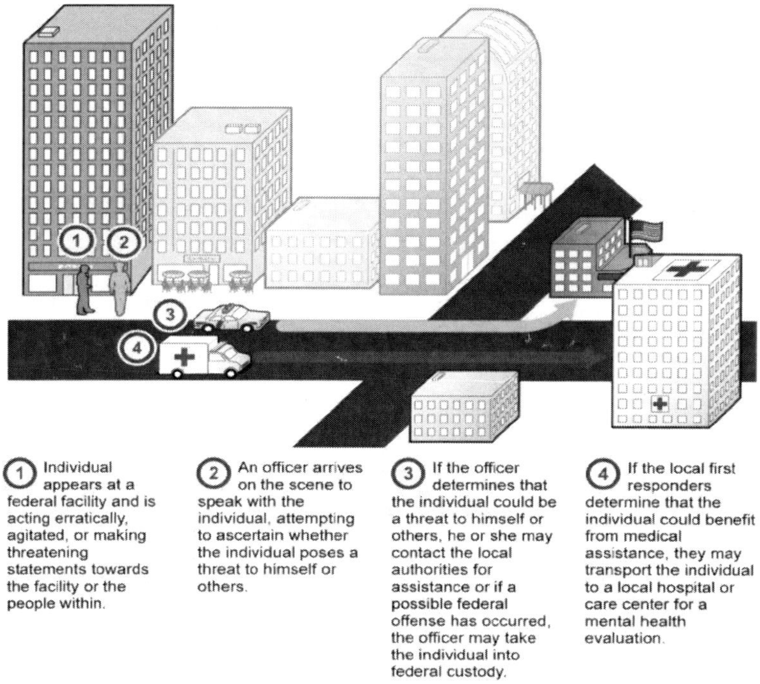

Source: GAO summary of comments from law enforcement officials: Art Explosion (clip art). | GAO-18-229.

Note: The figure above is a general illustration of how a federal law enforcement officer or agent might respond to and resolve a disturbance at or near a federal facility. It is not intended to address a "typical" incident for any of the components in our review because the missions and activities of each component vary significantly and officers and agents interact with the public in different capacities. For example, Federal Protective Service or Secret Service officers and agents might be more likely to experience this type of incident when protecting federal facilities than Bureau of Prisons correctional officers operating within prisons or than Federal Bureau of Investigations agents conducting investigations would be.

Figure 1. Illustrative Example of an Incident at a Federal Facility Involving Federal Law Enforcement and an Individual Displaying Signs of a Mental Illness.

---

[13] PERF is an independent research organization that seeks to identify best practices on issues such as reducing police use of force; developing community and problem-oriented policing; and evaluating crime reduction strategies. CSG JC is a national nonprofit organization that serves policymakers at the local, state, and federal levels from all branches of government. It aims to provide practical, nonpartisan advice and consensus-driven strategies, informed by available evidence, to increase public safety and strengthen communities.

[14] BJA aims to provide leadership and services in grant administration and criminal justice policy development to support local, state, and tribal justice strategies to achieve safer communities. BJA supports programs and initiatives in the areas of law enforcement, justice information sharing, managing offenders, combating drug crime and abuse, crime prevention, and protecting vulnerable populations, among other things.

Federal law enforcement officers and agents may interact with individuals displaying signs of mental illness in a number of different types of incidents while performing their various missions, such as protecting federal property or officials or when apprehending subjects of an investigation. Figure 1 provides one example of a possible incident an officer or agent might experience and the response options available. Generally, when federal officers and agents encounter individuals displaying signs of mental illness—and there is no evidence of a federal crime—they may refer them to local law enforcement or health care providers to assess their mental health and determine whether they need further health care.[15] If local providers determine that such care is needed, it is generally provided through a voluntary or involuntary commitment to a local mental health services provider. One exception to this is for correctional officers and other staff within BOP, as these staff interact with individuals with a diagnosed mental illness as part of their daily duties in ensuring a secure prison environment.[16] BOP pre-designates all inmates entering its institutions and assigns initial mental health and medical screen assignments.[17] Throughout an inmate's incarceration, BOP's psychologists, psychiatrists, and qualified mid-level practitioners can determine a new mental health care level following a review of records and a face-to-face clinical interview.

Relevant Legislation and Departmental Efforts

Under section 504 of the Rehabilitation Act of 1973, as amended, discrimination on the basis of disability in federally funded and federally conducted programs and activities is prohibited.[18] A person with a disability includes anyone who has a physical or mental impairment that substantially limits one or more major life activities, has a record of such impairment, or is regarded as having such an impairment.

DHS and DOJ both currently have efforts underway, in various stages of development, to have their components review their existing policies, guidance, and training in response

[15] The nature of these interactions by federal law enforcement officers and agents may vary greatly depending on the nature of each component's mission. For example, according to FBI officials, FBI Special Agents apprehending a subject displaying signs of mental illness do not refer that individual to local law enforcement or health care providers, but would carry out the arrest warrant or arrest on probable cause.

[16] By statute, BOP is required to provide for suitable housing and the safekeeping, care, and subsistence of all persons charged with or convicted of offenses against the United States. *See* 18 U.S.C. § 4042(a)(2).

[17] After inmates enter an institution, and within timeframes dependent upon the mental health screen assignment, BOP completes a psychology intake screening and assigns inmates a mental health care level ranging from 1 to 4, depending on the inmates' level of mental health care needs. Mental health care level 1 inmates show no significant level of functional impairment associated with mental illness and demonstrate no need for regular mental health interventions, while mental health care level 4 inmates are those requiring acute care in a psychiatric hospital. We have previously reported on mental health care and general medical care in BOP. See GAO, *Bureau of Prisons: Timelier Reviews, Plans for Evaluations, and Updated Policies Could Improve Inmate Mental Health Services Oversight*, GAO-13-1 (Washington, D.C.: July 17, 2013), and *Bureau of Prisons: Better Planning and Evaluation Needed to Understand and Control Rising Inmate Health Care Costs*, GAO-17-379 (Washington, D.C.: June 29, 2017).

[18] 29 U.S.C. § 794. "Federally conducted programs and activities" include those of federal law enforcement agencies.

to departmental guidance on addressing individuals with disabilities and obligations under section 504. Pursuant to departmental guidance, after completing their reviews, components are to determine areas that could be enhanced. Within DHS, components have been asked to report on the status of their efforts to DHS' Office for Civil Rights and Civil Liberties (CRCL).[19] Within DOJ, the Office of the Deputy Attorney General (ODAG) is overseeing components' efforts.[20]

In addition, the 21st Century Cures Act requires the Attorney General to provide direction and guidance for the following by December 13, 2017:

- "Programs that offer specialized and comprehensive training, in procedures to identify and appropriately respond to incidents in which the unique needs of individuals who have a mental illness are involved, to first responders and tactical units of—(A) Federal law enforcement agencies; and (B) other Federal criminal justice agencies, such as [BOP] and the Administrative Office of the United States Courts, and other agencies that the Attorney General determines appropriate."
- "The establishment of, or improvement of existing, computerized information systems to provide timely information to employees of Federal law enforcement agencies, and Federal criminal justice agencies to improve the response of such employees to situations involving individuals who have a mental illness." [21]

Discussion Groups Identified Several Challenges that Officers and Agents Encounter When Responding to Incidents Involving Individuals with Mental Illness

According to the DHS and DOJ law enforcement officers and agents we interviewed, they are not positioned to diagnose any specific mental health condition that an individual might have, as they are not trained mental health professionals.[22] However, responding to incidents involving individuals with mental illness can be challenging for multiple reasons, including determining whether the person is suffering from a mental illness or from another issue, such as drug addiction, and communicating with the person, for example, when a person may be suffering from delusions. These officers and agents face these challenges

[19] DHS CRCL promotes civil rights and civil liberties in policy creation and implementation by advising DHS leadership and personnel, communicates with individuals and communities whose civil rights and civil liberties may be affected by DHS activities, and leads DHS equal employment opportunity programs, among other things.

[20] DOJ ODAG advises and assists the Attorney General in formulating and implementing DOJ policies and programs and in providing supervision and direction to all organizational units of DOJ.

[21] Pub. L. No. 114-255, § 14025, 130 Stat. at 1310.

[22] BOP employs mental health professionals such as psychologists or psychiatrists at each of its institutions. These staff are trained to diagnose mental illness and share their assessments with correctional officers and other staff. In addition, each institution has medical and mental health profiles of each inmate in its care.

while also being responsible for ensuring their own safety and that of others in the area. Some of the common challenges officers and agents identified during our discussion groups follow.

Identifying Whether an Individual Has a Mental Illness

Some officers and agents in our group discussions stated that when encountering individuals displaying erratic behavior (e.g., rapid or nonsensical speech, paranoid or delusional statements), it can be difficult to determine if that behavior is attributable to a mental illness or the influence of drugs. Specifically, Border Patrol agents—who are broadly responsible for preventing the illegal entry or exit of people and goods at places other than ports of entry—stated that determining whether someone has a mental illness or is experiencing other issues is challenging and may be complicated by language barriers. Border Patrol agents may at times encounter large groups of people attempting to cross the border at one time and thus have limited time to make that determination. ATF officers—who may encounter individuals with a mental illness who are targets of an investigation—commented that incidents may involve an individual who could suffer a mental illness (treated or untreated), or be under the influence of alcohol or drugs. Unless the individual discloses his or her condition, or family or friends are there to explain the condition, officers would not know the cause of the individual's behavior. They explained that if mental health information about a suspect is known in advance of an operation, officers can adjust their approach; however, they told us that most of the time they do not know if someone has a mental health condition and how it might present itself.

Similarly, an FBI police officer—who may encounter individuals displaying signs of mental illness if those individuals enter an FBI office—told us that it can be challenging to deal with an individual who is acting erratically, not knowing precisely whether the behavior is attributable to a mental illness, and there may be limited time available to address an individual posing a safety risk. BOP corrections officers also echoed this challenge. They said that despite having back-up mental health staff on call, their initial reaction to an inmate exhibiting some type of erratic behavior has to be fairly quick to secure the safety of the staff and other inmates. Officers and agents across components and departments made clear that they are not mental health professionals or psychologists and, as such, are charged with responding to the behaviors that are exhibited to secure the scene.

Communicating with Individuals with a Mental Illness

Some of the officers and agents in our discussion groups stated that communicating effectively with someone exhibiting signs of a mental illness and understanding what he or she may be going through or how he or she sees reality can be challenging. One officer told us that trying to make individuals who may have a mental illness understand that their reality is not everyone else's reality is particularly challenging. This was very difficult, for example, for Secret Service Uniformed Division officers who explained that they encounter individuals when providing security along the White House fence and for FPS officers, who often encounter individuals displaying signs of mental illness near or in federal buildings that they are assigned to protect. As the Secret Service officers explained, even if individuals exhibit delusional behavior, so long as they have not broken any laws, then they are free to be near protected federal venues and the officers are limited in any actions they can take.

> One officer, discussing the challenges in speaking with someone with a mental illness who may be experiencing delusions, stated that the person is "wholeheartedly convinced that what he or she perceives is the true reality."
>
> Source: GAO observation. | GAO-18-229.

Officers and agents who we met with in CBP reported that they rely on common sense to dictate appropriate action and use reasonable efforts to protect themselves and others. They noted that additional training on communicating effectively with individuals suffering from mental illness could be beneficial.

The challenges noted above in identifying causes of erratic behavior or effectively communicating with individuals with a mental illness can make it difficult for officers to resolve a tense situation or apprehend an individual (if necessary) as securely or peacefully as possible. For example, Border Patrol agents stated that ensuring that such encounters are resolved safely for the individuals involved and other members of the public is their biggest challenge. It might require removing someone in distress from a group of individuals that he or she may be traveling with or keeping him or her calm. When someone is in an extreme state of panic, emotional distress, or anger, officers try to remove the person from the group to prevent a potential incident from escalating quickly.

Operating with Limited Access to Mental Health Resources

Officers and agents also stated that a limited number of mental health professionals available within their components or through local agencies can pose a challenge in helping persons with mental illness receive necessary treatment. As such, they must rely on state and local entities in the area (e.g., law enforcement, hospitals) to provide assistance for individuals. Federal Air Marshals—who provide protection at airports and other transportation modes—we spoke with explained that since they do not have holding facilities to secure individuals with mental illness, they are reliant on local law enforcement and mental health professionals to manage an incident.[23] Officers and agents highlighted the importance of maintaining close relationships with state and local partners and added that trained mental health professionals provide an excellent resource.

In addition, officers and agents in some discussion groups noted there may be training offered by state or local agencies related to understanding and responding to individuals with mental illness that could be leveraged by federal agencies.[24] Officers and agents reported, however, that it can be difficult for the components to find the time and resources to send officers to the trainings. According to USMS officers— who provide security at federal courthouses and oversee transport of federal prisoners—this is particularly challenging in small offices where there may be very few staff.

Frequently Encountering the Same Individuals

Another common challenge noted in discussion groups was that officers and agents repeatedly encounter the same individuals with mental illness. Officers and agents explained that they can sometimes apprehend individuals who are creating a disturbance, but these individuals often cannot be charged with a federal crime. As such, following the apprehension, the officers and agents release these individuals to local or state authorities who may transport them to local providers for a mental health evaluation. Typically, if the local providers determine a commitment is necessary, they will hold these individuals at a hospital or clinic for up to 72 hours. According to the officers and agents in our discussion groups, many of these individuals return after they are released and the officers and agents encounter them time and again, with very little that they can do to provide these individuals with assistance. According to the officers and agents, incidents involving frequent encounters with the same individuals can take time away from performing other important activities.

---

[23] The Federal Air Marshals instructors with whom we met largely train Visible Intermodal Prevention and Response teams that consist of Federal Air Marshals, Behavioral Detection Officers, Transportation Security Specialists-Explosives, Transportation Security Inspectors, and Canine teams who work closely with federal, state, and local law enforcement partners and stakeholders in the aviation and surface transportation sectors.

[24] Training courses that focus on mental health awareness offered by other entities, such as state and local law enforcement agencies, may be available to federal officers and agents. Generally, federal officers and agents are made aware of internal and external training opportunities through their internal component learning systems and email notifications.

Secret Service Uniformed Division officers told us they repeatedly encounter the same individuals with mental illness and know some of these individuals very well. For example, Secret Service officers stated that when performing their duties in patrolling the grounds of the White House, they have had frequent encounters with a woman who believes she has family members living in the White House. The officers have turned her away from the scene on multiple occasions, but she continues to return.

COMPONENTS HAVE SOME TYPE OF TRAINING, POLICIES, AND GUIDANCE RELATED TO MENTAL ILLNESS, AND REVIEWS TO ENHANCE PRACTICES ARE UNDERWAY

DHS and DOJ Components Offer, Receive, or Are Developing Some Type of Training Related to Mental Illness

All of the law enforcement components in our scope offer training directly, receive training through FLETC, or are developing some training on responding to incidents involving individuals with mental illness. Agency and FLETC training includes courses on communication, de-escalation, and suicide prevention (related to federal inmates). Since these components have varying missions and operational needs and interact with the public in different capacities, the nature and scope of this training, as well as the number of courses and the duration of courses offered varies. For example, BOP's staff—including food service workers and nurses, as well as correctional officers—have daily contact with inmates with mental illness and can act as "first responders" when situations merit. According to BOP officials, training is offered to all staff in all of its institutions on mental health and working with the mentally ill, along with courses on communication, de-escalation, suicide prevention, and use of force. As another example, ATF's agents told us they have less routine contact with individuals with mental illness, but ATF offers a course to its agents on de-escalation concepts and tactics, which addresses responding to incidents involving individuals with mental illness, as well as crisis intervention training to its cadre of crisis negotiators. Further, some of the components' training is mandatory and offered annually through class instruction or online portals. These courses may be offered to new hires or available to tenured officers. In addition, some components' training courses are delivered as stand-alone sessions, while others may be modules within a larger course exploring other law enforcement topics.

Training DHS Components Offer

Three DHS operational components in our scope, in addition to FLETC, offered some type of training specifically for their officers and agents.

Another one (TSA) has training in development as of October 2017, on topics related to responding to incidents involving individuals with mental illness.

FLETC explained that it provides basic training to all DHS law enforcement officers through one of three basic program categories— Center Basic, Center Integrated Basic, and Agency Specific Basic—which vary in length.[25] Two Center Basic training programs include a 2-hour module titled Managing Abnormal Behavior, which covers how to identify common signs of mental disorders (among other things) and how to handle people exhibiting abnormal behavior. Specifically, this module examines basic human behavior that may be classified as abnormal, differentiates between mental disorders, and also covers physical and organic causes that may be related to abnormal behavior with the appropriate officer responses. In addition, FLETC informed us that it has developed scenario-based training in these programs, allowing the officers or agents to develop decision-making skills in situations involving people exhibiting abnormal behavior. See appendix II for more information on FLETC's training programs.

In addition to this module provided to all DHS agents and officers, the components in our review also offer or are preparing component-specific training courses. Table 2 lists illustrative examples of DHS training.

U.S. Secret Service Training

We observed Secret Service training on Protective Intelligence Questioning for First Line Officers, which is offered to Uniformed Division Officers. The course instructor played the role of three different individuals with schizophrenia, bipolar disorder, and sociopathic personality disorder and trained agents on interacting and interviewing subjects who attempt to breach the White House fence.

Source: GAO observation. | GAO-18-229.

In addition, TSA has developed a mandatory course entitled Awareness Training on Mental Health Conditions to be delivered in the classroom and through scenarios and exercises during fiscal year 2018. This course is designed to introduce Federal Air Marshals to the fundamentals of predominant mental disorders, such as schizophrenia or psychosis.

[25] According to DHS officials, one exception would be for training provided to Border Patrol agents. While this training takes place at FLETC venues, according to CBP, the Border Patrol itself conducts nearly all of the training provided to its agents.

Table 2. Examples of Department of Homeland Security (DHS) Operational Components' Training Content Related to Officers' Response to Incidents Involving Individuals with Mental Illness, as of October 2017

DHS component	Name of course	Officers taking course	General description	Format / duration
Federal Protective Service (FPS)a	Mentally Ill Persons	Law Enforcement Officers	Covers characteristics of mental illness, emotionally disturbed persons (EDP), and excited delirium syndrome;[b] how to manage EDPs; steps needed for subjects to be committed voluntarily or involuntarily for a mental health evaluation; and becoming familiar with various cases regarding EDPs.	Class/1 hour
U.S. Customs and Border Protection (CBP)	Detecting Excited Delirium Syndrome	Customs and Border Protection Agents and Officers	Covers how to identify excited delirium syndrome and the implications for a sudden in-custody death.	Online/1 hour
U. S. Secret Service (Secret Service)	Protective Intelligence Questioning for First Line Officers	Uniformed Division	Provides approaches and strategies to use when interviewing subjects who may be mentally ill, including symptoms that may be commonly exhibited, and how to obtain useful and actionable information. This is followed up with a practical exercise in which officers conduct three separate interviews of role players who act as if they are suffering from schizophrenia, bipolar disorder, and paranoid personality disorder respectively.	Class/5 hours

Source: GAO analysis of documentation provided by components | GAO-18-229.

Note: Officials reported that in addition to the training courses above, some components, such as CBP, have officers who are also trained as emergency medical technicians. Part of basic emergency medical technician training addresses how to respond to individuals who may be displaying signs of mental illness. Also, U.S. Immigration and Customs Enforcement, which does not provide mental health training generally to all of its agents or officers, employs health services medics who screen apprehended individuals for medical conditions to include mental illness and provides those health services medics with suicide prevention training.

[a] In addition, FPS officials informed us that they are developing further training on familiarizing officers with local resources available and anticipate offering this training beginning in March 2018.

[b] Excited delirium syndrome is a set of symptoms such as disorientation, violent or bizarre behavior, insensitivity to pain, elevated body temperature, or superhuman strength that results in a temporary state of wild excitement or mental confusion.

Training DOJ Components Offer

All of the DOJ components in our review provide some type of training to their officers on topics related to responding to incidents involving individuals with mental illness—as illustrated in Table 3.

Table 3. Examples of Department of Justice (DOJ) Components' Training Content Related to Officers' Response to Incidents Involving Individuals with Mental Illness, as of October 2017

DOJ components	Name of course	Officers taking course	General description	Format / duration
Alcohol, Tobacco, Firearms and Explosives (ATF)	Understanding De-Escalation Concepts and Tactics	Agents	Addresses the importance and process of de-escalation, communication, and use of force and response to resistance, including practical exercise scenarios and video demonstrations.	Class/8 hours
Drug Enforcement Administration (DEA)	Use of Force	Agents	Covers one scenario based on a court case pertaining to the reasonableness of the use of force during a situation involving a mentally ill suspect.	Class/20 minutes
Federal Bureau of Prisons (BOP)	Mental Health Annual Training	All Staff	Covers stigma associated with mental illness, characteristics and symptoms of serious mental illness, and inmates who have been diagnosed with a mental illness/disorder.	Class/1 hour
Federal Bureau of Investigation (FBI)	Mental Health First Aid for Public Safety Officersa	Agents	Covers abnormal behavior, communication, intellectual and developmental disabilities, deescalation, mental health awareness, suicide prevention, trauma crisis response, use of force, and practical exercises and simulations.	Virtual/8 hours
U.S. Marshals Service (USMS)	Mental Illness and Human Behavior	Protective Intelligence Investigators, District Threat Investigators[b]	Covers mental illness and abnormal behavior; cause of serious mental illness; mental health statistics; stress; common mental, mood, anxiety, and personality disorders; post-traumatic stress disorder (PTSD); and substance abuse.	Class/2 hours

Source: GAO analysis of documentation provided by components | GAO-18-229.

[a] This course is currently offered at only one FBI field office; FBI has no component-wide training specific to mental illness.

[b] Protective Intelligence Investigators are Senior Criminal Investigators who conduct protective investigations to identify and mitigate potential threats to USMS protectees. District Threat Investigators are Deputy U.S. Marshals who, as a collateral duty, identify security threats or incidents and assist Protective Intelligence Investigators with developing a strategy to mitigate the threat.

DHS and DOJ Components Have Existing Policies or Guidance That Addresses Responding to Individuals with Mental Illness

The law enforcement components within our scope at DHS and DOJ have policies or guidance in place that addresses responding to incidents involving individuals with mental illness. Some components' policies or guidance specifically addresses mental illness, while others touch on the issue as part of larger policies on other topics (such as use of force)—as illustrated in Table 4.

Table 4. Examples of Policies and Guidance at Departments of Homeland Security (DHS) and Justice (DOJ) Components Related to Officers' Response to Incidents Involving Individuals with Mental Illness, as of October 2017

	Policy/Guidance Name	General Description
DHS component		
Federal Protective Service (FPS)	Incidents Involving Mentally Ill Persons	This policy provides official guidance on responding to incidents involving individuals with mental illness. It covers communication, use-of-force, interviews, excited delirium syndrome,[a] voluntary and involuntary mental health evaluations, as well as suicide prevention.
Transportation Security Administration (TSA)	Access and Communication for Individuals with Disabilities	This guidance is designed to help ensure that interactions with the public are accessible to individuals with a disability, which includes mental illness.
U.S. Customs and Border Protection (CBP)	National Standards on Transport, Escort, Detention, and Search	Prior to transporting or escorting an individual, officers and agents are to conduct an assessment of the individual's safety and known or reported medical or mental health issues, among other things, and provide reasonable accommodations for such issues.
U.S. Immigration and Customs Enforcement (ICE), Enforcement and Removal Operations	Identification of Detainees with Serious Mental Disorders or Conditions	This policy memo assists ICE and detention facility personnel in identifying detainees with serious mental disorders or conditions in order to assess appropriate facility placement and treatment.
U. S. Secret Service (Secret Service)	Use of Force Policy	This policy mentions that officers and agents may take into account the mental health history of the subjects to determine a reasonable level of force necessary to control them.
DOJ Components		
Alcohol, Tobacco, Firearms and Explosives (ATF)	Memo on Resources for Dealing with Persons in Crisis	Instructs all special agents in charge to identify and be familiar with local resources (e.g., crisis intervention teams)b that can provide assistance when they encounter a member of the public who may suffer from mental illness or may be in crisis.

	Policy/Guidance Name	General Description
Federal Bureau of Prisons (BOP)	Suicide Prevention Program Statement	One of several policies in place that addresses interaction with inmates with a mental illness, this policy directs each prison warden to implement a prison-specific suicide prevention program detailing what the program must contain, including but not limited to, training for all staff on suicide prevention, suicide risk assessments, suicide watch procedures, and identification of at-risk inmates.
Federal Bureau of Investigation (FBI)	FBI Police Manual for Police Operations, Section 31-Unsolicited Contact/Mentally Ill	Provides general safety and communication guidelines for FBI police officers when responding to an incident involving individuals with mental illness.
Drug Enforcement Administration (DEA)	Use of Force, Section S. Deadly Force Against Mentally Ill Subject	Provides federal case law regarding police conduct in responding to individuals with a mental illness, particularly use of deadly force.
U.S. Marshals Service (USMS)	Procedures for Movement of Prisoners w/ Psychological or Medical Conditions	Includes a medical guide that the transportation specialist, Justice Prisoner and Alien Transportation System staff,[c] or Public Health Services nurse can use to determine the proper mode of transportation, coordination with the holdover facility, and the provision of medicines, if applicable, to detainees or prisoners during transport.

Source: GAO analysis of documentation provided by components | GAO-18-229.

[a] Excited delirium syndrome is a physiological and mental state often characterized by extreme physical and mental agitation, bizarre behavior, hyperthermia, hostility, exceptional strength, and endurance without apparent fatigue.

[b] Crisis intervention teams are used in community policing efforts and bring together law enforcement, mental health providers, hospital emergency departments and individuals with mental illness and their families to improve responses to people in crisis.

[c] USMS's Justice Prisoner and Alien Transportation System transports prisoners in federal custody between federal judicial districts to hearings, court appearances and detention facilities. USMS houses and transports all federal prisoners from the time they enter federal custody until they are either acquitted or convicted and delivered to their designated federal Bureau of Prisons facility.

All DHS and DOJ Components Are Reviewing Policies, Guidance, and Training to Align with Departmental Guidance

DHS Efforts to Review Policies, Guidance, and Training

DHS has guidance in place to help ensure that its components have policies and training that ensure their alignment with section 504 of the Rehabilitation Act. In 2013 and

2015, respectively, DHS issued a directive[26] and implementing instruction[27] to its components intended to strengthen compliance with section 504. These documents required DHS components to conduct a self-evaluation and prepare a component plan identifying any policies or practices that may result in a qualified individual with a disability being excluded from participation in, or being denied the benefits of, a program or activity.

In 2016, DHS's CRCL office issued guidance and a self-evaluation tool to DHS components on the steps to take in performing the self-evaluation of their facilities, programs, policies, and practices (to include training). The guidance also addresses the development and execution of the components' plans intended to remedy any areas deemed insufficient in permitting individuals with disabilities—including mental illness—to participate fully in the components' programs and activities.[28]

Department of Homeland Security (DHS) Component Self-Evaluation Tool

The self-evaluation tool that DHS's Office of Civil Rights and Civil Liberties developed requires components to—among other things—describe whether there is an established policy ensuring equal treatment for individuals with disabilities, how the component's personnel and procedures ensure that individuals with disabilities are treated in a nondiscriminatory manner, and the component's process for providing auxiliary aids and services to ensure effective communication. The tool also provides examples of interactions in the areas of customer service, security, and custody activities that would likely be compliant, or possibly noncompliant, with section 504 of the Rehabilitation Act.

Source: DHS. | GAO-18-229.

Disability Access Coordinators, who are representatives from each component charged with overseeing their components' responses to DHS Rehabilitation Act guidance, are leading the components' efforts in conducting the self-evaluations. CRCL set a deadline for components to submit all self-evaluations to CRCL for review by the end of August 2017. As of September 2017, all five components had submitted selfevaluations.[29] CRCL officials explained that as they review self-evaluations, they are looking to see if policies or training for law enforcement officers' and agents' responses to individuals with mental illness have been identified or otherwise addressed. If not, the officials indicated that they will request the components identify and address this topic in their plans for aligning with

[26] DHS Office for Civil Rights and Civil Liberties, *Component Self-Evaluation and Planning Reference Guide,* Guide 065-01-001-01, June 6, 2016.

[27] FPS's efforts were included in the submission of the plan for the National Protection and Programs Directorate, which houses FPS.

[28] DHS Office for Civil Rights and Civil Liberties, *Component Self-Evaluation and Planning Reference Guide,* Guide 065-01-001-01, June 6, 2016.

[29] FPS's efforts were included in the submission of the plan for the National Protection and Programs Directorate, which houses FPS.

Rehabilitation Act guidance. The remaining steps in CRCL's effort to review and comment on component plans as of September follow:

- December 31, 2017: CRCL provides comments to components on the content of their self-evaluations.
- February 28, 2018: the components develop and submit their draft plans for aligning with the Rehabilitation Act guidance.
- April 30, 2018: CRCL reviews and provides comments on the components' draft plans.
- May 31, 2018: the components address CRCL's comments and submit their final plans for alignment with Rehabilitation Act guidance for approval.

DOJ Efforts to Review Policies, Guidance, and Training

DOJ has directed components to review and implement guidance on addressing individuals with disabilities—including mental illness—and obligations under section 504. Specifically, in January 2017, DOJ's then-Deputy Attorney General issued a memo with attached guidance directing components to review their policies and training and, where necessary, modify or develop policies and training to implement legal requirements and principles related to section 504.[30] This guidance identified, among other things, DOJ's law enforcement components' legal obligations under section 504 as well as the policies and procedures that components must have so that officers and agents can anticipate and plan for encounters with members of the public with disabilities. For example, the guidance states that law enforcement components must train officers and agents on different types of commonly encountered disabilities; how to identify, without medical or psychological training, analysis, or diagnosis, common characteristics and behaviors most often associated with disabilities; and appropriate responses to the challenges that an encounter with a member of the public with a disability may present. Training for officers and agents in effective communication with members of the public with a mental illness is explicitly referenced in the guidance as well.

To date, officials from DOJ's Office of the Deputy Attorney General (ODAG)—who are overseeing the components' efforts—have maintained communication with the components to confirm that they have begun reviewing their policies and training to identify any deficiencies or necessary enhancements pursuant to the January 2017 guidance. During the course of our review and in part due to our inquiries, in the fall of 2017, ODAG notified the components that they should complete their reviews by December 2017. ODAG also notified the components that they should begin implementing any new policies or training identified by September 2018.

---

[30] DOJ Memorandum from the Deputy Attorney General, "Department Guidance in Interactions with Members of the Public with Disabilities in Traditional Law Enforcement Programs and Activities," January 6, 2017.

In addition, a provision of the 21st Century Cures Act—section 14025— requires DOJ to provide direction and guidance to federal law enforcement agencies and federal criminal justice agencies on training programs and improved technologies related to responding to individuals with mental illness, by December 13, 2017. ODAG officials told us that the January 2017 guidance addresses the requirement to provide direction and guidance on training for the DOJ components, but acknowledged that it does not respond to all of the requirements for the Attorney General under section 14025 of the 21st Century Cures Act. In particular, section 14025 requires the Attorney General to provide direction and guidance to federal law enforcement agencies and federal criminal justice agencies beyond DOJ in the areas of specialized and comprehensive training programs to identify and respond to individuals with mental illness. Section 14025 also calls for direction and guidance on the establishment and improvement of computerized information systems to provide timely information related to situations involving individuals with mental illness.

As a result of our questions about whether such efforts would be developed, on December 7, 2017, DOJ sent a letter from the Principal Deputy Assistant Attorney General for the Office of Justice Programs to federal law enforcement partners outlining resources available for federal law enforcement when considering training or procedures appropriate for their missions. Specifically, DOJ sent the letter to executive officers within DOJ, DHS, the Administrative Office of the United States Courts, and other executive departments that DOJ deemed appropriate. Some examples of resources that the letter highlights include (1) the Police-Mental Health Collaboration Toolkit, which provides resources to assist law enforcement agencies in partnering with mental health providers (and is discussed later in this chapter) and (2) a forthcoming "roadmap" planned for release in 2018 that the Office of Justice Programs and BJA are developing that will help law enforcement agencies as they plan for engagement with mental health entities.

Stakeholders Cited Leading Practices and Tools for Effective Law Enforcement Responses, and Components Have Generally Leveraged Information from Other Knowledgeable Parties

Two Leading Practices and Four Tools Can Enhance Officer Responses to Individuals with Mental Illness

Of the six stakeholders in the field of law enforcement-mental health we interviewed, all six considered the Crisis Intervention Team Model to be a leading practice and five considered the Co-responder Model to be a leading practice—see Figure 2.These practices are typically implemented at local and state law enforcement agencies. Nevertheless, certain aspects and associated benefits could be considered in other settings, such as federal law enforcement operations.

In addition, stakeholders cited four key tools that may assist law enforcement agencies in responding to individuals with mental illness. These tools can include training guides, summary reports, or model policies, among other things, as shown in table 5.

Crisis Intervention Team (CIT) model		Potential benefits	Examples
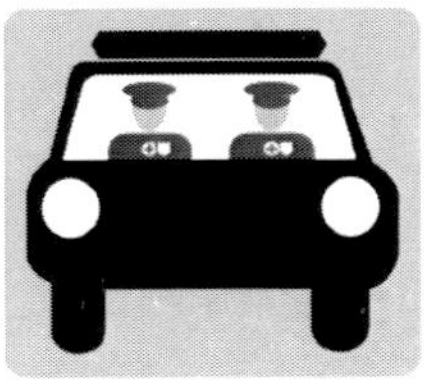	A model for community policing where law enforcement agencies partner with mental health providers and other community stakeholders to provide crisis intervention for persons experiencing mental illnesses. CIT programs typically provide selected officers with 40 hours of training on several topics including: signs and symptoms of mental illnesses, mental health treatment, co-occurring disorders, and de-escalation techniques, among others. After completing the 40-hour CIT training, these police officers are typically dispatched to mental health-related calls.	Aims to enhance communication, identify mental health resources for assisting people in crisis and ensure that officers receive the training and support that they need.	**Salt Lake City Police Department's CIT Model** Although the implementation of a CIT program can vary by jurisdiction and locality, the Council of State Governments, Justice Center in collaboration with the Bureau of Justice Assistance (BJA) has designated the Salt Lake City Police Department as a national learning site for its implementation of the CIT Model.[b] Salt Lake City's CIT Model includes a 40-hour training curriculum, small city and rural collaboration across jurisdictions, and a CIT Investigative Unit.
Co-responder model			
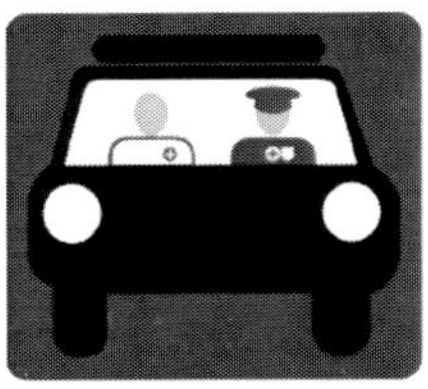	An approach that pairs specially trained police officers with mental health workers to respond to calls involving individuals in crisis. The co-responder teams may link individuals with mental illnesses to appropriate mental health services or provide other appropriate responses. Typically, co-responder teams ride together in the same vehicle for an entire shift and respond to mental health-related calls.	Attempts to divert individuals with a serious and persistent mental illness from the criminal justice system by helping them find appropriate services to meet their needs.	**Los Angeles Police Department's Co-Responder Model** Although the implementation of this model can differ greatly across jurisdictions and localities, the Council of State Governments, Justice Center in collaboration with BJA has designated the Los Angeles Police Department as a national learning site for its implementation of the Co-responder Model. The Los Angeles Police Department's Co-responder Model includes 40-hour mental health intervention training, co-responder teams, and a crisis response advisory board.

Source: GAO review of available documents; Art Explosion. | GAO-18-229.

[a] For the purposes of our review, a "leading" practice is one that is generally effective when officers apply it to their interactions with individuals with mental illness, (for example, it helps the officers de-escalate a given situation or better positions them to assist the individuals in receiving care) even if robust evaluations of such a practice's effectiveness have not been conducted or have shown mixed results.

[b] CSG JC through a cooperative agreement with the BJA, selected six police departments to act as national law enforcement-mental health learning sites. Located across the country, these learning sites are dedicated to helping other jurisdictions improve their responses to people with mental illness.

Figure 2. Stakeholder-Cited Leading Practices[a] for Effective Law Enforcement Responses to Incidents Involving Individuals with Mental Illness.

Table 5. Stakeholder-Cited Tools that May Enhance Law Enforcement Responses to Incidents Involving Individuals with Mental Illness

Tools	Description
Police Executive Research Forum's (PERF)[a] Integrating Communications, Assessment, and Tactics Training Guide	PERF developed this guide in October 2016 to help officers assess situations, make safe and effective decisions, and learn from their actions. The training guide aims to provide police officers with additional tools, skills, and options for handling different types of critical incidents, especially those that involve subjects who act erratically due to a mental illness and who are unarmed or armed with a weapon other than a firearm.
The Bureau of Justice Assistance's (BJA)[b] Police-Mental Health Collaboration Toolkit	BJA developed the toolkit in fiscal year 2017 in partnership with Council of State Governments, Justice Center (CSG JC). The toolkit provides resources to assist law enforcement agencies in establishing partnerships with mental health providers to effectively respond to calls for service and improve outcomes for people with mental illness.
Council of State Governments Justice Center's (CSG JC)[c] reports	These reports, such as Law Enforcement Responses to People with Mental Illnesses: A Guide to Research-Informed Policy and Practice (2009)—produced with BJA funding and guidance—summarize available research on law enforcement encounters with people with mental illness and describe strategies to improve these interactions.
International Association of Chiefs of Police's (IACP)[d] One Mind Campaign	IACP began this campaign in October 2016 to promote successful interactions between police officers and persons affected by mental illness. The campaign highlights four practices that IACP has labeled as promising: establishing a partnership with local mental health organization(s), developing a model policy, training officers in mental health first aid,[e] and providing crisis intervention team training to 20 percent of an agency's officers.

Source: GAO review of available documents | GAO-18-229.

[a] PERF is an independent research organization that seeks to identify best practices on issues such as reducing police use of force, developing community and problem-oriented policing, and evaluating crime reduction strategies.

[b] BJA, within the Department of Justice's Office of Justice Programs, aims to provide leadership and services in grant administration and criminal justice policy development to support local, state, and tribal justice strategies to achieve safer communities. BJA supports programs and initiatives in the areas of law enforcement, justice information sharing, managing offenders, combating drug crime and abuse, crime prevention, and protecting vulnerable populations, among other things.

[c] CSG JC is a national nonprofit organization that serves policymakers at the local, state, and federal levels from all branches of government. It aims to provide practical, nonpartisan advice and consensus-driven strategies, informed by available evidence, to increase public safety and strengthen communities.

[d] IACP is a professional association for law enforcement, representing more than 30,000 members in more than 150 countries. IACP aims to advance the law enforcement profession through advocacy, outreach, education, and programs.

[e] According to IACP, Mental Health First Aid for Public Safety is an eight-hour course focused on mental illness and addictions as well as providing law enforcement with effective response options in order to de-escalate incidents without compromising safety.

Components Have Generally Leveraged Information from Other Knowledgeable Parties, and BJA Is Standing Up a Training and Technical Assistance Center

DHS and DOJ law enforcement components generally leveraged information from knowledgeable parties within their departments on efforts to respond to incidents involving individuals with mental illness. To enhance information sharing among DHS components, CRCL has implemented an interagency collaboration mechanism.[31] Specifically, CRCL officials reported that since June 2016 they have led monthly coordination conference calls with component Disability Access Coordinators to collaborate on their respective efforts to complete their self-evaluations. According to the Disability Access Coordinators, these sessions have provided a forum to share ideas and lessons learned across the DHS components. In addition, according to CRCL officials, once their office receives the components' self-evaluations and plans, it aims to disseminate information on lessons learned and effective practices to all the components.

Coordination efforts to leverage information also exist within DOJ. Specifically, through the efforts to review policies and training under the January 2017 guidance and provisions of the 21st Century Cures Act discussed earlier, DOJ's components have reported taking efforts to collaborate with one another and share information on training, best practices and lessons learned. For example, officials from ATF reported holding meetings with other components to discuss their efforts to implement the January 2017 guidance.

Additionally, BJA officials told us they took part in the ODAG's working group in early 2016 when the then-Deputy Attorney General's January 2017 guidance was in development. Along with BJA, this ODAG working group included DOJ's law enforcement components and other offices within the department. The working group provided a forum to advise ODAG in developing the January 2017 guidance and discuss issues surrounding disabilities, which involved responses to individuals with mental illness. BJA officials told us that they provided to components a compendium of all its resources available to assist law enforcement's response to incidents involving individuals with mental illness. BJA officials said they later took the most promising of these and folded them into its Police-Mental Health Collaboration Toolkit. Further, BJA officials told us that they make all of the resources it develops, including the Toolkit, publicly available on the BJA website. According to the officials, these resources are available for all law enforcement agencies, including federal entities, to review and consider implementing as they deem appropriate.

In addition to these online resources, which facilitate information sharing, BJA is also planning to release a national CIT curriculum in 2018 that will serve as a resource that can

---

[31] GAO has previously reported on different mechanisms used by federal agencies to implement interagency collaborative efforts. See *Managing for Results: Key Considerations for Implementing Interagency Collaborative Mechanisms*, GAO-12-1022 (Washington, D.C.: September 27, 2012).

be tailored to reflect mental health training and collaboration under development or underway at the local level. The Office of Justice Programs is supporting a partnership between the IACP and a research organization to deliver the curriculum to law enforcement agencies. In addition, BJA—as one of DOJ's grant-making entities—is standing up the National Training and Technical Assistance Center to Improve Law Enforcement Responses to Individuals with Mental Health Disorders and Intellectual and Developmental Disabilities.[32] BJA officials reported that in September 2017, BJA selected the awardee to design and operate the center. Once the center is operational, it will benefit state, local, and tribal law enforcement entities. In addition, BJA envisions that the center will facilitate better collaboration between law enforcement agencies and their mental health partners. A BJA official also acknowledged that the center could serve as an additional resource for federal law enforcement agencies to consult as they review their trainings, policies, and guidance relevant to responding to incidents involving individuals with mental illness.

AGENCY COMMENTS

We provided a draft of this chapter to DOJ and DHS for their review and comment. The departments did not provide us with formal written comments, but did provide technical comments, which we incorporated as appropriate.

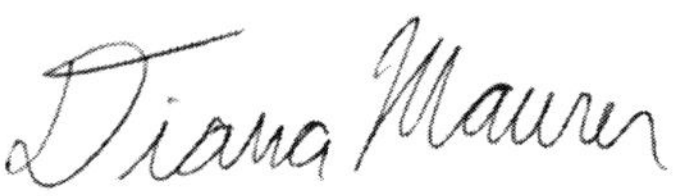

Diana Maurer
Director, Homeland Security and Justice Issues

List of Committees

The Honorable Charles E. Grassley
Chairman

[32] The Consolidated Appropriations Act, 2017, Pub. L. No. 115-31, provided $2,500,000 to DOJ/Office of Justice Programs "for a national training initiative to improve police-based responses to people with mental illness or developmental disabilities."

The Honorable Dianne Feinstein Ranking Member
Committee on the Judiciary
United States Senate

The Honorable Ron Johnson
Chairman

The Honorable Claire McCaskill
Ranking Member
Committee on Homeland Security and Governmental Affairs
United States Senate

The Honorable Lamar Alexander
Chairman

The Honorable Patty Murray
Ranking Member
Committee on Health, Education, Labor and Pensions
United States Senate

The Honorable Bob Goodlatte Chairman

The Honorable Jerrold Nadler
Ranking Member
Committee on the Judiciary House of Representatives

The Honorable Michael McCaul Chairman

The Honorable Bennie Thompson Ranking Member
Committee on Homeland Security House of Representatives

The Honorable Greg Walden Chairman

The Honorable Frank Pallone, Jr.
Ranking Member
Committee on Energy and Commerce
House of Representatives

APPENDIX I: OBJECTIVES, SCOPE AND METHODOLOGY

This chapter addresses the following key questions: (1) What challenges, if any, do federal law enforcement officers at selected Department of Homeland Security (DHS) and Department of Justice (DOJ) components face when responding to incidents involving individuals with mental illness? (2) What type of training, policies, and guidance, if any, are in place at selected DHS and DOJ components to prepare federal law enforcement officers for responding to incidents involving individuals with mental illness? (3) What leading practices or tools have relevant stakeholders cited for effective responses to incidents involving individuals with mental illness, and how have DHS and DOJ components leveraged information from other knowledgeable parties?

We focused our review on the training, policies, and guidance put forth by the DHS and DOJ components listed in table 6 below because they comprise nearly all of the federal law enforcement officers in these agencies.

To identify challenges that federal law enforcement officers and agents at our selected DHS and DOJ components face when responding to incidents involving individuals with mental illness, we held discussion groups of six to eleven agents or officers within each component in our scope. We worked with officials at each component to identify officers and agents with varied tenures and experiences. We held semi-structured in-person and telephone discussion groups using a script and set of questions. Discussion groups are not designed to provide generalizable or statistically reliable results; they are instead intended to generate in-depth information about the reasons for the discussion group participants' attitudes on specific topics and to offer insight into their concerns. During the discussion groups, we asked officers and agents what challenges they face when responding to incidents involving individuals with mental illness, among other topics. We moderated each discussion to keep participants focused on the specified issues within discussion time frames. Participants identified challenges when we explicitly asked them to do so, or during the course of the discussion. We took detailed notes on each discussion and documented the perspectives participants raised in each discussion group. We then summarized the information collected and identified common themes. Because our questions were open-ended and designed to allow participants to discuss any challenges they may have experienced, we cannot determine whether the absence of a particular concern or challenge by a group of officers or agents is an indication that they did not experience the concern or that they did not raise it when asked broadly about the topic.

While these participants' perspectives cannot be generalized to their entire component or all law enforcement components, their views provided insights into the challenges federal law enforcement officers and agents face when responding to incidents involving individuals with mental illness.

Table 6. Department of Homeland Security and Department of Justice Federal Law Enforcement Components Selected for Review and Their Missions

Component	Mission
Department of Homeland Security	
Federal Law Enforcement Training Centers (FLETC)[a]	Provides career-long training to law enforcement professionals to help them fulfill their responsibilities safely and proficiently. Under a collaborative training model, FLETC's federal partner organizations deliver training unique to their missions, while FLETC provides training in areas common to all law enforcement officers, such as firearms, driving, tactics, investigations, and legal training.
Federal Protective Service (FPS)	Provides integrated security and law enforcement services, such as conducting facility security assessments; responding to crimes and other incidents to protect life and property; and detecting, investigating, and mitigating threats to more than 9,500 federal facilities nationwide.
Transportation Security Administration (TSA)	Protects the nation's transportation systems to ensure freedom of movement for people and commerce. TSA does this by, among other things, deploying Federal Air Marshals on U.S. aircraft worldwide. Our review focuses on TSA's Federal Air Marshals, who are to detect, deter, and defeat criminal and terrorist activity targeting transportation systems.
U.S. Customs and Border Protection (CBP)	Protects the borders of the United States from dangerous people and materials, while facilitating lawful international travel and trade.
U.S. Immigration and Customs Enforcement (ICE)	Protects the United States from cross-border crime and illegal immigration that threaten national security and public safety. ICE executes this mission through enforcement of federal statutes and focuses on immigration enforcement, preventing terrorism, and combating the illegal movement of people and goods. Our review focuses on ICE's Homeland Security Investigations office, which investigates cross-border criminal activity, and Enforcement and Removal Operations, which identifies and apprehends removable aliens, detains them when necessary, and removes illegal aliens from the United States.
U.S. Secret Service	Provides physical protection to the nation's highest elected leaders, visiting foreign dignitaries, facilities and major events, and safeguards the payment and financial systems of the United States from a wide range of financial and computer-based crimes.
Department of Justice	
Bureau of Alcohol, Tobacco, Firearms and Explosives (ATF)	Responsibilities include the investigation and prevention of federal offenses involving the unlawful use, manufacture, and possession of firearms and explosives; acts of arson and bombings; and illegal trafficking of alcohol and tobacco products.
Federal Bureau of Prisons (BOP)	Confines offenders in the controlled environments of prisons and community-based facilities that are safe, humane, cost-efficient, and appropriately secure, and that provide work and other self-improvement opportunities to assist offenders in becoming law-abiding citizens. As part of its duties, BOP is responsible for delivering medically necessary health care to inmates in accordance with proven standards of care, including medical, dental and mental health.

Table 6. (Continued)

Component	Mission
Federal Bureau of Investigation (FBI)	Protects the nation from terrorism, espionage, cyber attacks, and major criminal threats through intelligence-gathering and law enforcement responsibilities. Our review focuses on the FBI's Special Agents, who are primarily responsible for executing this mission, as well as FBI Police Officers, who provide security at FBI facilities.
U.S. Drug Enforcement Administration (DEA)	Enforces the controlled substances laws and regulations of the United States and brings to the criminal and civil justice system of the United States, or any other competent jurisdiction, those organizations and principal members of organizations involved in the growing, manufacture, or distribution of controlled substances appearing in or destined for illicit traffic in the United States.
U.S. Marshals Service (USMS)	Provides federal judicial security; apprehends fugitives and non-compliant sex offenders; secures and transports federal prisoners from arrest to incarceration; executes federal court orders; seizes and manages assets acquired through illegal means; and assures the safety of endangered government witnesses and their families.

Source: GAO summary of information from components. | GAO-18-229.

Note: According to data the departments provided to us, as of the end of fiscal year 2016, the DHS components above—excluding FLETC—employed 42,823 of 43,222 law enforcement officers within DHS, and the DOJ components above employed 43,502 of 43,639 law enforcement officers within DOJ.

[a] FLETC information is presented in this table as they provide various types of training to a number of federal law enforcement agencies. However, we do not consider them an operational law enforcement component for our subsequent discussions of training in place at components.

We have relied on the observations gathered during these discussion groups to answer this reporting objective as the officers and agents are uniquely positioned to speak to their experiences, and any challenges they face, responding to incidents involving individuals with mental illness. To identify the training, policies, and guidance in place, we reviewed documents from each of our selected law enforcement components, when available, to examine their nature and scope. We further reviewed information on the duration, requirements, and delivery mechanism of the training. We then summarized and verified this training information with each component through email documentation. For the policies, we reviewed the documentation to determine whether it was specific to responding to incidents involving individuals with mental illness or whether mental illness was contained within a larger directive. We also reviewed 2018 budget justification documents for each component in order to identify changes in staffing levels or training plans that might be related to officers' and agents' response to incidents involving individuals with mental illness. We also interviewed officials responsible for the development or delivery of training, policies, or guidance from the components in our scope to gather additional information that could help prepare federal law enforcement officers and agents to respond to incidents involving individuals with mental illness. In addition, since section 504 of the Rehabilitation Act of 1973, as amended, prohibits discrimination on the basis of disability, which includes mental illness, in federally funded and federally conducted programs and activities,[36] we took steps to understand the section's applicability to federal law enforcement operations.[37] Specifically, we reviewed departmental guidance related to section 504 and reviewed the selected components' documentation of efforts to review their training, policies, and procedures in accordance with that guidance. We also interviewed officials from the departmental offices overseeing these component efforts—DHS's Office of Civil Rights and Civil Liberties (CRCL) and DOJ's Office of the Deputy Attorney General (ODAG).

To identify leading practices or tools stakeholders cited for effective law enforcement responses to incidents involving individuals with mental illness, we used a multi-stage process[38] Specifically, we:

1. conducted a search of databases, such as ProQuest and Scopus, and organizational websites, such as those from the Council of State Governments, Justice Center (CSG JC) and Police Executive Research Forum (PERF), to identify published work related to law enforcement responses to individuals with mental illness that had been published on or after January 1, 2007 (the last 10 years).
2. reviewed the 96 published research papers and articles that our initial search yielded and then refined our selection criteria to include only those that were literature reviews, meta-analyses, or summary papers published by academics, think tanks and advocacy groups, or government agencies. We reviewed summary articles rather than all the primary research articles to balance breadth, depth, and efficiency. After refining our search, there were 16 documents that met our selection criteria.
3. reviewed the 16 to identify any potential leading practices. We determined that a practice was potentially leading if it was found in at least one of the remaining 16 articles and was a law enforcement – mental health program. Using these criteria, we identified two potential leading practices.[39]
4. asked individual and organizational stakeholders to validate whether these were leading practices and to identify any additional leading practices that we might

---

[36] 29 U.S.C. § 794. A person with a disability includes anyone who has a physical or mental impairment that substantially limits one or more major life activities, has a record of such impairment, or is regarded as having such an impairment. The definition of disability for purposes of § 504 of the Rehabilitation Act is derived from the Americans with Disabilities Act. 29 U.S.C. § 705(9); 42 U.S.C. § 12102.

[37] DOJ and DHS regulations and guidance provide that section 504 applies to all programs and activities of the department. For example, DOJ guidance states that DOJ's obligations under section 504 and implementing regulations "apply to all members of the public with disabilities whom the Department serves or encounters as part of the Department's traditional law enforcement programs and activities." However, according to this same guidance, "[e]xigencies, dangers, and safety considerations, however, play a significant role in determining whether and to what extent an accommodation [for a member of the public with a disability] is reasonable."

[38] For the purposes of our report, stakeholders are either academic or independent researchers or advocacy groups that are known to have substantial knowledge or expertise in the area of law enforcement responses to individuals with mental illness.

[39] By using the term "leading practices," we refer to practices that are generally effective when officers or agents apply them when responding to interactions with individuals with mental illness even if robust evaluations of such practices' effectiveness have not been conducted or have shown mixed results.

have missed. In order for us to consider an independent researcher as a stakeholder, the individual needed to have (a) authored or co-authored at least 2 of the 16 documents that met our search criteria as outlined earlier and (b) been recommended by another stakeholder. These criteria yielded two independent researchers from whom to solicit views. In order for us to consider an organization as a stakeholder, the organizations needed to have either (a) conducted research on law enforcement responses to individuals with mental illness; (b) administered law enforcement-mental health collaborative programs; or (c) launched a national campaign on law enforcement responses to individuals with mental illness. After reviewing the websites of organizations that potentially met these criteria, we selected four organizations from which to solicit views. In addition, we selected individuals within the organizations as knowledgeable stakeholders if they were either (1) recommended by another stakeholder; or (2) managed a law enforcement-mental health program or national campaign. As a result of these steps, we identified and interviewed six stakeholders (two independent researchers and four organizations) to gather their broad views of the dynamic between law enforcement and individuals with mental illness; to obtain their observations of any practices or tools, such as training guides or reports that have been used to enhance officer response; and to provide feedback on leading practices. The six selected stakeholders were:

- Amy Watson, PhD: Professor at the Jane Addams College of Social Work, University of Illinois at Chicago.
- Melissa Reuland, MS: Research Fellow at the Police Foundation and Senior Research Program Manager at Johns Hopkins School of Medicine, Department of Psychiatry.
- Council of State Governments, Justice Center (CSG JC): a national nonprofit organization that serves policymakers at the local, state, and federal levels from all branches of government. It aims to provide practical, nonpartisan advice and consensus-driven strategies, informed by available evidence, to increase public safety and strengthen communities.
- International Association of Chiefs of Police (IACP): a professional association for law enforcement, representing more than 30,000 members in more than 150 countries. IACP aims to advance the law enforcement profession through advocacy, outreach, education, and programs.
- National Alliance on Mental Illness: a national grassroots mental health organization dedicated to building better lives for the millions of Americans affected by mental illness.

- Police Executive Research Forum (PERF): an independent research organization that seeks to identify best practices on issues such as reducing police use of force; developing community and problem-oriented policing; and evaluating crime reduction strategies.

After reaching out to each researcher and organization, we then sent a follow up written request to each of them to attempt to achieve consensus on whether or not the two practices we identified through our search—the Crisis Intervention Team (CIT) Model and the Co-responder Model— should be considered leading. We also took note of any tools they mentioned and probed further to understand their origins and intent. We confirmed with all six of the selected stakeholders that the CIT Model met our definition of leading practice and confirmed with five out of the six stakeholders that the Co-responder Model met our definition. Some stakeholders also identified other practices as leading; however, none of those practices had at least two other stakeholders confirm it as a leading practice.

In addition, to determine how DOJ and DHS components leverage information from other knowledgeable parties, such as experts, associations, or colleagues in other components, we reviewed relevant documentation on these efforts, as available. We also interviewed agency officials from the components in our scope who are responsible for the development or delivery of training or policies.

We conducted this performance audit from February 2017 through February 2018 in accordance with generally accepted government auditing standards. Those standards require that we plan and perform an audit to obtain sufficient, appropriate evidence to provide a reasonable basis for our findings and conclusions based on our audit objectives. We believe that the evidence obtained provides a reasonable basis for our findings and conclusions based on our audit objectives.

Appendix II: Description of the Federal Law Enforcement Training Centers (FLETC) Basic Training Programs

FLETC provides basic training to all Department of Homeland Security (DHS) law enforcement officers through one of three basic program categories, which vary in length, described as follows:[40]

- Center Basic is a FLETC training program category in which personnel from various agencies are provided with the critical competencies of a specific job, job

[40] One exception would be for training provided to Border Patrol agents. While this training takes place at FLETC venues, according to U.S. Customs and Border Protection (CBP), the U.S. Border Patrol itself conducts nearly all of the training provided to its agents.

series, or a group of closely related job series. FLETC provides all instruction. Training is offered in three basic training programs: Criminal Investigator Training Program, Uniformed Police Training Program and the Land Management Police Training Program.[41]

- Center Integrated Basic is a FLETC training program category that provides entry-level law enforcement officers or direct law enforcement support personnel from a single partner organization with the core competencies of a specific job series or a group of closely related job series. FLETC provides all common and basic core foundational instruction (i.e., firearms, physical techniques, etc.). This category of training includes eight specific programs.[42]
- Agency-Specific Basic is a training program category designed to provide entry-level law enforcement officers or direct law enforcement support personnel with instruction necessary to meet a single agency's mission-specific basic training needs. Generally, Agency-Specific Basic courses precede or follow a Center Basic training program, with partner organizations providing the majority of the instruction. Agency-Specific Basic covers an additional 59 training programs.

---

[41] The Criminal Investigator Training Program provides, on an interagency basis, a program of instruction for all basic criminal investigative training requirements necessary for all investigators. The Land Management Police Training Program is designed to meet the entry level training needs of law enforcement officers responsible for protecting natural resources and public lands. The Uniformed Police Training Program provides a study of the basic law enforcement concepts that a new officer should understand and/or be able to perform upon employment in a federal law enforcement organization. According to FLETC, it maintains contact with partner organizations to keep abreast of their changing needs and to provide current information to students concerning federal laws, jurisdiction, policies, procedures and basic operations.

[42] Of the eight Center Integrated Basic programs, five are specific to the components in our review: CBP Air and Marine basic training, CBP Officer basic training, Federal Air Marshal training, Immigration and Customs Enforcement basic immigration enforcement training, and U.S. Border Patrol basic police training.

In: Focus on Mental Health and Illness
Editor: Isaac Banks
ISBN: 978-1-53615-081-0

Chapter 6

REVIEW OF THE FEDERAL BUREAU OF PRISONS' USE OF RESTRICTIVE HOUSING FOR INMATES WITH MENTAL ILLNESS*

Office of the Inspector General
U.S. Department of Justice

EXECUTIVE SUMMARY

Introduction

The Federal Bureau of Prisons (BOP) is responsible for confining offenders in environments that are safe, humane, cost-efficient, and appropriately secure. To do so, the BOP utilizes various forms of Restrictive Housing Unit (RHU) to confine certain inmates, including those with mental illness. However, according to recent research and reports, as well as the BOP's own policy, confinement in RHUs, even for relatively short periods of time, can adversely affect inmates' mental health and can be particularly harmful for inmates with mental illness.

As of June 2016, of the 148,227 sentenced inmates in the BOP's 122 institutions, 9,749 inmates (7 percent) were housed in its three largest forms of RHU: Special Housing Units (SHU) in 111 institutions; 2 Special Management Units (SMU) at the U.S. Penitentiaries

* This is an edited, reformatted and augmented version of Office of the Inspector General; U.S. Department of Justice, Evaluation and Inspections Division 17-05, dated July 2017.

(USP) in Lewisburg and Allenwood, Pennsylvania; and the USP Administrative Maximum Security Facility (ADX) in Florence, Colorado.[1]

The Office of the Inspector General conducted this review to examine the BOP's use of RHUs for inmates with mental illness, including trends in the use of restrictive housing and the screening, treatment, and monitoring of inmates with mental illness who are housed in RHUs. We found significant issues with the adequacy of the BOP's policies and its implementation efforts in this critical area.

Results in Brief

BOP Policies Do Not Adequately Address the Confinement of Inmates with Mental Illness in RHUs, and the BOP Does Not Sufficiently Track or Monitor Such Inmates

BOP guidance and policies do not clearly define "restrictive housing" or "extended placement." Although the BOP states that it does not practice solitary confinement, or even recognize the term, we found inmates, including those with mental illness, who were housed in single-cell confinement for long periods of time, isolated from other inmates and with limited human contact. For example, at the ADX, we observed an RHU that held two inmates, each in their own cell, isolated from other inmates. The inmates did not engage in recreation with each other or with other inmates and were confined to their cells for over 22 hours a day. Also, in five SHUs, we observed single-celled inmates, many with serious mental illness.

One inmate, who we were told was denied ADX placement for mental health reasons, had been single-celled for about 4 years.

Although the BOP generally imposes a minimum amount of time that inmates must spend in RHUs, it does not limit the maximum amount of time and does not monitor inmates' cumulative time in RHUs.[2] The BOP also does not track its housing of inmates in single-cell RHU confinement, nor does it account for their confinement in all RHUs throughout BOP institutions. As a result, inmates, including those with mental illness, may spend years and even decades in RHUs. For example, we learned of an inmate with serious mental illness who spent about 19 years at the ADX before being transferred to a secure residential mental health treatment program. In addition, our sample of inmates with mental illness showed that they had been placed in the ADX for an average of about 69 months. Similarly, we found that between fiscal years (FY) 2008 and 2015, inmates with mental illness averaged about 896 consecutive days, or about 29 months, in the SMU. We further found that inmates with mental illness spend disproportionately longer periods of time in

---

[1] The USP Allenwood SMU closed in October 2016, during the course of our review. USP Lewisburg is the only remaining BOP institution that maintains the SMU program.

[2] In August 2016, the BOP issued a revised SMU policy that now limits the duration of time an inmate can spend in the SMU. We discuss the revised SMU policy throughout the report.

RHUs than their peers. Equally concerning, our review showed that 13 percent of the inmates with mental illness in our sample were released by the BOP directly into the community after spending nearly 29 months in the SMU prior to their release.

By contrast, officials in six of the eight state departments of corrections told us that they limit the length of time inmates with mental illness can be placed in restrictive housing. In 2015, three states (Massachusetts, Mississippi, and New York) had at least a 30-day limit, while three other states (Colorado, Maine, and Pennsylvania) no longer placed inmates with serious mental illness in RHUs at all.

Mental Health Staff Do Not Always Document Inmates' Mental Disorders, Leaving the BOP Unable to Accurately Determine the Number of Inmates with Mental Illness and Ensure that It Is Providing Appropriate Care to Them

BOP data showed that, as of 2015, only 3 percent of the BOP's sentenced inmate population was being treated regularly for mental illness. Yet, the BOP's *FY 2016 Performance Budget Congressional Submission* cited an internal BOP study, which suggested that approximately 19 percent of federal inmates had a history of mental illness. Moreover, a 2006 Bureau of Justice Statistics report concluded that 45 percent of federal inmates had symptoms or a recent history of mental illness.

We found that the BOP cannot accurately determine the number of inmates who have mental illness because institution staff do not always document mental disorders. The BOP's FY 2014 data estimates that approximately 12 percent of inmates have a history of mental illness; however, in 2015, the BOP's Chief Psychiatrist estimated, based on discussions with institutions' Psychology Services staffs, that approximately 40 percent of inmates have mental illness, excluding inmates with only personality disorder diagnoses. Similarly, one institution's Deputy Chief Psychologist estimated that 50 percent of that institution's inmates may have Antisocial Personality Disorder; nevertheless, we found that this disorder was documented for only about 3.3 percent of the BOP's total inmate population. Because mental health staffs do not always document inmates' mental disorders, the BOP is unable to ensure that it is providing appropriate care to them.

Since the BOP Adopted Its New Mental Health Policy, BOP Data Shows a 30 Percent Reduction in Inmates Who Receive Regular Mental Health Treatment

The BOP adopted a new mental health policy in 2014, increasing the standards of care for inmates with mental illness. However, since the policy was issued, the total number of inmates who receive regular mental health treatment decreased by approximately 30 percent, including 56 percent for inmates in SMUs, and about 20 percent overall for inmates in RHUs during the scope of our review. Based on our review, it appears that mental health staff may have reduced the number of inmates, including those in RHUs, who must receive regular mental health treatment because they did not have the necessary staffing resources to meet the policy's increased treatment standards. Indeed, we found that, as of October 2015, the BOP had filled only 57 percent of its authorized full-time Psychiatrist positions nationwide and that it had significant staffing issues with regard to Psychologist positions as well.

This treatment trend was particularly pronounced among SMU inmates at USP Lewisburg, which confined over 1,100 SMU inmates as of June 2016. Based on our sample of SMU inmates, we found that, prior to the new policy, the number of inmates (16) whose mental health care level was increased equaled the number of inmates (16) whose care level was decreased. In contrast, after the new policy was adopted, all 27 inmates whose care level changed had a decrease and therefore ostensibly required less treatment. By May 2015, only about 2.5 percent of SMU inmates at USP Lewisburg were categorized as requiring regular treatment, compared to about 11 percent of ADX inmates and 7 percent of SHU inmates nationwide, which we believe raises treatment concerns for inmates in USP Lewisburg's SMU.

While the BOP Has Taken Recent Steps to Mitigate Mental Health Concerns for Inmates in RHUs, Additional Actions Can Be Taken

The BOP has taken a number of steps to mitigate the mental health concerns for inmates in RHUs. These efforts include diverting inmates with serious mental illness from placement in traditional RHUs (i.e., SHUs, the SMUs, and the ADX) and into alternative programs such as secure residential mental health treatment programs. While these are positive BOP initiatives, limited inmate capacities, slow inmate progression through the programs, high staffing needs, and a lack of formal performance metrics with which to measure the effectiveness of these programs limit their utility and the BOP's ability to expand their use to other institutions.

Recommendations

We make 15 recommendations to the BOP to improve its screening, treatment, and monitoring of inmates with mental illness housed in RHUs.

INTRODUCTION

Background

The Federal Bureau of Prisons (BOP) is responsible for confining offenders in environments that are safe, humane, cost -efficient, and appropriately secure. To ensure safc and orderly environments for inmates and staff, the BOP utilizes various forms of Restrictive Housing Unit (RHU) for the confinement of some inmates, including inmates with mental illness. The U.S. Department of Justice (Department, DOJ) defines restrictive housing as "any type of detention that includes removal from the general inmate population, whether voluntary or involuntary; placement in a locked room or cell, whether alone or with another inmate; and inability to leave the room or cell for the vast majority of the day, typically 22 hours or more."[3] In recent years, studies have suggested that the frequency, duration, and conditions of confinement of restrictive housing, even for short periods of time, can cause psychological harm and significant adverse effects on these inmates' mental health. For example, research suggests that "isolation can be psychologically harmful to any prisoner — psychological effects can include anxiety, depression, anger, cognitive disturbances, perceptual disorders, obsessive thoughts, paranoia, and psychosis" — some of which may be long lasting.[4] According to some experts, inmates who have spent long periods in isolation are more likely to recidivate and have a more difficult time creating the lasting social bonds that are necessary for reintegration into society.[5] The BOP's own policy also recognizes that "an inmate's mental health may deteriorate during restrictive housing placement."[6]

As of June 2016, of the 148,227 sentenced inmates in the BOP's 122 institutions, 9,749 inmates (7 percent) were housed in its 3 largest forms of RHU: Special Housing Units (SHU) in 111 institutions; 2 Special Management Units (SMU) at the U.S. Penitentiaries (USP) in Lewisburg and Allenwood, Pennsylvania; and the USP Administrative Maximum Security Facility (ADX) in Florence, Colorado.

In this review, the Office of the Inspector General (OIG) examined the BOP's use of restrictive housing for inmates with mental illness in these RHUs and analyzed trends in the BOP's placement of inmates with mental illness in restrictive housing. We also evaluated the BOP's policies and procedures related to its screening, treatment, and monitoring of inmates with mental illness in RHUs. In the following sections and Appendix 2, we discuss the three primary types of RHU that the BOP uses, as well as the prevalence of mental illness among BOP inmates; we explain how the BOP determines an inmate's mental health needs, as well as trends in the placement of inmates with mental illness in RHUs; we describe previous reports related to the use of RHUs and inmates with mental illness; and we summarize the BOP's RHU and mental health policies.

---

[3] DOJ, *Report and Recommendations concerning the Use of Restrictive Housing* (January 2016), 3. While the BOP has taken several corrective actions in response to the recommendations in this report, we found that several issues remain unresolved and require the BOP's immediate attention.

[4] Jeffrey L. Metzner, MD, and Jamie Fellner, Esq., "Solitary Confinement and Mental Illness in U.S. Prisons: A Challenge for Medical Ethics," *Journal of the American Academy of Psychiatry and the Law,* 38 (March 2010): 104–08.

[5] Craig Haney, Professor of Psychology at the University of California, Santa Cruz, before the Judiciary Subcommittee on the Constitution, Civil Rights, and Human Rights, U.S. Senate, concerning "Reassessing Solitary Confinement: The Human Rights, Fiscal, and Public Safety Consequences" (June 19, 2012), 10–11. The Office of the Inspector General (OIG) separately reviewed the BOP's Release Preparation Program. See DOJ OIG, *Review of the Federal Bureau of Prisons' Release Preparation Program,* Evaluation and Inspections Report 16-07 (August 2016).

[6] BOP Program Statement 5310.16, Treatment and Care of Inmates with Mental Illness (May 1, 2014), 16.

Types of Restrictive Housing Units

There are three primary types of RHU within BOP institutions. As of January 2016, 111 institutions have a SHU to house inmates for both disciplinary reasons and non-disciplinary reasons, such as for their own protection.[7] In two BOP institutions, a SMU houses inmates who present unique security and management concerns.[8] The ADX houses inmates who have demonstrated violent, disruptive, and/or escape-prone behavior at other BOP institutions or those who cannot be safely housed in the general population of other BOP institutions. We further discuss the three primary types of RHU below, and we then discuss the prevalence of mental illness among BOP inmates generally, followed by the availability of mental health services for inmates housed in the different types of RHU. See Appendix 2 for more information on SHUs, the SMUs, and the ADX.

Special Housing Units

Institution SHUs are securely separated from general inmate population housing. In August 2015, the BOP's former Director stated that, on average, inmates spend about 65 days (about 2 months) in the SHU BOP-wide.[9] In June 2016, the BOP housed about 5 percent (8,065 inmates) of its total population of sentenced inmates in SHUs. Eighty-three percent of all BOP inmates in RHUs are housed in SHUs; though some inmates are placed in a SHU for disciplinary reasons, most are held there for non-disciplinary reasons, including for their own protection.

Special Management Units

The BOP established SMUs in 2008 as a program to house inmates who require greater management of their interactions with others to ensure the safety, security, or orderly operation of BOP institutions and to protect the public.[10] Most SMU inmates are transferred

---

[7] In November 2016, the BOP issued a revised SHU policy in response to the recommendations detailed in the Department's January 2016 report on the use of restrictive housing. See DOJ, *Use of Restrictive Housing*, which we discuss below. See also BOP Program Statement 5270.11, Special Housing Units (November 23, 2016). We did not evaluate this new policy, as it was issued after completion of our fieldwork. However, we note throughout this report examples of changes to the SHU policy as they relate to our findings during the course of our review. See Appendix 2 for more information on the revised SHU policy.

[8] BOP Program Statement 5217.01, Special Management Units (November 19, 2008), provides guidance and procedures for operation of the SMU.
In August 2016, the BOP issued a revised SMU policy. See BOP Program Statement 5217.02, Special Management Units (August 9, 2016). We did not evaluate this new policy, as it was issued after the completion of our fieldwork. However, we note throughout this report examples of changes to the SMU policy as they relate to our findings on the SMU program during the course of our review. See Appendix 2 for more information on the revised SMU policy.

[9] Former BOP Director Charles E. Samuels, Jr., before the Homeland Security and Governmental Affairs Committee, U.S. Senate, concerning "Oversight of the Bureau of Prisons: First Hand Accounts of Challenges Facing the Federal Prison System" (August 4, 2015).

[10] By 2012, the SMU program had expanded to 5 institutions with a population of over 1,700 inmates. However, as of June 2016, the BOP maintained its SMU program within two institutions, USP Lewisburg (1,166) and USP Allenwood (124), both in Pennsylvania, which together house 1,290 inmates. According to the former Deputy Assistant Director for the Correctional Programs Division, the BOP condensed the SMU program to two institutions because the need for the program had diminished. He cited fewer inmate assaults, staff assaults, and

from USPs. Inmates assigned to the SMUs are expected to complete a four-phase program, which means they have demonstrated a sustained ability to coexist and interact appropriately with other inmates and staff, within 18 to 24 months, after which they may be designated to another appropriate facility.[11]

U.S. Penitentiary Administrative Maximum Security Facility

Activated in November 1994 in Florence, Colorado, the ADX has a rated capacity of 490 inmates and confines inmates under close control. As of November 2013, the BOP determined that the average length of stay for inmates at the ADX was 1,376 days (about 45 months, or 3.8 years).[12] At the time of our review, the ADX housed the majority (about 70 percent) of its inmates in general population, while the remaining 142 inmates, who require closer control and increased levels of security, are housed in the ADX's Control Unit or its Special Security Unit.[13] All inmates in the ADX are in single-occupant cells and can receive programming through a closed-circuit television system.

Mental Illness among BOP Inmates

Reports citing statistics on the prevalence of mental illness, both within the BOP's inmate population and nationally, vary based on sources of data and mental health information, the definition of mental illness used, and the research methodology employed. For example, the BOP's fiscal year (FY) *2016 Performance Budget Congressional Submission* cited an internal BOP study that suggested that approximately 19 percent of federal inmates had a history of mental illness.[14] In comparison, a 2006 Bureau of Justice

---

protective custody cases throughout the BOP. In October 2016, Psychology Services Branch officials told us that USP Allenwood's SMU has since closed and, currently, USP Lewisburg is the only remaining institution that maintains the SMU program.

[11] In August 2016, as a result of recommendations made in the Department's January 2016 restrictive housing report, the BOP issued a revised SMU policy that, among other things, reduced the intended time frame for inmates' completion of the program to 9–13 months. See DOJ, *Use of Restrictive Housing*. See Appendix 2 of this report for more information on the revised SMU policy.

[12] This was the most recent data the BOP had at the time that a Center of Naval Analysis and Solutions (CNA) analysis was done, which we discuss further below. CNA, *Federal Bureau of Prisons: Special Housing Review and Assessment* (December 2014), 58.

[13] The ADX's Control Unit provides housing for inmates who are unable to function in a less restrictive environment without posing a threat to others. This unit typically houses inmates who have assaulted or killed staff or other inmates or who have escaped or attempted escape from other institutions. The ADX's Special Security Unit houses inmates who are subject to Special Administrative Measures, which are restrictions on communications that the U.S. Attorney General imposes, typically for reasons related to national security.

[14] This study was limited to 2,855 inmates who were new court commitments to the BOP's custody, spoke either English or Spanish fluently, could read at a fourth grade level, and were physically and mentally able to complete self-reporting instruments. Philip R. Magaletta et al., "Estimating the Mental Illness Component of Service Need in Corrections, Results from the *Mental Health Prevalence Project*," *Criminal Justice and Behavior* 36, no. 3 (March 2009).

Statistics report concluded that 45 percent of federal inmates had symptoms or a recent history of mental illness.[15]

According to the BOP, inmates with diagnosed mental illness, including inmates with serious mental illness, may be housed in each of the RHUs described above "due to safety and/or security needs for any length of time."[16] BOP policy defines a mental disorder (illness) as:

> A syndrome characterized by clinical significant disturbance in an individual's cognition, emotional regulation, or behavior that reflects a dysfunction in the psychological, biological, or developmental processes underlying mental functioning. Mental disorders are usually associated with significant distress or disability in social, occupational, or other important activities.[17]

In determining whether an inmate should be classified as having serious mental illness, BOP policy states that mental health staff will consider the inmate's diagnosed mental illness or illnesses, the severity and duration of the symptoms, the degree of functional impairment associated with the illness or illnesses, and the inmate's treatment history and current treatment needs. BOP policy lists specific diagnoses that are generally classified as serious mental illnesses, as well as specific diagnoses that may be classified as serious mental illnesses.[18]

According to BOP policy, when inmates with serious mental illness are placed in restrictive housing, they should continue to receive mental health care commensurate with their treatment needs.[19] The BOP limits the placement of inmates with serious mental

---

[15] DOJ Office of Justice Programs, Bureau of Justice Statistics, *Mental Health Problems of Prison and Jail Inmates*, Special Report (revised December 14, 2006), https://www.bjs.gov/content/pub/pdf/mhppji.pdf (accessed June 27, 2017). This report was based on data collected from structured clinical interviews of federal inmates during 2004. It was limited to inmates' self-reported symptoms or recent history of mental illness that must have occurred during the 12 months prior to the interview. It did not exclude symptoms due to medical illness, bereavement, or substance abuse.

By contrast, this report also stated that about 11 percent of persons age 18 or older in the U.S. general population displayed symptoms of mental disorder, while in 2015 the National Institute of Mental Health estimated that 17.9 percent of all adults in the United States had experienced mental illness within the previous year. See National Institute of Mental Health, "Any Mental Illness (AMI) among U.S. Adults," https://www.nimh.nih.gov/health/statistics/prevalence/any-mental-illness-ami-among-us-adults.shtml (accessed June 27, 2017).

[16] BOP Program Statement 5310.16, 15. The BOP's definition of mental illness is derived from the American Psychiatric Association's *Diagnostic and Statistical Manual for Mental Disorders*, 5th ed. (Arlington, Va.: American Psychiatric Association, 2013) (DSM-5), which is a classification and diagnostic tool used throughout the field of psychology.

[17] BOP Program Statement 5310.16, 1.

[18] BOP policy lists Schizophrenia Spectrum and other Psychotic Disorders, Bipolar and related disorders, and Major Depressive Disorders as diagnoses that are generally classified as serious mental illnesses. The policy lists Anxiety Disorders, Obsessive-Compulsive and related disorders, Trauma and Stressor-Related Disorders, Intellectual Disabilities and Autism Spectrum Disorders, Major Neurocognitive Disorders, and Personality Disorders as diagnoses that are often classified as serious mental illnesses, especially if the condition is sufficiently severe, persistent, and disabling. See BOP Program Statement 5310.16, 1–2.

[19] BOP policy specifies that if an inmate with a serious mental illness must be placed in restrictive housing, he/she will continue to receive mental health care commensurate with his/her treatment needs. See BOP Program Statement 5310.16, 15, 19.

illness in the SMUs and the ADX to those inmates who present extraordinary security needs that cannot be managed elsewhere. Below, we discuss how the BOP categorizes inmates' mental health, as well as its policies to address inmates with mental illness in RHUs.

BOP Mental Health Care Levels

The BOP classifies inmates into four Mental Health Care Levels (MHCL), which are determined by the resources and services an inmate needs as opposed to the inmate's diagnosed mental illness. The BOP policy classifies inmate MHCLs as follows:

- **MHCL 1:** The inmate shows no significant level of functional impairment associated with a mental illness and demonstrates no need for regular mental health intervention. Or, if a history of mental illness is present, the inmate has consistently demonstrated appropriate help-seeking behavior in response to any reemergence of symptoms.
- **MHCL 2:** The inmate requires routine outpatient mental health care on an ongoing basis and/or brief, crisis-oriented mental health care of significant intensity, e.g., placement on suicide watch or behavioral observation status.
- **MHCL 3:** The inmate requires enhanced outpatient care (i.e., weekly mental health intervention) or residential mental health care (i.e., placement in a residential Psychology Treatment Program).
- **MHCL 4:** The inmate may require inpatient psychiatric care and acute care in a psychiatric hospital if the inmate is gravely disabled and cannot function within the general population at an institution having the mission and resources to house MHCL 3 inmates.

According to BOP Psychology Services Branch officials, MHCLs are based on resource utilization and, as such, the BOP tries to assess what type of resources an inmate needs to function effectively.[20] Inmates at both MHCL 3 and MHCL 4 are considered to have serious mental illness. However, inmates at all MHCLs may have a serious mental illness. For example, an inmate with a history of psychosis could be designated at MHCL 1 or 2 despite having a serious mental illness, as long as he or she faithfully takes medication and does not need further staff intervention to function effectively. MHCLs do not necessarily correspond to specific diagnoses, although this is a factor that the BOP

[20] Similar to how MHCLs delineate the mental health needs of inmates, the BOP also designates institutional care levels to delineate the varying levels of medical and mental health care that can be provided to inmates at its institutions. For example, an MHCL 4 inmate should be housed only at a Care Level 4 institution because only Care Level 4 institutions have the resources needed to address that inmate's intensive mental health needs.

takes into consideration. Rather, MHCLs correspond to treatment requirements and how often inmates need intervention. The BOP directs its clinicians to assess inmates who are asking for services and inmates who could benefit from services. For example, the BOP would typically classify an inmate with Schizophrenia at MHCL 2, 3, or 4, even if the inmate does not require reoccurring mental health interventions for a prolonged period of time, because such services may be required in the future.

Recent MHCL Trends

BOP data indicates that a smaller percentage of inmates are being treated for mental illness than the percentage that the BOP's *Mental Health Prevalence Project* reported as having mental health needs. Specifically, BOP data showed that as of 2015 only 3 percent of the BOP's total sentenced inmate population was designated at MHCL 2, 3, or 4, thus requiring recurring treatment, as opposed to nearly 4.3 percent in 2010.[21] From the end of FY 2010 through May 2015, the number of inmates designated at MHCL 2, 3, or 4 decreased by over 30 percent, from 6,853 inmates to 4,768 inmates, while the number of inmates designated at MHCL 1 increased slightly (2 percent). Most notably, the number of inmates designated at MHCL 4 decreased by almost 60 percent. Table 1 below shows the total number of inmates across all institutions, by MHCL, from FY 2010 through May 2015.[22]

Table 1. Inmate MHCLs, FY 2010 – May 2015

Inmates Designated at All MHCLs	FY 2010	May 2015	Percent Change (+/-)
MHCL 1	147,907	150,884	2.01%
MHCL 2	5,701	3,971	-30.35%
MHCL 3	578	551	-4.67%
MHCL 4	574	246	-57.14%
Total	154,760	155,652	0.57%

Note: This table does not include inmates who had undergone an initial mental health records review, were given a tentative MHCL designation by the BOP's Designation and Sentence Computation Center, but had yet to be examined, in person, by a mental health clinician.

Source: OIG analysis of BOP data.

Over this same period, the BOP decreased its use of restrictive housing for inmates in general by nearly 20 percent and for inmates designated at MHCL 2, 3, or 4 by slightly more. Specifically:

---

[21] Later in this report, we discuss what BOP officials estimated as the percentage of the BOP's inmate population with mental illness.

[22] In response to a working draft of this report, the BOP cited disparities following an MHCL analysis of its inmate population at the end of FY 2010. While the BOP found the same ratio of its inmate population who required recurring treatment in FY 2010 (4.3 percent) and May 2015 (3.0 percent), the BOP did not include 17,269 inmates in its FY 2010 numbers that we included in Table 1 (below). According to the BOP, it did not include these inmates in its analysis because the MHCL system was formally adopted in December 2009 and many inmates at the end of FY 2010 did not have a MHCL yet assigned to them. However, the raw data the BOP provided to us for the end of FY 2010 showed that, with few exceptions, all inmates had MHCLs assigned to them. We based our analysis on this data.

- The number of inmates housed in SHUs decreased 22.3 percent, with a corresponding decrease of 26.3 percent in the number of MHCL 2, 3, or 4 inmates housed in SHUs.
- The number of inmates placed in the SMU program increased 11.3 percent, from 1,157 to 1,288. However, the number of MHCL 2, 3, or 4 inmates placed in the SMU program decreased 13.9 percent overall (from 36 to 31).[23]
- The number of inmates at the ADX decreased 7.6 percent (from 447 to 413) and the number of MHCL 2, 3, or 4 inmates at the ADX increased by nearly 40 percent (from 33 to 46).

BOP policy currently prohibits the placement of MHCL 4 inmates in the SMUs or the ADX. Similarly, under the BOP's 2014 policy, most MHCL 3 inmates are diverted from SMU or ADX placement, except when extraordinary security needs prevent them from being housed anywhere else. Later in this chapter, we discuss further the 30 percent reduction in the number of inmates who receive regular mental health treatment, including those in RHUs.

BOP Policies Impacting Inmates in RHUs, Including Those with Mental Illness

In 2014, the BOP adopted a new national mental health care policy that detailed enhanced standards of care for all inmates with mental illness. The BOP supplements this policy with its longstanding Psychology Services Manual, which, among other things, specifies national mental health screening requirements for all inmates.[24] To govern the operation of RHUs, the BOP maintains national policies for institutions' use of both SHUs and SMUs. Meanwhile, the ADX has local policies and guidelines establishing an institution's daily operating procedures, including supplementing BOP policy regarding the care and treatment of ADX inmates with mental illness. We discuss the policies below and provide additional detail in Appendix 2.

National Mental Health Care Program

The BOP's Psychology Services Branch, located within the Reentry Services Division, and its Health Services Division develop policy and oversee the overall psychology, psychiatry, and medical services provided at institutions. Within institutions, psychology, psychiatry, and medical staff provide mental health services to inmates with mental illness. Psychologists have the primary responsibility for diagnosing inmates' mental illness,

[23] We note that the number of MHCL 2, 3, or 4 inmates in the SMU increased by 294 percent (from 36 to 142) from 2010 to 2012 and has since decreased by 78 percent (from 142 to 31).

[24] For more information about the Psychology Services Manual, see Appendix 2.

treating inmates with diagnosed mental illness, and monitoring the mental health of inmates, including all inmates housed in RHUs.[25] Psychologists share these responsibilities with Psychiatrists, particularly for inmates diagnosed with serious mental illness, for whom Psychiatrists may prescribe psychotropic medications.[26] General practitioners may also diagnose inmates' mental illness and prescribe psychotropic medications.[27]

Mental Health Care Policy

In May 2014, the BOP issued a national policy requiring that all inmates receive mental health care commensurate with their needs, even while they are in restrictive housing. The policy seeks to ensure that inmates with mental illness are identified and receive treatment to assist their progress toward recovery and to reduce or eliminate the frequency and severity of symptoms and associated negative outcomes of mental illness, such as placement in restrictive housing. According to the policy, any BOP staff member who observes unusual behavior that may indicate mental illness must report such observations to the institution's Chief Psychologist or Mental Health Treatment Coordinator. The policy also redefines MHCLs, as we described above, and incorporates additional diagnostic, impairment, and intervention-based criteria for inmates designated at MHCL 2, 3, or 4.[28] Additionally, the policy increases the frequency of psychosocial interventions that institution Psychologists are required to provide to inmates with mental illness, mandating that such interventions occur at least monthly for MHCL 2 inmates and at least weekly for MHCL 3 and 4 inmates. The policy requires that these interventions be consistent with the goals of the inmate's treatment and be conducted out of cell, face to face, and in a private setting to the extent possible based on security and safety considerations.[29] Further, the policy establishes a Care Coordination and Reentry (CCARE) team, which is a multidisciplinary team that meets no less than once a month to share information on the treatment needs of inmates with mental illness.[30]

---

[25] Psychologists are not medical doctors, but they attend graduate school and earn a doctorate degree in psychology. They are trained to apply psychological assessments, testing for mental health diagnoses, and various types of treatment; but they generally are not licensed to prescribe medications without additional, specialized training.

[26] Research refers to psychotropic medication as "any drug capable of affecting the mind, emotions, and behavior" of an individual. See MedicineNet.com, "Medical Definition of Psychotropic drug," http://www.medicinenet.com/script/main/art.asp?articlekey=30807 (accessed June 27, 2017).

[27] Both General Practitioners and Psychiatrists attend medical school and become medical doctors who are licensed to diagnose mental illness and prescribe medications, including psychotropic medications. Psychiatrists generally receive more extensive and specialized mental health training than do General Practitioners.

[28] Prior to May 2014, MHCL 1 inmates "required clinical intervention no more frequently than every 3 to 6 months." Under the 2014 policy, MHCL 1 inmates are not required to be evaluated other than during their initial mental health screening but inmates have the option to pursue mental health services on an as-needed basis.

[29] According to the BOP, psychosocial interventions are treatment interventions between mental health staff and inmates and can include different types of psychotherapy, psycho education, self-help and support groups, as well as skills training aimed at providing treatment, education, and support to inmates with mental illness. According to BOP policy, the mental health staff's psychosocial interventions and individualized treatment plans must rely on evidence-based clinical practices that have been demonstrated to reduce the symptoms of mental illness. See BOP Program Statement 5310.16.

[30] According to BOP policy, a CCARE team meets to identify potential issues for inmates with mental illness, such as an inmate who presents mental health symptoms that are unreported or have gone unidentified or who

Finally, the policy requires that all MHCL 2, 3, or 4 inmates have an individualized mental health treatment plan, which Psychology Services staffs are supposed to develop in collaboration with the inmate. Each plan identifies the inmate's individual and/or group programming needs and describes the inmate's mental health conditions and goals and the interventions planned to help the inmate reach them. The policy requires plans to be reviewed and updated every 12 months for MHCL 2 inmates, every 6 months for MHCL 3 inmates, and every 90 days for MHCL 4 inmates.

The policy requires Psychology Services staff to conduct an Extended Restrictive Housing Placement Review for each inmate housed in an RHU for an extended period of time to determine whether he or she has mental issues that preclude placement in this setting. The policy requires that Psychology Services staff conduct these reviews when an inmate is housed in the SHU continuously for 6 months, in the ADX for 12 months, or in the SMU for 18 months.[31]

Restrictive Housing Units

As discussed earlier, to ensure safe and orderly environments for inmates and staff, the BOP utilizes various forms of RHUs to confine some inmates, including inmates with mental illness. The BOP has established policies to govern how inmates are confined in each of the three primary types of RHU.

Special Housing Units

According to the BOP's SHU policy, inmates may be placed in the SHU for disciplinary segregation or administrative detention, but the SHU policy does not specifically address conditions of confinement for inmates with mental illness.[32] All inmates placed in the SHU on administrative detention status receive a segregation review within 3 workdays of placement. All inmates placed in the SHU, regardless of the reason for their placement, receive a formal review within 7 calendar days of placement, with subsequent reviews every 7 continuous days thereafter. In addition, the SHU policy states that after every 30 calendar days of continuous placement, each SHU inmate receives a mental health examination, including a personal interview, and emergency mental health care must always be available.[33]

---

demonstrates escalating patterns of destructive or dangerous behavior. Per policy, the CCARE team must include, at a minimum, the Mental Health Treatment Coordinator (CCARE team co-leader), psychiatric services provider (CCARE team co-leader), treating Psychologist, institution Social Worker (if applicable), and Pharmacist. See BOP Program Statement 5310.16.

[31] BOP Program Statement 5310.16, 16.

[32] Administrative detention status removes the inmate from the general population when necessary to ensure the safety, security, and orderly operation of correctional facilities or to protect the public. Administrative detention status applies only to SHU inmates, is non-punitive, and can occur for a variety of reasons. See BOP Program Statement 5270.10, Special Housing Units (August 1, 2011), 2.

[33] See BOP Program Statement 5270.10, 5–6.

Special Management Units

The BOP's mental health policy excludes the placement of inmates with serious mental illness in the SMU unless there are extraordinary security concerns that prevent their placement elsewhere.[34] According to the BOP's SMU policy, the BOP designates an inmate to a SMU when greater management of the inmate's interaction is necessary to ensure the safety, security, or orderly operation of BOP institutions, or for the protection of the public.[35] Conditions of confinement are more restrictive for SMU inmates than for general population inmates, though the conditions become less restrictive as the inmate progresses through the phases of the SMU program. Each inmate is evaluated by mental health staff every 30 days, and emergency mental health care must always be available at the institution or from the community.

Administrative Maximum Security Facility

The BOP's mental health policy also excludes inmates with serious mental illness from ADX placement unless there are extraordinary security concerns that cannot be met elsewhere.[36] Seriously mentally ill inmates who are to remain at the ADX must have an individualized mental health treatment plan and be provided with at least 10, and as many as 20, hours of out-of-cell time per week, consistent with their treatment plan.[37] In July 2015, the ADX issued local policy for the care and treatment of its inmates with mental illness. The policy establishes that all ADX inmates will receive psychotropic medications as clinically indicated and requires that inmates receiving psychotropic medications be seen by a Psychiatrist, Physician, or Psychiatric Nurse every 90 days, or more often if clinically indicated, for at least the first year of ADX placement. When in-person psychiatry services are not available, private tele-psychiatry is to be provided. In addition to private group counseling and treatment, ADX inmates ordinarily have access to in-cell therapeutic and recreation activities, including access to Psychology Services programming through closed-circuit television.

For all types of restrictive housing, staff members are required to make themselves available to RHU inmates for brief conversations and to demonstrate their concern and availability to help. Qualified health practitioners and one or more responsible officers the Warden designates (ordinarily the Institution Duty Officer) are required to visit each inmate daily, including on weekends and holidays. After every 30 calendar days of continuous placement in an RHU, each inmate, including those with mental illness, is required to be examined by mental health staff. The examination must include a personal

---

[34] See BOP Program Statement 5310.16, 19.

[35] National policy for the operation of the SMU is found in BOP Program Statement 5217.01. As stated earlier, in August 2016 the BOP issued a revised SMU policy. See Appendix 2 for more information.

[36] See BOP Program Statement 5310.16, 19.

[37] U.S. Penitentiary, Administrative Maximum, Institution Supplement FLM 5310.16A, Treatment and Care of Inmates with Mental Illness (July 22, 2015).

interview to evaluate the inmate's adjustment to his or her surroundings and to determine whether the inmate poses any threat to himself or herself, staff, or other inmates.[38]

Prior Reports on the BOP's Use of Restrictive Housing and Inmates with Mental Illness

As part of our review, we examined the following reports published by other agencies related to restrictive housing and mental illness:

The Government Accountability Office's Review of BOP Segregated Housing

In May 2013, the U.S. Government Accountability Office (GAO) issued a report on the BOP's segregated housing unit practices. The GAO found that from FY 2008 through February 2013, the population of SHUs, SMUs, and the ADX had increased 17 percent compared to just 6 percent growth in the BOP's total inmate population during the same period.[39] The GAO also found that the BOP's monitoring of its segregated housing units varied greatly by type of unit, with some institutions' documentation related to conditions of confinement and inmate placement being incomplete and with oversight of ADX-specific conditions of confinement notably lacking. Further, the GAO determined that the BOP had not evaluated the effects of long-term segregation on inmates' mental health, despite BOP policy acknowledging the risks. The GAO recommended that the BOP develop ADX-specific monitoring requirements and that any BOP study to assess segregated housing units also assess the extent that segregated housing contributes to institutional safety and the impact of long-term segregation on inmates in SHUs, SMUs, and the ADX.

The Center of Naval Analysis and Solutions' Review of BOP SHUs

In 2013, the BOP funded an independent assessment of its operation of restrictive housing following a June 2012 Senate Judiciary Committee hearing on solitary

---

[38] BOP Program Statement 5270.10, 11–12.

[39] GAO, *Bureau of Prisons: Improvements Needed in Bureau of Prisons' Monitoring and Evaluation of Impact of Segregated Housing*, GAO-13-429 (May 2013). The GAO also issued *Bureau of Prisons: Timelier Reviews, Plan for Evaluations and Updated Policies Could Improve Inmate Mental Health Services Oversight*, GAO-13-1 (July 2013). Although not specifically related to restrictive housing, the GAO found that the BOP had not evaluated the effectiveness of most mental health treatment programs, that the most common deficiencies cited in Psychology Services program reviews were related to care provided in residential treatment programs, and that delays in completing BOP internal program reviews were most often due to institution staffing issues. The GAO recommended that the BOP update Program Statements 5310.13, Institutional Management of Mentally Ill Inmates (March 31, 1995), and 5310.12, Psychology Services Manual (March 7, 1995).

confinement.[40] During the hearing, the former BOP Director stated that SHUs and the SMU are forms of solitary confinement but that the BOP had no internal studies or policies to evaluate the effects of solitary confinement. Following the hearing (and the release of the GAO's May 2013 report discussed above), the BOP contracted with the Center of Naval Analysis and Solutions (CNA), which issued a report with 9 findings and 11 recommendations specifically related to the diagnosis, care, and treatment of inmates with mental illness in the BOP's RHUs.[41] Most notably, the CNA disagreed with the BOP's mental health diagnoses of inmates in nearly two-thirds of the cases it reviewed and concluded that the treatment the BOP provided was insufficient or inappropriate in over half of the cases it reviewed.

The CNA also found inmates in RHUs whose mental conditions should have precluded them from assignment to these units; that most RHUs had no mental health programming, including out-of-cell programming for inmates; that almost all institutions reported a shortage of staff to provide mental health treatment; and that a number of inmates in RHUs had symptoms of serious mental illness that BOP psychology staff had failed to detect. The BOP concurred with some of the CNA's key findings, but also expressed concern with some recommendations and key points the BOP believed the CNA report had omitted.

The Department of Justice's Report and Recommendations Concerning the Use of Restrictive Housing

In January 2016, the Department issued a report on the use of restrictive housing within the U.S. criminal justice system.[42] The Department's report included "Guiding Principles" to serve "as best practices for correctional facilities within the American criminal justice system" to implement if resources allow. The report defined the term restrictive housing as "any type of detention that includes removal from the general inmate population, whether voluntary or involuntary; placement in a locked room or cell, whether alone or with another inmate; and inability to leave the room or cell for the vast majority of the day, typically 22 hours or more." The Department recommended that the BOP expand its ability to divert inmates with serious mental illness to mental health treatment programs, by increasing the capacity of existing secure mental health units, and provided the BOP with an estimated cost of this expansion. The Department also recommended that the BOP expand its ability to divert "protective custody" inmates to less restrictive forms of housing by building "Reintegration Housing Units" at multiple BOP institutions. The Department further recommended that the BOP cut the duration of the SMU program by half, direct Wardens

---

[40] U.S. Senate, Hearing before the Subcommittee on Constitution, Civil Rights and Human Rights of the Committee on the Judiciary, "Reassessing Solitary Confinement: The Human Rights, Fiscal, and Public Safety Consequences," June 19, 2012.

[41] CNA, *Federal Bureau of Prisons: Special Housing Unit Review and Assessment* (December 2014). The CNA report was issued just prior to the start of the OIG's review. Our review did not seek to support or refute the CNA's findings.

[42] DOJ, *Use of Restrictive Housing.*

to develop plans for expanding out-of-cell time for inmates in restrictive housing, and finalize upgrades in data collection software to improve tracking of inmates in restrictive housing.

A Department official provided the OIG with the Department's "180-day Status Report" on steps the BOP had taken in response to the Department's recommendations.[43] According to the Department, the BOP implemented new training for staff; ended the placement of juveniles and pregnant women in restrictive housing; and limited the length of investigations and maximum penalties for disciplinary violations, as well as the length of stay in SMUs. The BOP also created new "protective custody" units, increased transparency by releasing monthly data on restrictive housing, expanded a mental health pilot program, and enhanced officer-to-inmate communication. Finally, the BOP revised its SHU and SMU policies to address a number of the Department's recommendations. We did not assess the steps that the BOP took in response to the Department's recommendations as part of this review. However, throughout this chapter we provide additional information on steps the BOP has taken as they relate to findings resulting from our review.

Scope and Methodology of the OIG Review

We examined BOP program statements, policies, and other guidance related to the screening, treatment, and monitoring of inmates with mental illness and those related to the SHUs, the SMUs, and the ADX. Our fieldwork occurred from April 2015 through October 2016 and consisted of document review, case file reviews, data analysis, interviews, site visits, and observations. We analyzed BOP population data, mental health data, and restrictive housing data from FY 2010 through May 30, 2015. We also analyzed how the BOP collects and analyzes mental health and RHU data at BOP-managed institutions. We interviewed officials with the Office of the Deputy Attorney General, the Civil Rights Division, BOP officials in the Central Office, institution staff, and representatives from eight state departments of corrections about reforms and policies related to the treatment of inmates with mental illness. We also interviewed inmates with a history of mental illness. See Appendix 1 for more information about the OIG's methodology.

In this chapter, we discuss our concerns related to the confinement of inmates with mental illness in RHUs, including single-cell confinement or conditions that could be considered "solitary confinement," as well as the screening, treatment, and monitoring of

---

[43] DOJ, "Report and Recommendations concerning the Use of Restrictive Housing: 180-day Status Report" (September 2016). The status report also discusses steps taken in response to recommendations directed to the U.S. Marshals Service and the Office of Justice Programs, as well as reforms at the state and local law enforcement levels.

inmates with mental illness, including but not limited to those in restrictive housing.[44] We also discuss steps that the BOP has taken to address concerns with inmates in RHUs, including inmates with mental illness, and additional steps the BOP might take to build on them.

RESULTS OF THE REVIEW

BOP Policies Do Not Adequately Address the Confinement of Inmates with Mental Illness in RHUs, and the BOP Does Not Sufficiently Track or Monitor Such Inmates

During the OIG team's visits to BOP institutions, we found inmates who had been housed in traditional Restrictive Housing Units (RHU), including Special Housing Units (SHU), Special Management Units (SMU), and the U.S. Penitentiary Administrative Maximum Security Facility (ADX), as well as in other conditions of confinement that could be considered solitary confinement. However, the BOP does not have explicit guidance and policy to define or address solitary confinement, extended placement, or restrictive housing. While our review focused on traditional RHUs, including the SHU, the SMU, and the ADX, we found that existing policies do not account for the broad variation of RHUs throughout BOP institutions. In addition, while the BOP recognizes that inmates' mental health can deteriorate if they are held in restrictive housing for long periods of time, BOP policy does not limit the length of time inmates spend in restrictive housing. In contrast, we found that state departments of corrections do limit the length of time inmates spend in restrictive housing. We also found that the BOP does not track inmates' single - cell confinement or assess cumulative time in RHUs. The lack of specificity in BOP policy for RHUs can potentially affect the mental health services provided to all inmates, to include those in RHUs, which is particularly concerning for inmates with mental illness.[45]

---

[44] For the purposes of our analysis, we considered solitary confinement to be an inmate alone in a cell for 22 hours or more per day with limited human contact.

[45] In response to a working draft of this report, the BOP stated that the report cites only research findings with negative outcomes for inmates in restrictive housing. The BOP also said the science in this area is not settled and that credible research with different findings should also be included. The BOP cited as an example a DOJ Office of Justice Programs, National Institute of Justice (NIJ) study on the Colorado Department of Corrections, "One Year Longitudinal Study of the Psychological Effects of Administrative Segregation," https://www.ncjrs.gov/pdffiles1/nij/grants/232973.pdf (accessed June 27, 2017). We note that the NIJ's study states that there may have been other negative consequences of administrative segregation that the study did not evaluate.

Though Policies Do Not Specifically Define "Solitary Confinement," the BOP Houses Inmates in Restrictive Conditions of Confinement that Could Be Considered Solitary Confinement

Neither the BOP nor the Department has a definition for the term solitary confinement. When the OIG asked the BOP for its definition of solitary confinement, the BOP responded: "The Bureau does not recognize the term solitary confinement. Therefore, the Bureau does not have a definition or a reference to provide." The former Correctional Programs Division Administrator told us that "solitary confinement does not exist within the BOP."

However, in testimony at a congressional hearing on solitary confinement, the former BOP Director acknowledged its use in the BOP, stating, "we believe with solitary confinement for the inmates who pose the most violence and disruption within the facility that we utilize it as a deterrent to correct the behavior."[46] Even the former Attorney General acknowledged in early 2016 that solitary confinement does exist within the BOP, stating that she would require from the BOP an "across-the-board reduction of maximum penalties for punitive segregation to curb excessive use of restrictive housing and solitary confinement as punishment."[47] The Department's 2016 report on the use of restrictive housing used restrictive housing as a "general corrections term" to describe various restrictive conditions of confinement but did not use the term "solitary confinement."[48] Rather, it described housing inmates in cells alone as "single-celled," such as the case at the ADX. However, we observed inmates, including inmates with mental illness, housed in similar conditions within BOP institutions that we visited. Research indicates that prolonged exposure to conditions of solitary confinement can result in psychological and psychiatric conditions, such as irritability, anger, aggression, and rage.[49] Inmates could also experience chronic insomnia, loss of control, panic attacks, paranoia, and hypersensitivity to noise, light, and smells.[50]

At the ADX, we observed an RHU that held two inmates on "Range 13," each in his own cell, isolated from other inmates. The inmates did not engage in recreation with each other or with other inmates and were confined to their cells for over 22 hours a day. When

---

[46] Charles E. Samuels, Jr., Director, BOP, before the Subcommittee on Constitution, Civil Rights, and Human Rights of the Committee on the Judiciary, U.S. Senate, concerning "Reassessing Solitary Confinement: The Human Rights, Fiscal, and Public Safety Consequences" (June 19, 2012).

[47] Loretta E. Lynch, U.S. Attorney General, Prepared Remarks (presented at the American Correctional Association Winter Conference, New Orleans, Louisiana, January 26, 2016), https://www.justice.gov/ opa/speech/attorney-general-loretta-e-lynch-delivers-remarks-american-correctional-association (accessed June 27, 2016).

[48] The Department's report defines restrictive housing as having three elements: (1) removal from the general inmate population, whether voluntary or involuntary; (2) placement in a locked room or cell, whether alone or with another inmate; and (3) the inability to leave the room or cell for the vast majority of the day, typically 22 hours or more. See DOJ, *Report and Recommendations concerning the Use of Restrictive Housing* (January 2016), 3.

[49] Craig Haney, Professor of Psychology at the University of California, Santa Cruz, before the Subcommittee on Constitution, Civil Rights, and Human Rights, Committee on the Judiciary, U.S. Senate, concerning "Reassessing Solitary Confinement: The Human Rights, Fiscal, and Public Safety Consequences" (June 19, 2012), 10–11.

[50] Haney, "Reassessing Solitary Confinement."

we asked whether placement on Range 13 could be considered a form of solitary confinement, a Psychologist at the ADX said, "you have no contact, you don't speak to anybody, and it's a form of torture on some level.... [Inmates] still talk to officers and stuff like that, but they don't really get a chance to see anybody.... They rec[reate] alone; we don't even have to be back there to rec them. So, yes, I would say that they are in fact in solitary confinement." Also, an RHU at U.S. Penitentiary (USP) Terre Haute, known as the Special Confinement Unit, houses "death row" inmates in single-cell confinement for an average of 23 hours a day. We interviewed two inmates in this unit who were designated at Mental Health Care Level (MHCL) 2 at the time of our visit. One inmate told us that, since his placement in this RHU 10 years ago, he has been out of his cell for only 3 hours a week, no more than 1 hour a day, and spends the remaining 4 days alone in his cell, 24 hours a day.[51] Another inmate, who has been in this RHU since 2010, stated that, due to the nature of his crime, BOP policy restricts him from recreating or participating in leisure activities with other inmates.[52] Due to these restrictions, he believes that his confinement constitutes solitary confinement.[53]

Further, in five SHUs we observed single-celled inmates, many of whom had a serious mental illness. One inmate, who Staff Psychologists told us was denied placement at the ADX for mental health reasons, had been single-celled for about 4 years because staff believed he posed a serious threat to other inmates given his violent history.[54] While we did not observe inmates celled alone in Federal Correctional Complex (FCC) Petersburg's SHU, a Staff Psychologist told us that single-celling inmates does occur in the institution's SHU and that she did not always know why some inmates were single-celled. She stated that single-celling inmates can be an added risk (to an inmate's mental health) and that, in the past, she has annotated the SHU Application, a computer program, to request that correctional staff refrain from single-celling specific inmates who had mental illness.[55]

---

[51] There are three phases of restriction in the Special Confinement Unit, with Phases 1 and 3 representing the most restrictive levels and Phase 2 representing the least restrictive level. According to BOP policy, inmates will remain at Phase 1 for at least 1 year and may be managed at this level for an indefinite period of time. BOP policy also states that, in addition to recreation, inmates managed at Phase 2 may also participate in out-of-cell leisure activities with up to two other approved inmates; but this time is considered a privilege that is limited to the availability of the common area. We do not know what phase(s) the BOP has used to manage this inmate since his arrival to this RHU. See BOP Institution Supplement THX-5217.01K, Operation and Security of the Special Confinement Unit (June 25, 2015).

[52] This inmate was convicted with his co-defendant of murdering another inmate while in BOP custody. BOP policy states that, "Phase 1 inmates will recreate alone" and that "inmates who have committed murder or attempted to kill anyone while incarcerated will not normally be considered for Phase II." See BOP Institution Supplement THX-5217.01K.

[53] The inmate also told us that he prefers this unit to the SHU at this institution. During our fieldwork, BOP officials, staff, and other inmates told us that inmates sometimes prefer to be housed in RHUs, including single-cell confinement, as opposed to placement in the general population.

[54] Institution staff told us that the inmate had declined to go to the secure residential treatment program, which at that time was pending activation. However, the institution's mental health staff told us that they did not believe that he was seriously mentally ill and thus he was suitable for ADX placement.

[55] We discuss the SHU Application later in this report.

SMU Conditions of Confinement

We found that the conditions of confinement, including the size and ventilation of cells, could result in harm to SMU inmates with mental illness. For example, an unknown number of SMU cells at USP Lewisburg in Pennsylvania do not meet the American Correctional Association's (ACA) minimum standards for restrictive housing cell sizes. ACA standards stipulate that all restrictive housing cells provide a minimum of 80 square feet, of which 35 square feet is to be unencumbered. According to the BOP, some SMU cells at USP Lewisburg are only 58.5 square feet in size. When we asked BOP officials whether USP Lewisburg's SMU cells met ACA standards, they provided conflicting responses. Additionally, a senior official from the BOP's Program Review Division told us that the ACA standards for restrictive housing cell size are not mandatory.

We observed a lack of air conditioning at USP Lewisburg, which was the only one of the seven institutions we visited that relied on ceiling fans instead of air conditioning to ventilate inmates' cells and cellblocks. This is especially troubling since psychotropic medications can hinder the body's ability to sweat. These conditions can make inmates who take psychotropic medications more prone to heat stroke and heat-related illnesses.

Sources: OIG observations; BOP Program Statement 5217.01, Special Management Units (November 19, 2008), 6–7; ACA, *Standards for Adult Correctional Institutions,* 4th ed. (Lanham, Md.: American Correctional Association 2003), 39; Human Rights Clinic, University of Texas School of Law, *Reckless Indifference: Extreme Heat in Texas Prisons* (March 2015), 20.

Although most inmates in the SMU have a cellmate, inmates, including inmates with mental illness, may also be placed in single-cell confinement and in conditions that may jeopardize their mental health. At USP Lewisburg, the only remaining SMU institution, we observed infrastructure issues that were particularly concerning in light of the fact that inmates may be placed in these conditions for years. See the text box below regarding our observations and the concerning conditions of confinement for inmates, including those with mental illness, at USP Lewisburg.

In addition, most inmates placed in RHUs, including those with mental illness, have limited out-of-cell opportunities.[56] For instance, inmates placed in the SHUs do not have out-of-cell programming opportunities and inmates' participation in general population group therapy would be discontinued during their SHU placement, according to Psychology Services Branch officials.[57] These officials indicated that the BOP is looking to provide inmates in restrictive housing with group therapy opportunities but stated that

---

[56] After the completion of our fieldwork, the BOP issued a revised SHU program statement in November 2016. Although we did not evaluate this policy, we note throughout this report examples of changes to the SHU policy as they relate to our findings during the course of our review. For example, to enhance inmates' out-of-cell time, the BOP's revised SHU policy requires that staff at each institution locally develop plans for increasing inmates' recreation and that institutions with the necessary resources should do so. See BOP Program Statement 5270.11, Special Housing Units (November 23, 2016), 12.

[57] We further discuss disruptions to inmate's continuity of care later in this report.

not every institution has the resources to do so. Also, while BOP policy requires that inmates have the opportunity to exercise outside their individual quarters at least 5 hours per week, ordinarily on different days in 1-hour periods, it also states that inmates, including those in single- cell confinement, may have recreation privileges suspended.[58] According to policy, an institution's Warden can deny exercise privileges for a week at a time if it is determined that an inmate's use of recreation threatens the safety, security, and orderly operation of a correctional facility, or public safety. Further, the BOP does not provide recreation on weekends to inmates in RHUs and, consequently, inmates are confined to their cell for approximately 72 consecutive hours every weekend without any out-of-cell opportunities. The BOP's Correctional Programs Division (CPD) officials told us that the BOP does not have the correctional staffing resources to offer recreation to inmates during the weekend. Psychology Services Branch officials also recognized this resource limitation but acknowledged that out-of-cell opportunities during the weekend would be beneficial for inmates, including those with mental illness. We recognize the challenges in providing inmates in RHUs with out-of-cell opportunities; however, confining inmates, particularly those in single-cell confinement, in cells for prolonged periods of time with limited human contact, could potentially harm their mental health.

We found a discrepancy between what we observed at BOP institutions and what Department and BOP policies stated regarding single-cell confinement. The former Acting Chief of Staff for the Office of the Deputy Attorney General told us that the Department did not consider specific policies for double-celling or single-celling inmates when developing its report. He added that the corrections and advocacy communities define solitary confinement differently and that in reality restrictive housing and solitary confinement are the same.[59]

While the Department's report does not define solitary confinement, it does reference Civil Rights Division investigations that, in some cases, define solitary confinement more specifically. A May 2013 Civil Rights Division investigation of the Pennsylvania State Institution at Cresson defined "isolation," or "solitary confinement," as "the state of being confined to one's cell for approximately 22 hours per day or more, alone or with other prisoners, that limits contact with others."[60] In February 2014, the Civil Rights Division completed a system-wide investigation of the Pennsylvania Department of Corrections (PDOC) after having found that prisoners with serious mental illness and intellectual

[58] BOP Program Statement 5270.10, Special Housing Units (August 1, 2011), 8–9.

[59] The Department's report stated that the term solitary confinement is disfavored by correctional officials because, in part, it conjures a specific and in some cases misleading image of the practice. The Department also stated that not all segregation is truly "solitary" because many prisons, including the BOP's, often house two segregated inmates together in the same cell, a practice known as "double-celling." The Department adopted the terms restrictive housing and segregation to avoid this confusion. See DOJ, *Use of Restrictive Housing,* 3.

[60] Thomas E. Perez, Assistant Attorney General, DOJ Civil Rights Division, and David J. Hickton, U.S. Attorney, Western District of Pennsylvania, letter to the Honorable Tom Corbett, Pennsylvania Governor's Office, May 31, 2013, https://www.justice.gov/sites/default/files/crt/legacy/2013/06/03/cresson_findings_5-31-13.pdf (accessed June 27, 2017).

disabilities at Cresson were routinely subjected to solitary confinement under conditions that violated their constitutional rights and their rights under Title II of the *Americans with Disabilities Act of 1990.*[61]

The Mandela Rules

The United Nations' Standard Minimum Rules for the Treatment of Prisoners, Rule 44 states: "For the purpose of these rules, solitary confinement shall refer to the confinement of prisoners for 22 hours or more a day without meaningful human contact. Prolonged solitary confinement shall refer to solitary confinement for a time period in excess of 15 consecutive days." Rule 45 states: "The imposition of solitary confinement should be prohibited in the case of prisoners with mental or physical disabilities when their conditions would be exacerbated by such measures."

According to an official of the U.S. Department of State, the United States "whole-heartedly" endorses all of the United Nations Rules and is proud to have participated in the collaborative process that produced them.

Sources: United Nations, Standard Minimum Rules for the Treatment of Prisoners, September 29, 2015 (Mandela Rules); Sarah Sewall, Under Secretary for Civilian Security, Democracy, and Human Rights, U.S. Department of State, Prepared Remarks (presented at a High Level Presentation of the Nelson Mandela Rules — the Draft Revised Standard Minimum Rules on the Treatment of Prisoners, October 2015).

The February 2014 investigation referred to solitary confinement as "the state of being confined to one's cell for approximately 23 hours a day or more."[62] Since BOP and Department policies do not specifically recognize the term solitary confinement, to help us evaluate actual conditions of confinement in BOP institutions, we considered the Civil Rights Division's definition, as well as the United Nations' "Mandela Rules." According to a March 2016 report from the National Institute of Justice, the United Nations passed the Mandela Rules in May 2015, which represented the first modification to the United

[61] For the purposes of the investigation, the Civil Rights Division used the state's definition of serious mental illness as "a substantial disorder of thought or mood that significantly impairs judgment, behavior, or capacity to recognize reality or cope with the ordinary demands of life."

[62] Jocelyn Samuels, Acting Assistant Attorney General, DOJ Civil Rights Division, and David J. Hickton, U.S. Attorney, Western District of Pennsylvania, letter to the Honorable Tom Corbett, Pennsylvania Governor's Office, February 24, 2014, https://www.justice.gov/sites/default/files/crt/legacy/2014/02/25/pdoc_finding_2-24-14.pdf (accessed June 27, 2017).

A Civil Rights Division Deputy Chief and a Trial Attorney associated with both the Cresson and PDOC investigations told us that they did not know why the definition of solitary confinement changed between their May 2013 and February 2014 findings letters. They also told us that the Civil Rights Division had not directly decided to change the hours from 22 to 23, but rather had done so in collaboration with the BOP and other DOJ components. In the case of the Cresson and PDOC investigations, and other investigations related to corrections, the Civil Rights Division works with the BOP to ensure it does not conflict with BOP policies or practices and that factual distinctions are made before the findings letters are released publicly. The Deputy Chief told us:

We couldn't say anything in a blanket way that if you lock people up for 23 hours a day, for months or even years, that that violates the Constitution. We couldn't say that, because BOP locks people up for 23 hours a day for months and years.... So, therefore, we made factual distinctions [between the BOP and Cresson or PDOC], because we had to.

Nations' standards on the treatment of prisoners in 60 years.[63] The United Nations describes solitary confinement in the Mandela Rules as "confinement of prisoners from 22 hours or more a day without meaningful human contact."[64] (See the text box above).

While the Department's definition of restrictive housing acknowledges the placement of an inmate in a locked room or cell alone, it does not specify how contacts between staff and inmates housed in such conditions are to take place.[65] During our visits to BOP institutions throughout this review, we found that the BOP houses inmates, including those with mental illness, for long periods of time isolated from other inmates and with limited human contact — conditions of confinement that could constitute solitary confinement according to the Civil Rights Division's definition, as well as the Mandela Rules.[66] The Office of the Deputy Attorney General's former Acting Chief of Staff told us that it was clear that restrictive housing usually involved someone being in isolation for 22 hours a day without being able to leave and that focusing on the definition of the term solitary confinement detracts from ensuring that inmates housed in restrictive housing for long periods of time receive meaningful contact. BOP CPD officials told us that meaningful contact was a "pretty broad term" and "hard to define." Finally, officials with the BOP's Psychology Services Branch told us that the BOP has outlined for staff what meaningful contacts should look like, through training and during rounds; however, the BOP does not have policy to describe meaningful contact or the monitoring of inmates in a cell alone.[67]

While we acknowledge that BOP policies require contacts between staff and inmates, not all contacts are specified in BOP policies nor are they specific for inmates housed in a cell alone. By not acknowledging such conditions in policy and establishing when they may be appropriate procedures for the management and care of these inmates, including appropriate contacts for those with mental illness, all inmates in such conditions are potentially subjected to long periods of time in forms of confinement that could exacerbate existing mental illness or create the onset of mental disorder.

The BOP Needs to Improve Its Tracking of Inmates Placed in Single-Cell Confinement

In addition to finding that the BOP's policies are inadequate to address conditions amounting to solitary confinement, we found that the BOP is unaware of how many of its

---

[63] According to an NIJ report, "Rule 43 of the Mandela Rules prohibits both *indefinite* solitary confinement and *prolonged* solitary confinement (defined as lasting more than 15 days)." See NIJ, *Administrative Segregation in U.S. Prisons* (March 2016), 1

[64] United Nations, Mandela Rules.

[65] See DOJ, *Use of Restrictive Housing,* 14.

[66] For the purposes of our analysis, we considered solitary confinement to be an inmate alone in a cell for 22 hours or more a day with limited human contact.

[67] Throughout our review, BOP staff and officials described several forms of contact for inmates in SHUs, including rounds made by Correctional Officers every 30 minutes, a supervisor seeing an inmate during every shift, a Captain seeing inmates every week, and regular visits from inmates' unit team, medical team, and a Chaplain. Also, inmates are fed three times a day and Psychology Services visits each inmate every 30 days. Though communication is through a small window, a Segregation Review Official sees an inmate every 7 days. After 30 days, an inmate will have the opportunity to come out of his or her cell to speak to the Lieutenant.

inmates in RHUs (other than at the ADX or in secure residential mental health treatment programs) are housed alone in a cell (single-cell confinement) because the BOP does not track this information. The former Deputy Assistant Director for the CPD told us that while institution staff review the placement of inmates in the SHU on a weekly basis, there is no national database that identifies inmates who are celled alone or tracks the duration of such placement. He added that there are legitimate reasons why inmates may be single-celled, such as for a contagious disease, disability, protective custody, medical recovery, or because they are a danger to other inmates. Still, in light of mental health concerns, Psychology Services Branch officials told us that they prefer inmates to be double-celled in RHUs; but they acknowledged that some institution staff are not receptive to this practice.

We recognize that some inmates with mental illness may be celled alone for legitimate reasons, such as being too dangerous to house with others. However, we question why the BOP does not separately track inmates who have been in prolonged periods of single-cell confinement because, by most accounts, these inmates are held in conditions of confinement that mirror conditions in the ADX, which can have a detrimental effect on their mental health. Moreover, unlike the ADX, most RHUs are not intended for long-term placement and thus lack the staffing and infrastructure suitable for this type of prolonged confinement. Since the BOP does not specifically track inmates placed in single-cell confinement, BOP officials cannot easily identify inmates celled alone or ascertain the duration of such placement and, consequently, cannot intervene when single-cell confinement may not be necessary or may be unduly harmful to the inmate.

The BOP Does Not Have Adequate Policy to Address the Needs of Inmates with Mental Illness in All RHUs

In addition to inadequate policies addressing single- cell confinement, we found that the BOP's SHU policy, issued in 2011, does not differentiate among the various types of RHUs throughout BOP institutions. Also, neither it nor the mental health policy issued in 2014 adequately addresses the mental health needs of inmates housed in these RHUs. The BOP told the OIG that it defines restrictive housing as "those situations when an inmate is placed in confinement, outside of the general population for the safety, security, and orderly operation of our correctional facilities." The former CPD Deputy Assistant Director said that there are RHUs at all BOP facilities and that the SHU policy sets the standard that all RHU programs have to meet.[68]

---

[68] The BOP's SHU Program Statement (5270.10) provides that alternative segregation housing must be proposed by the Warden to the Regional Director, and ultimately approved by the Assistant Director, CPD, before activation. These alternative housing units will be approved only as SHU overflow for inmates in administrative detention or disciplinary segregation status. Operation of such alternative segregation housing requires compliance with all BOP rules, policies, staffing, and post orders for operating SHUs. See also BOP Program Statement 5310.16, Treatment and Care of Inmates with Mental Illness (May 1, 2014).

Concerns regarding Inmates with Mental Illness in M3

We found at FMC Carswell a unit, known as "M3," which has been used since at least 1999 to house the most volatile and decompensating female inmates (predominately MHCL 4 inmates), with the intent to eventually return them to a less restrictive environment. The Warden told us that inmates with serious mental illness may be placed in this unit for administrative and disciplinary segregation in lieu of traditional SHU placement. We observed that the majority of inmates in this RHU were single-celled, with no designated recreation area. A Correctional Officer who has worked extensively in this unit told us that he has seen a few inmates housed in this unit for about a year. He also told us that when the institution's SHU is full, SHU inmates may also be housed in this unit.

The BOP's SHU policy states that inmates should "receive the opportunity to exercise outside [their] individual quarters at least five hours per week." The Chief Psychologist told us of the challenges, including Correctional Officer staffing, which have hindered the institution from having an outdoor recreation area for inmates in this unit. While the unit has an indoor recreation cell, the Chief Psychologist told us that it is "important for the mental and physical well-being of a person to get sun and fresh air and you cannot do that indoors." In addition, according to BOP's new mental health policy, all inmates in the SHU must receive an extended placement review every 6 months. We found that although the psychology staff conducts monthly SHU reviews for the inmates in this unit, according to the Chief Psychologist these inmates do not receive extended placement reviews because the unit is not considered to be a SHU. We discuss Extended Restrictive Housing Placement Reviews later in this chapter.

Sources: OIG observation and analysis, interviews with BOP staff.

During our site visits, we found forms of restrictive housing in which inmates with mental illness experience conditions of confinement contrary to the BOP's SHU and mental health policies. (See the text box for an example of an RHU at Federal Medical Center (FMC) Carswell in which the practices appear to be contrary to BOP policies).

We also observed another RHU at FMC Carswell, the Administrative Unit, with its own SHU that houses inmates, including those with mental illness, with histories of escape, chronic behavioral problems, repeated incidents of assaultive or predatory behavior, or other special management concerns. As of June 2016, this unit housed 17 total inmates, including 6 inmates at MHCL 2 and 1 inmate at MHCL 3 (the remaining 10 inmates were at MHCL 1). Institution staff said they do not consider this unit to be an RHU but rather a "self-contained, open unit."[69]

However, the unit's local policy establishes, among other things, procedures for the placement of inmates in the unit for "Administrative Detention" or "Disciplinary

---

[69] The Unit Manager told us that all services, including recreation, education, mental health, dentistry, unit team, psychology, and psychiatry, are provided within that unit. The Chief Psychologist told us that in the rare instances when inmates are required to leave the unit, the entire institution is placed on lockdown.

Segregation." Also, the Chief Psychologist told us that the unit "functions like the ADX."[70] Specifically, the institution uses a five-level classification system to manage inmates within the unit and those designated at the highest level are confined to their cells for up to an average of 23 hours per day. The Chief Psychologist told us that although inmates within the unit's SHU receive more frequent clinical contacts from mental health staff than what is required in the SHU policy, none of the inmates in this unit receive SHU reviews, despite the fact that the SHU policy states that all inmates in restrictive housing must be given a SHU review every 30 calendar days to monitor their mental health.

CPD officials told us that the BOP does not maintain a centralized list or otherwise track how many of these other forms of restrictive housing exist. With the exception of SHUs, SMUs, and the ADX, the BOP does not know how many inmates are housed in these units. For example, none of the inmates from FMC Carswell's Administrative Unit, including inmates with mental illness in this unit's SHU, were accounted for in FMC Carswell's SHU population data that the BOP provided to us. However, at time of our visit in August 2015, we observed inmates with mental illness placed in this unit's SHU, including one inmate designated at MHCL 3 and two inmates designated at MHCL 2.

The OIG believes that not recognizing certain types of housing conditions as restrictive housing may prevent inmates with mental illness from receiving appropriate reviews, which has the potential to exacerbate the inmates' mental illnesses. The BOP should identify all forms of restrictive housing throughout its institutions and ensure that all local policies reflect standards established in national policies.[71]

The BOP Does Not Limit the Length of Time Inmates Spend in Restrictive Housing, Including Single-Cell Confinement, Which May Affect Inmates' Mental Health

During the scope of our review, in addition to not accounting for the various types of RHU throughout BOP institutions, no BOP policy limited the length of time inmates can be assigned to an RHU.[72] The BOP's mental health policy states that "inmates referred for

---

[70] In November 2016, the BOP issued a revision to its 1997 Management of Female Offenders policy (see BOP Program Statement 5200.02, Female Offender Manual). We note that this new policy acknowledges this unit and states that, "female offenders will receive mental health screening prior to placement on this unit consistent with the procedures for male inmates referred to the Administrative Maximum Penitentiary (ADX) described in the Program Statement Treatment and Care of Inmates with Mental Illness."

[71] The Department's "Report and Recommendations concerning the Use of Restrictive Housing: 180-day Status Report" (September 2016) states that in May 2016 the BOP began posting data on restrictive housing on its public website, "Statistics," http://www.bop.gov/about/statistics (accessed June 27, 2017). Our review of data posted to the BOP's public website found that the BOP provides data only on those inmates housed in SHUs, SMUs, and the ADX. The Department also reported that the BOP was implementing new software to better track inmates as they progress through restrictive housing and that testing on this software was expected to begin in the fall of 2016.

[72] The ACA manual defines restrictive housing as "a placement that requires an inmate to be confined to a cell at least 22 hours per day." ACA, *Restrictive Housing Performance Based Standards*, 4th ed. (American Correctional Association, August 2016), 3. In addition, the BOP issued a revised SMU policy in August 2016 that, among other things, restricts all inmates' length of time in the SMU to 24 consecutive months. However, it is important to note that this limit applies only to the SMU and that no BOP policy prohibits inmates' continued placement

extended placement in restrictive housing (i.e., SMU, ADX) must be reviewed by Psychology Services staff to determine whether mental health issues exist that preclude placement in this setting."[73] However, neither the BOP nor the Department defines "extended placement."[74] Rather, the BOP policy requires that an inmate receive an Extended Restrictive Housing Placement Review after being continuously housed in the SHU for 6 months, in the ADX for 12 months, or in the SMU for 18 months.[75] Moreover, these are only minimum intervals, after which the staff must review the inmate's placement. The policy does not limit the amount of time an inmate can ultimately spend in an RHU. The former CPD Deputy Assistant Director told us that there is no limit to the amount of time an inmate can be placed on extended placement. He further stated that the length of an inmate's placement in restrictive housing depends on the behavior of the inmate and that RHUs are used in an effort to change or regulate negative behavior. According to BOP data, one MHCL 3 inmate was housed in the SHU for 5 years (1,912 consecutive days).[76] Another inmate with mental illness, who previously had been designated MHCL 2, had spent over 6 years (2,326 consecutive days) in the SMU and was still there at the time of our site visit.[77] Additionally, an MHCL 3 inmate had spent about 19 years (6,874 consecutive days) at the ADX before being transferred to a secure residential mental health treatment program in 2014.[78]

---

in other RHUs (SHUs, ADX, etc.) following 24 months of placement in the SMU. See BOP Program Statement 5217.02, Special Management Units (August 9, 2016).

73 During the scope of our review, BOP policy did not preclude the placement of inmates with serious mental illness in SHUs. While SHU inmates received Extended Restrictive Housing Placement Reviews, BOP policy did not prevent their placement in SHUs. See BOP Program Statement 5310.16, 16, 20–21. We discuss Extended Restrictive Housing Placement Reviews later in Results of the Review.

Since the completion of our fieldwork, the BOP issued a revised SHU policy that prohibits SHU placement for inmates whom mental health staff have designated at MHCL 3 or 4, who have a psychology alert in SENTRY (the BOP's primary mission support database), or who have been identified on the monthly SHU advisory (Hot List) unless the inmate presents an immediate or serious danger to self, staff, or the orderly operation of a facility. In the event that an inmate who meets one of these criteria is placed in the SHU, Psychology Services staff must be notified and must conduct a mental health evaluation within 24 hours of the inmate's placement. See BOP Program Statement 5270.11, 15–16.

74 The ACA defines extended restrictive housing as "housing that separates the offender from contact with general population while restricting an offender/inmate to his/her cell for at least 22 hours per day and for more than 30 days for the safe and secure operation of the facility." ACA, *Restrictive Housing Performance Based Standards*, 3.

The Department's report briefly discusses Extended Restrictive Housing Placement Reviews, replicating language from the BOP's Program Statement 5310.16; but the Department does not define extended placement. See DOJ, *Use of Restrictive Housing*, 51.

75 Institution Psychologists complete Extended Restrictive Housing Placement Reviews, which include records reviews, behavioral observations, a clinical interview, and psychological testing if clinically indicated. See BOP Program Statement 5310.16, 16.

76 According to BOP data, in October 2011 the BOP diagnosed this inmate with Antisocial Personality Disorder and Schizophrenia. The number of consecutive days in the SHU for this inmate was valid as of October 2012, and he was an MHCL 3 inmate as of September 2012.

77 From as early as 2005, the BOP diagnosed this inmate with Oppositional Defiant Disorder, Borderline Intellectual Functioning, Borderline Personality Disorder, Malingering, Antisocial Personality Disorder, and Exhibitionism. The number of consecutive days in the SMU for this inmate was valid as of September 2015, and he was an MHCL 1 inmate at that time. However, he had been designated at MHCL 2 from December 2012 until January 2014.

78 The inmate's diagnoses date to as early as 2006. The BOP has since diagnosed this inmate with Borderline Personality Disorder, Antisocial Personality Disorder, Personality Disorder Not Otherwise Specified, Major

Despite Concerns, the BOP Has Released Mentally Ill Inmates into the Community Directly from RHUs

Based on a sample of 239 SMU inmates with mental illness, we found that 31 inmates (13 percent) were released directly into the community from the SMU. We also found that, on average, these 31 inmates had spent nearly 29 months in the SMU prior to their release. The former CPD Deputy Assistant Director said it is "troubling" to release someone from that status into the community. Some institution staff told us that they are aware of inmates with mental illness who have been released from their institution's SHU directly into the community. One Psychologist stated that within the previous 2 years she could recall an MHCL 3 inmate who was in the SHU for at least 6 months and was then released directly into the community. Both she and the institution's Chief Psychologist told us that releasing inmates from the SHU directly into the community has become increasingly rare in recent years as the BOP has improved its efforts to prevent it. We did not find that inmates at the ADX had been released directly into the community. The Deputy Chief Psychologist over the ADX told us that this does not occur and that inmates will be transferred to and released from other institutions. However, she also stated that until a couple of years ago the BOP used to transfer ADX inmates with upcoming release dates to a U.S. Penitentiary that would then place the inmates in its SHU until they were released into the community. She stated that this practice was "no different than releasing from the ADX."

Sources: OIG analysis.

These cases show that inmates, including those with mental illness, may in effect be placed in an RHU for an unlimited amount of time. Not only may inmates be placed in restrictive housing, including in single-cell confinement, for what essentially could amount to an unlimited amount of time; but, equally concerning, inmates may be placed in these conditions for long periods of time and then be released directly into the community, as we discuss in the text box below.[79] Research shows that "time spent in solitary confinement contributes to elevated rates of recidivism" and that many inmates released into the community from RHUs "come out of these units damaged and functionally disabled," which can be a public safety concern.[80]

Depressive Disorder-Recurrent, and Anxiety Disorder Not Otherwise Specified. At the time of his departure from the ADX, he was designated at MHCL 3 and transferred to a secure residential treatment program. We discuss these programs later in this report.

[79] In August 2016, the OIG released a report on the BOP's Release Preparation Program, which seeks to prepare inmates for the challenges they will face when they are released into the community. DOJ OIG, *Review of the Federal Bureau of Prisons' Release Preparation Program,* Evaluation and Inspections Report 16-07 (August 2016). Also see DOJ OIG, *Audit of the Federal Bureau of Prisons' Management of Inmate Placements in Residential Reentry Centers and Home Confinement*, Audit Report 17-01 (November 2016).

In November 2016, the BOP issued its revised SHU policy, which stated that, ordinarily, inmates nearing the end of their term of incarceration will not be placed in SHU, except when their presence in the general population threatens the safety, security, or the orderly operation of a BOP institution, and that every effort will be made to prevent inmates' direct release from the SHU into the community. See BOP Program Statement 5270.11, 16.

[80] Haney, "Reassessing Solitary Confinement," 15.

State Departments of Corrections Do Limit the Length of Time that Inmates Spend in Long-term Restrictive Housing

The OIG found that, unlike the BOP, at least some state departments of corrections do limit the length of time inmates are placed in restrictive housing. We interviewed officials from eight state departments of corrections (Colorado, Maine, Massachusetts, New York, Virginia, Mississippi, Washington, and Pennsylvania) to better understand their initiatives to limit or prohibit the placement of inmates with serious mental illness in restrictive housing.[81] Corrections officials from three states (Massachusetts, New York, and Mississippi) told us that their states have at least a 30-day limit on housing inmates with serious mental illness in RHUs.[82] We also found that three other states (Pennsylvania, Colorado, and Maine) no longer place inmates with serious mental illness in RHUs at all. We found that states are implementing alternatives to long-term segregation by placing inmates with serious mental illness in residential treatment programs. We discuss these state programs, as well as the BOP's secure residential mental health treatment programs, later in this chapter.

The BOP Does Not Monitor Inmates' Cumulative Time in All RHUs

Inmates' Cumulative Time in the SHU May Be Extensive

As we discussed in the Introduction, studies have shown that the frequency, duration, and conditions of confinement of restrictive housing, even for short periods of time, can cause psychological harm and significant adverse effects on inmates' mental health. While the BOP tracks and monitors inmates' time in SHUs, we found that the BOP does not monitor inmates' cumulative time in SHUs. According to officials with the BOP's Psychology Services Branch, assessing such information could be clinically relevant for some inmates. As a result of the BOP's failure to track such information, the BOP cannot determine the number of inmates who frequent the SHUs in multiple, shorter durations or may have longer overall periods in such conditions of confinement. BOP policy now requires that all inmates receive an Extended Restrictive Housing Placement Review after 180 consecutive days in the SHU.[83] To assist institutions in meeting this requirement, the BOP developed a dashboard that each month notifies institutions of inmates who have been in the SHU for at least 150 consecutive days and may be due for their review during the upcoming month.[84] However, Psychology Services Branch officials and staff told us that

---

[81] We found that each state department of corrections has a different definition of serious mental illness and a different inmate mental health classification system.

[82] In response to a working draft of this report, an official with Mississippi's Department of Corrections told us that, since the time of our fieldwork in 2015, Mississippi no longer limits the placement of inmates with serious mental illness in restrictive housing.

[83] BOP Program Statement 5310.16, 20.

[84] While BOP policy requires that all inmates receive an Extended Restrictive Housing Placement Review after every 180 consecutive days in the SHU, the BOP staff must still check the report to verify which inmates are due for review by the end of each month. For example, the dashboard may identify inmates who have been in the SHU

the clock resets if an inmate has a 24-hour break in SHU housing placement.[85] Consequently, an inmate theoretically could spend up to 363 days of the year in the SHU, up to 179 days at any time and, per policy, not warrant an Extended Restrictive Housing Placement Review. In addition, a Staff Psychologist said that when an inmate leaves the SHU, his or her record in the SHU Application is "completely erased."[86] This includes the Psychology Services staff's mental health notes for SHU correctional staff, which can be comprehensive for inmates with serious mental illness. Collectively, these limitations may compromise the BOP's ability to monitor inmates who have been in SHUs for multiple, shorter durations that add up to extensive periods of time and can limit the Psychology Services staff's ability to detect deteriorations in mental health that would make continued SHU placement inappropriate.

Inmates with Mental Illness Are in the ADX Significantly Longer Than Their Peers

As with the cumulative time that inmates spend in the SHU, the BOP does not monitor the cumulative time in the ADX for inmates, including inmates with mental illness, who have been placed there on multiple occasions. Psychology Services Branch officials told us that they would not normally be aware of an inmate's prior placement in the ADX unless the inmate had previously been removed from the ADX for mental health reasons.[87] Rather than assessing cumulative time, the BOP monitors the number of consecutive days that inmates are placed in the ADX. Based on the most recent data available, from November 2013, the BOP determined that inmates had been confined in the ADX for an average of 1,376 consecutive days (about 45 months, or 3.8 years).[88]

We analyzed data for a judgmental sample of 82 ADX inmates with mental illness to determine the average number of consecutive days they had spent at the facility.[89] We found that 59 inmates from our sample, as of November 23, 2013, had spent an average of 1,906 consecutive days (about 63 months, or 5.25 years) in the ADX. Our analysis showed

---

for 9 months but do not require their second Extended Restrictive Housing Placement Review until they reach 1 year in the SHU.

[85] BOP officials told us that while the dashboard is useful, it has limitations and that ultimately it is the responsibility of institutions' SHU staff to ensure that all inmates who require an Extended Restrictive Housing Placement Review receive one, whether or not the dashboard identifies them. For example, institution staff told us of an inmate who had been housed in the SHU for approximately 4 years as of August 2015. Based on our analysis of dashboard reports, at the end of FY 2014 this inmate was reported as having been in the SHU for only 290 days.

[86] As referenced above, the SHU Application is a computer program that the SHU staff uses to manage, record, and track daily activities in the SHU. Although the SHU Application does not preserve the notes mental health staff document for SHU correctional staff once the inmate's placement in the SHU concludes, clinical notes documented by mental health staff in the BOP's mental health system (the Bureau's Electronic Medical Record System and Psychology Data System (BEMR-PDS)) are preserved, regardless of the inmate's housing assignment.

[87] CPD officials told us that they would be aware of an inmate's previous placement in the ADX but this would not be a consideration for them in deciding whether the inmate should be re-admitted to the ADX.

[88] Center of Naval Analysis and Solutions (CNA), *Federal Bureau of Prisons: Special Housing Review and Assessment* (December 2014).

[89] Our inmate sample includes all ADX inmates whom the BOP designated at MHCLs 2–4 from the end of FY 2010 through May 30, 2015.

that inmates with mental illness were housed at the ADX for an average of more than 17 months longer than what the BOP reported for all ADX inmates (See Table 2).

Table 2. BOP ADX Statistics vs. OIG ADX Analysis

	BOP Statistics ADX Inmates	OIG Analysis ADX Inmates with Mental Illness
Total No. of ADX Inmates	415	59
Average No. of Days at the ADX	1,376	1,906
Median No. of Days at the ADX	941	1,213

Note: The data in this table was valid as of November 23, 2013.

Sources: BOP Office of Research and Evaluation and OIG analysis of BOP data.

In total, we found that our entire sample of inmates with mental illness had been placed in the ADX for an average of 2,109 consecutive days (about 69 months, or 5.8 years).[90] Thus, our analysis indicates that inmates with mental illness were housed at the ADX significantly longer than their peers.

Inmates with Mental Illness Are in the SMU Significantly Longer than the Program's Intended Duration

We also examined the length of time that inmates with mental illness spent in the SMU. Similar to the ADX, the BOP monitors consecutive days for inmates who are placed in the SMU, but not their cumulative time in such units. We also found that, even focusing on consecutive days in the SMU, inmates with mental illness spend, on average, about 5 to 11 months longer than the program's intended duration of 18 to 24 months.[91] Between FY 2008 and FY 2015, inmates with mental illness averaged about 896 consecutive days, or about 29 months, in the SMU program and 50 percent of stays in a SMU by inmates with mental illness were longer than 24 months.[92] (See Figure 1 below.) From our sample of SMU inmates, we also found that inmates with mental illness were housed in the SMU for almost 14 months longer than what the BOP reported for all SMU inmates. Specifically, in November 2013, the BOP reported that the average length of stay for all inmates in the SMU, including inmates with mental illness, was 277 days, or about 9 months.[93] However, we found that 151 SMU inmates with mental illness from our sample were still in the SMU

[90] This data was valid as of December 2015.

[91] BOP Program Statement 5217.01, Special Management Units (November 19, 2008), 1.

[92] Our sample included all 239 SMU inmates whom the BOP had designated as MHCL 2–4 at the end of FYs 2012, 2013, or 2014 or on May 30, 2015. "Stay" refers to the number of consecutive days the inmate spent in the SMU. See Appendix 1 for more information.

Although the OIG was able to determine that inmates with mental illness were placed in the SMU significantly longer than the program's intended duration, the OIG could not conduct a similar analysis for inmates with mental illness at the ADX because this RHU does not have an intended duration of placement for its inmates.

[93] The BOP's data was valid as of November 23, 2013, and was reported as part of the CNA's 2014 report on special housing.

at that time and had spent, on average, 698 days, or about 23 months, in the SMU.[94] (See Table 3 below.)

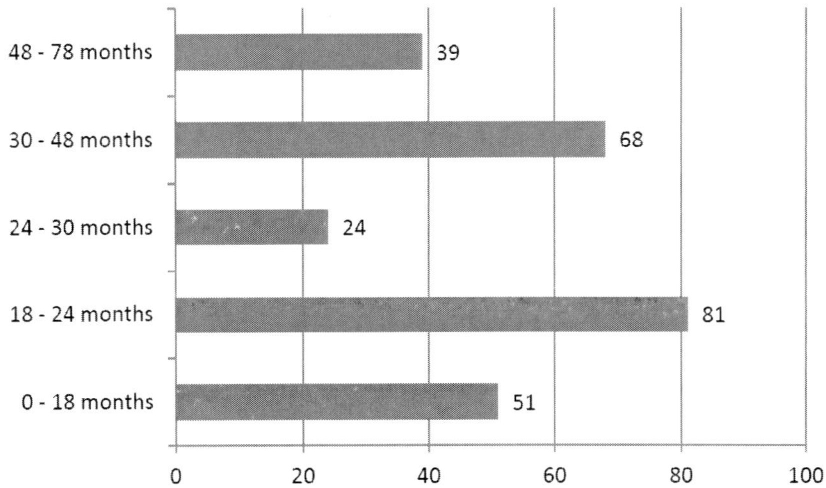

Note: The sample includes 239 inmates, and statistics are valid as of September 3, 2015. Because some sample inmates participated in the SMU program multiple times, this figure displays the lengths of 263 inmate stays in the SMU. The longest length of stay was 2,326 days, or about 76.5 months, by an inmate still in the SMU.

Source: OIG analysis of BOP data.

Figure 1. Months that Inmates with Mental Illness Spent in the SMU FY 2008 – FY 2015.

Perhaps even more concerning is that the most recent analysis from our SMU sample suggests that the length of time for inmates with mental illness who were still in the SMU was increasing. As of September 2015, 65 of the inmates from our SMU sample were still in the SMU and had been there for 935 consecutive days (about 31 months).[95] This is particularly troubling in light of other concerns we address later in this chapter regarding the mental health treatment provided to SMU inmates at USP Lewisburg, which now houses all SMU inmates.

---

[94] These 151 inmates included all SMU inmates whom the BOP had designated as MHCL 2, 3, or 4 at the end of FYs 2012, 2013, or 2014 or on May 30, 2015, and who were in the SMU as of November 23, 2013. See Appendix 1 for more information.

[95] After the completion of our fieldwork, the BOP issued a revised SMU policy, which now restricts all inmates' length of time in the SMU to 24 consecutive months (see BOP Program Statement 5217.02). However, even with the BOP's revised policy, inmates may still spend long periods of time in restrictive housing, without limit, before coming to the SMU or after leaving the SMU. One SHU Lieutenant we interviewed stated that, because of limited SMU capacity, approximately 30 inmates were in the SHU for over a year before finally being transferred to the SMU. Additionally, he stated that two of these inmates were still in the SHU awaiting transfer to the SMU at the time of our visit.

The Department's "180-day Status Report" stated that the BOP had reduced the SMU program to three phases that would take, on average, 9 to 13 months to complete. The report also stated that the BOP had established an incentive program for high-performing inmates to advance through the program on a faster timeline.

Table 3. Average Lengths of Stay for Inmates in the SMU

	BOP Statistics All SMU Inmates	OIG Analysis SMU Inmates with Mental Illness
Total No. of SMU Inmates	1,675	151
Average No. of Days in SMU	277	698
Median No. of Days in SMU	211	628

Note: The data in this table was valid as of November 23, 2013.
Source: BOP Office of Research and Evaluation and OIG analysis of BOP data.

Misleading Performance Metrics

We also found that misleading performance metrics in SMU program data could suggest that inmates with mental illness complete the SMU program at higher rates than they actually do. For example, CPD officials said that an inmate should be designated as "SMU Complete" in the BOP's program data only if the inmate has progressed through all phases of the SMU program and has returned to the general population. However, when we examined our sample of 239 inmates with mental illness, we found that 138 inmates were identified as SMU Complete, but 15 of the 138 (11 percent) were actually transferred out of the program for mental health reasons, not because they had completed the program.[96]

In addition, we found that BOP policy provides that an inmate can be designated as a "SMU Failure" if the inmate continues to exhibit disruptive conduct after spending 30 months in the SMU, 6 months beyond the program's maximum intended duration of 24 months.[97] The Warden at USP Lewisburg told us that when he arrived in June 2014 there were over 100 inmates designated as SMU Failures. He said that was no longer the case because inmates were "programming" and progressing through the SMU program's phases. At the time of our site visit in July 2015, this institution had only five inmates designated as SMU Failures. However, as discussed above, there were 65 inmates from our sample who were still in the SMU as of September 2015 and had spent, on average, 935 days, or about 31 consecutive months, there. Despite this, *none* of our sample inmates were designated as SMU Failures, including one inmate who had been in the SMU for almost

---

[96] During our fieldwork, in September 2015 the BOP stated that, "we are unaware of the existence of any data that would indicate the reason for removal from SMU, beyond the assignments of Complete or Fail." In response to a working draft of this report, the BOP stated that staff document a unique code in SENTRY for inmates who were removed from the SMU for mental health reasons.

The BOP cited a February 2017 memorandum from the Assistant Director of CPD to the Chief Executive Officers, which reflected the existence of an assignment code in SENTRY with a description for "SMU Removal Mental Health." While this code may exist today, the fact remains that none of the 15 inmates that we cited above should have been documented as having completed the SMU program.

[97] See BOP Program Statement 5217.01, 11. In this revised SMU policy, the BOP has reduced the intended duration of the SMU program to 9 to 13 months. In addition, the policy states that if an inmate fails to complete the SMU program within 24 consecutive months, which is the maximum amount of time for an inmate to be placed in the SMU, the inmate will be placed in SMU Failure status and the BOP will identify an appropriate institution for the inmate.

77 consecutive months. This data suggests that, contrary to BOP policy, the BOP may in effect rarely be designating inmates as SMU Failures, even though many inmates appear to meet this criteria and remain in the SMU well beyond the program's maximum intended duration. In October 2016, a CPD official confirmed that inmates who remained in the SMU 6 months longer than the program's maximum intended duration should be classified as a SMU Failure throughout the remainder of their placement.

Finally, many inmates with mental illness were given new SMU entry dates before ever leaving the program. We found that 53 of our sample of 239 SMU inmates with mental illness started the program multiple times, and 5 inmates restarted the program within 2 weeks of being designated as SMU Failures. While some of these inmates completed the program, transferred to other institutions, and were sent back to the SMU, more than half of the inmates who restarted the program did so before they had exited the program. CPD officials told us that SMU inmates may have received a new entry date when they transferred from different SMU institutions. However, by giving new entry dates to SMU inmates who restarted the program from the beginning, the BOP could artificially decrease the documented length of stay for these inmates. Consistent with our findings discussed earlier, this practice could prevent the BOP from accurately tracking inmates as they progress through the SMU program, and inmates with mental illness may linger in multiple iterations of the program much longer than what BOP data indicates.

Mental Health Staff Do Not Always Document Inmates' Mental Disorders, Leaving the BOP Unable to Accurately Determine the Number of Inmates with Mental Illness and Ensure that It Is Providing Appropriate Care to Them

We found that the BOP cannot accurately determine the number of its inmates who have mental illness, including inmates in RHUs, because institution staffs do not always document inmates' mental disorders. This could prevent the BOP from ensuring that it is caring for all of these inmates appropriately.

Based on our analysis of BOP FY 2014 data, 19,034 inmates, or approximately 12 percent of the BOP's total inmate population, had a history of mental illness.[98] However, this number appears too low to be accurate, according to BOP officials and institution staff. In 2015, the BOP's Chief Psychiatrist estimated, based on discussions with institutions'

---

[98] We determined the prevalence of inmates with a history of mental illness by quantifying those inmates who had at least one documented BOP diagnosis — either current, in remission, or resolved — provided in the BOP's data. This includes both psychotic disorders and personality disorders but excludes chemical dependency (substance abuse). This does not include inmates who had undergone an initial mental health records review, were given a tentative MHCL designation by the BOP's Designation and Sentence Computation Center, but had yet to be examined, in person, by a mental health clinician. See Appendix 1 for more information.

As discussed in the Introduction, according to the BOP's *Mental Health Prevalence Project*, approximately 19 percent of federal inmates entering the BOP had a history of mental illness.

Psychology Services staffs, that approximately 40 percent of inmates had a mental illness, excluding inmates with only personality disorder diagnoses. A Deputy Chief Psychologist estimated that 50 percent of inmates at her institution (which housed 961 total inmates as of May 2015) may have Antisocial Personality Disorder, which, according to staff we spoke with, is one of the most prevalent mental disorders among BOP inmates. Nevertheless, we found that this disorder was documented for only about 3.3 percent (5,272) of the BOP's total inmate population (157,872).[99] Psychology Services Branch officials told us that the BOP's mental health policy requires mental health staff to document mental disorders for inmates with an enduring pattern of behavior and for Antisocial Personality Disorder, a pervasive pattern of antisocial behavior may not necessarily be identified during an intake screening evaluation.[100] However, we believe that the underrepresentation of this disorder could also indicate that a significant number of inmate disorders are not formally documented and may as a result go untreated. The BOP's data indicates that approximately 22 percent of inmates in RHUs had a history of mental illness at the end of FY 2014.[101] Specifically, according to our analysis of BOP data, 37 percent of ADX inmates, 27 percent of SMU inmates, and 21 percent of SHU inmates had a history of mental illness.[102] (See Figure 2).

We believe that the BOP data used to determine the above numbers of inmates with mental illness in these RHUs may well be underinclusive. For example, in August 2015, during our site visit to the ADX, we observed a Care Coordination and Reentry (CCARE) meeting. Prior to this meeting, the ADX staff provided us with mental health documentation for 109 inmates whose cases the staff reviewed during the meeting. Based on this documentation, we found that 76 (70 percent) inmates had at least 1 mental health diagnosis. We also found that 71 (93 percent) of these 76 inmates were diagnosed with at least Antisocial Personality Disorder.[103] However, as of the date of this CCARE meeting,

---

[99] This includes both Antisocial Personality Disorder and Adult Antisocial Personality Disorder.

[100] In response to a working draft of this report, the BOP stated that an Antisocial Personality Disorder diagnosis would be given as a mental health diagnosis only if the inmate was functionally impaired in prison as a result of the condition (e.g., self-harm, poor emotional regulation, distress).

According to BOP policy, "all current mental health illnesses should be diagnosed in a Diagnostic and Care Level Formulation note in PDS, including personality disorders and intellectual disabilities. The cumulative effect of the disorders on functioning is taken into account when assigning a mental health care level." See BOP Program Statement 5310.16, 9.

[101] Using the BOP's unique inmate registration numbers, we cross-referenced SHU, SMU, and ADX population data as of September 30, 2014, with BEMR-PDS data as of September 30, 2014. See Appendix 1 for more information.

[102] The BOP's FY 2014 population data for the ADX included 936 total inmates, 46 of whom were designated at MHCLs 2–4. However, during our site visit to the ADX, the staff provided us with documentation that the ADX's rated capacity is 490 inmates. Further, many of the inmates provided in the BOP's population data had minimum, low, and medium security levels, which is inconsistent with inmates housed in the ADX. According to the BOP, this dataset included inmates housed in the Minimum Security Camp (Camp) as well as ADX inmates because, at the time, the ADX was responsible for the Camp and thus ADX staff counted its inmates. In March 2015, inmates in the Camp were realigned in the BOP's database to fall under FCC Florence's medium security institution. Therefore, we selected all 397 inmates with a high security level designation, which is consistent with inmates at the ADX. See Appendix 1 for more information.

[103] We included Adult Antisocial Personality Disorder diagnoses into this raw count and excluded chemical dependency (substance abuse).

99 of the 109 inmates (91 percent) were designated at MHCL 1 and the remaining 10 inmates (9 percent) were designated at MHCL 2.

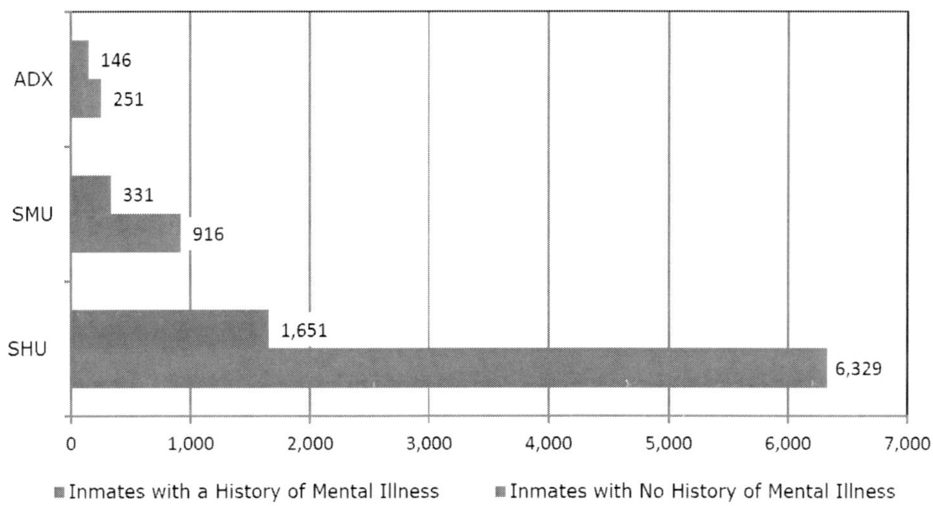

Source: OIG analysis of BOP data.

Figure 2. Inmates with a History of Mental Illness by RHU Type, FY 2014.

According to BOP policy, all inmates designated at MHCLs 2–4 must have been diagnosed with mental illness along with a Psychologist's rationale for the inmate's diagnosis and assigned care level.[104] However, based on our analysis of the BOP's FY 2014 data, 968 of 5,542 inmates (17 percent) designated at MHCLs 2–4 across BOP institutions did not have any documented diagnoses of mental illness. We also found that 74 of these 968 inmates (8 percent) were housed in RHUs.[105] The BOP's Chief of Mental Health Services told us that she had found a similar percentage of inmates who did not have a documented mental health diagnosis. Based on her review of a sampling of inmate records in the Bureau's Electronic Medical Record System and Psychology Data System (BEMR-PDS), she stated that BOP staff had not entered any mental health diagnoses in BEMR-PDS for "a few" of the 968 inmates. She said that the incomplete dataset was caused mostly by diagnoses that were not properly entered.[106] In response to a working draft of this chapter, the BOP stated that staff were not documenting diagnoses in the appropriate location in BEMR-PDS. To reconcile this issue, Psychology Services Branch officials told us that they had alerted institution staff about inmates designated at MHCL 2–4 who did not have a documented diagnosis in the system that was consistent with the *Diagnostic and*

[104] See BOP Program Statement 5310.16, 9.

[105] Of the 74 inmates, 1 inmate was in the ADX, 1 inmate was in the SMU program, and 72 inmates were in SHUs.

[106] The Chief of Mental Health Services elaborated that while staff entered diagnoses in BEMR-PDS, they either did not enter the appropriate diagnosis code or they manually entered diagnoses as free text rather than selecting diagnoses from a drop-down menu. As a result, she indicated that these inmates' diagnoses were not included in the data provided to the OIG. It was beyond our scope to further review them.

Statistical Manual for Mental Disorders (DSM).[107] In addition, these officials said that the BOP has since made changes in BEMR-PDS to ensure that mental health staff consistently enter DSM diagnoses.

Finally, we found that the BOP could improve its management and oversight of inmates with mental illness if it differentiated inmates at MHCL 1 who have mental illness and inmates who do not. According to BOP policy, inmates designated at MHCL 1 are not required to have a mental health diagnosis.[108] According to BOP data, over 90 percent of inmates are designated at MHCL 1, including most inmates with documented mental illness. However, as we indicate above, some inmates have undocumented mental illness and, as a result, the BOP cannot differentiate between inmates designated at MHCL 1 who may have undocumented mental health diagnoses and inmates who do not have any mental health diagnoses. To reconcile this issue, the BOP could reassess its MHCL system and use different classifications to differentiate between inmates who have some form of mental illness from inmates who do not have mental illness.

Since the BOP Adopted Its New Mental Health Policy, BOP Data Shows a 30 Percent Reduction in the Number of Inmates Who Receive Regular Mental Health Treatment

As noted in the Introduction, in May 2014 the BOP issued a new mental health policy intended to enhance the treatment of inmates with mental illness, including those in RHUs.[109] During our review, we found that the BOP has not provided sufficient resources, specifically with regard to the number of mental health staff, to implement the new policy. With no corresponding increase to mental health staff, we believe that mental health staff at institutions may have reduced the number of inmates designated at MHCLs 2–4 to help alleviate the increased work requirements associated with these care levels. Based on our analysis of BOP data, from the end of FY 2010 through April 2014, the number of inmates designated at MHCLs 2–4 remained relatively steady, decreasing by only 1 percent. However, as we describe in detail below, during the year after the new policy was issued, the number of inmates designated at MHCLs 2–4 decreased approximately 30 percent.[110] In addition, we found that the BOP's current mental health staffing challenges could result

---

[107] American Psychiatric Association, *Diagnostic and Statistical Manual for Mental Disorders,* 5th ed. (Arlington, Va.: American Psychiatric Association, 2013).

[108] BOP Program Statement 5310.16, 8.

[109] BOP Program Statement 5310.16.

[110] We requested that the BOP provide inmate population data for May 1, 2014. However, due to technical issues, the BOP instead provided us with inmate population data for April 26, 2014. We thus determined the BOP's decline in inmates' MHCLs from April 26, 2014, to May 30, 2015.

Additionally, while we indicate in the Introduction that the BOP reported a slightly smaller decline (about 20 percent) for inmates designated at MHCLs 2–4 from FY 2010 through May 2015, the BOP told us that it also had found a 30 percent reduction from April 2014 to May 2015.

in some inmates with mental illness, including those in RHUs, not receiving the appropriate treatment for their mental health needs. Finally, we found that mental health staffs disagree on the diagnoses of inmates with mental illness, and even more so for inmates in some RHU programs, which can affect the treatment and continuity of care of inmates with mental illness in RHUs.

Insufficient Resources to Implement the New Policy May Have Affected How Clinicians Determined the Mental Health Treatment Needs of Inmates

The BOP's new mental health policy requires staff to provide more comprehensive care and treatment for inmates with mental illness, including inmates with mental illness in RHUs. We found that mental health clinicians may have reduced, or been reluctant to increase, some inmates' MHCLs because of a lack of resources to implement the enhanced treatment standards. According to the Senior Deputy Assistant Director of the Reentry Services Division (RSD), which oversees the BOP's mental health services, the BOP's new policy "raised the bar" for the mental health care that the BOP wanted to provide to its inmates. The Chief of Mental Health Services told us that the BOP had expected to see an increase in inmates designated at MHCLs 2–4 under the new policy, and that its objective in developing the policy was to encourage staff to be "thoughtful and inclusive of the need for treatment when they see it." For example, the policy introduced the term "serious mental illness," which included personality disorders.[111] The Chief of Mental Health Services said that, prior to the new policy, mental health staff may not have considered personality disorders to be serious mental illness.[112] She added that personality disorders are very serious throughout the BOP's inmate population, are more prevalent in restrictive housing, and may require more frequent treatment than under the previous policy. [113] In light of this information, we believe that the inclusion of personality disorders in the criteria for serious mental illness certainly should have contributed to an overall increase in inmates designated at MHCLs 2–4 after adoption of the new policy in May 2014. According to BOP data, from the end of FY 2010 through April 2014, the number of MHCL 2–4 inmates

---

[111] According to the BOP staff we interviewed, personality disorders are among the most prevalent mental disorders throughout the BOP's inmate population.

[112] The Coordinator of a secure residential mental health treatment program told us that some mental disorders, such as personality disorders, do not involve psychosis, which may cause some staff to view these disorders as less severe forms of mental illness. We discuss secure residential mental health treatment programs later in the report and in Appendix 3.

[113] For example, as we discuss above, in August 2015 ADX staff provided us with mental health documentation for 109 inmates whose cases the staff reviewed during a CCARE meeting. Based on this documentation, we found that 76 (70 percent) inmates had at least 1 mental health diagnosis and that 71 (93 percent) of those were diagnosed with at least Antisocial Personality Disorder. In addition, a SMU Psychologist told us that approximately 90 percent of SMU inmates have mental illness, if personality disorders are included, and that over 90 percent of SMU inmates exhibit antisocial behavior.

had remained relatively steady, decreasing by only 1 percent.[114] Yet, from the end of April 2014 through May 2015, after the BOP issued its new mental health policy, the number of MHCL 2–4 inmates *decreased* about 30 percent, including a decrease in the number of MHCL 2–4 inmates at USP Hazelton by approximately 81 percent (from 238 to 46 inmates).[115]

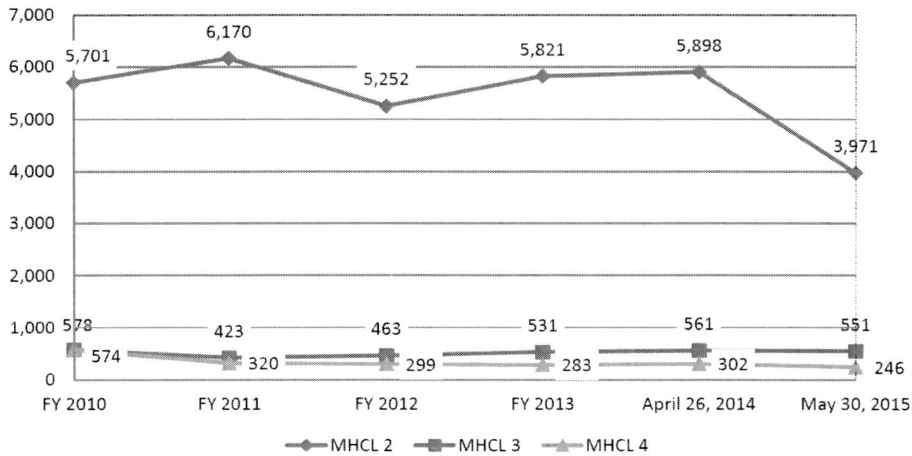

Source: OIG analysis of BOP data.

Figure 3. Number of MHCL 2–4 Inmates, September 2010 – May 2015.

Figure 3 below shows the BOP's total number of sentenced inmates designated at MHCLs 2–4 across all BOP institutions from the end of FY 2010 through May 2015. Based on a sample of 688 inmates in RHUs during the period of our review, we found that after May 2014 — when the new policy was implemented — the mental health staff was more likely to decrease and less likely to increase some inmates' MHCLs.[116] We found that prior to implementation of the new policy, for our sample of 688 RHU inmates, 178 inmates' MHCL increased, compared to 85 inmates whose MHCL decreased. Since the new policy, 45 inmates' MHCL increased, compared to 110 inmates whose MHCL decreased. Table 4 and Figure 4 below show the changes in the MHCLs for our sample of inmates in RHUs.[117]

---

[114] We based the percentage on the number of MHCL 2–4 inmates (6,853 out of the BOP's total of 154,760 inmates) at the end of FY 2010, compared to the number of MHCL 2–4 inmates (6,761 out of 159,284) as of April 26, 2014.

[115] We based the percentage on the number of MHCL 2–4 inmates (6,761 out of 159,284 total inmates) in April 2014, compared to the number of MHCL 2–4 inmates (4,768 out of 155,652) in May 2015. The median for our analysis is an MHCL reduction of approximately 28 percent.

[116] Our analysis is limited to a sample because it was not feasible to assess every inmate's MHCL history. We selected a sample of RHU inmates designated at all MHCLs and individually assessed the history of changes in their MHCLs before and after the new policy was issued. Our analysis does not account for every MHCL change that may have occurred between these times, but notes the inmate's MHCL change, when applicable, from FY 2010 through April 2014 and from late April 2014 through August 2015. See Appendix 1 for more detailed information on our methodology.

[117] Although the BOP established the MHCL system in December 2009, a few inmates in our sample had MHCLs initiated as early as October 2009, which explains why the scope of Table 4 and Figure 4 (below) predates when MHCLs were officially established.

Table 4. MHCL Changes for Sample RHU Inmates, October 2009 – August 29, 2015

BOP Policies	No. of Inmates with Increased MHCL	No. of Inmates with Decreased MHCL	No. of Inmates with the Same MHCL
Former Mental Health Treatment Policies (October 2009 – April 30, 2014)	178	85	425
New Mental Health Treatment Policy (May 1, 2014 – August 2015)	45	110	533
Percent Change (+/-)	-74.72%	29.41%	25.41%

Source: OIG analysis of BOP data.

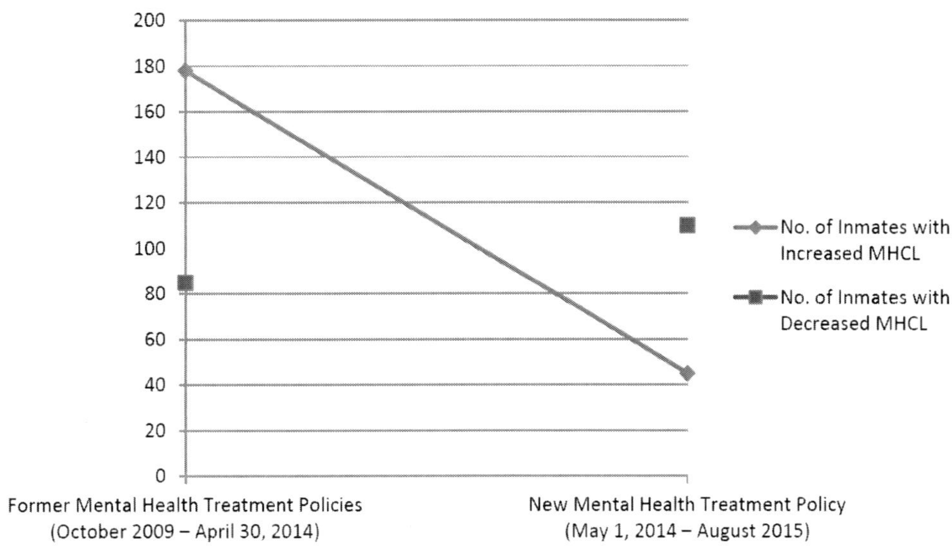

Source: OIG analysis of BOP data.

Figure 4. MHCL Changes for Sample RHU Inmates, October 2009 – August 29, 2015.

We discussed our analyses with BOP institution officials and staff, as well as Central Office officials.[118] Based on these discussions, we believe that the additional requirements established by the new policy, along with no increase in mental health staffing, resulted in institution mental health staffs reducing the number of MHCL 2–4 inmates, who are required to receive more frequent mental health care. A BOP Chief Psychologist told us:

[118] In May 2015, we asked BOP officials in the Psychology Services Branch to comment on the results of our data analyses showing a decrease in the number of BOP inmates designated at MHCLs 2–4. Both the Senior Deputy Assistant Director and the Chief of Mental Health Services had not anticipated our finding and were unaware of the reduction of inmates' MHCLs BOP-wide. They wanted to review the data to better understand this reduction before commenting. In October 2015, we re-interviewed these officials for their opinions on our results.

"If I have [an MHCL] 2, I've got to see them every month, they have a treatment plan, diagnostic formulation, I've got to update them, I've got to go to a [CCARE] meeting, ... that's a lot of dominoes to fall down. So what do you think human nature is? Well, I am going to lower my threshold and have less [MHCL] 2's.... I don't want to lower my threshold but I know that when staff are overwhelmed ... there may have been sometime where people are reducing care levels in order to survive." In light of staffing challenges, he suggested that the BOP could add another care level to the MHCL system that would allow Psychologists to treat on a quarterly basis those inmates who do not clinically need monthly treatment. Another Staff Psychologist told us that since the new policy she has encountered more transferred inmates with reduced MHCLs with which she disagreed. She believes that many institutions are pressed for staffing and were making such efforts to meet the new policy's standards.

The Increased Mental Health Staff at the ADX May Have Contributed to an Increased Number of Inmates at MHCLs 2–4

We found that despite decreases in the ADX's overall inmate population since FY 2010, the BOP has significantly increased the ADX's mental health staffing. We found that, as of May 2015, the number of ADX inmates designated at MHCLs 2–4 had increased by nearly 40 percent (from 33 inmates to 46 inmates). According to the Department, between 2012 and 2013, the BOP hired three additional full-time Psychologists, one Psychiatric Nurse, and one Psychology Technician for the ADX while also adding one Deputy Chief Psychologist to help manage mental health services throughout FCC Florence, including the ADX. We found that during this time, the BOP began to decrease the ADX's inmate population, in part due to a number of inmates with serious mental illness who were transferred to the BOP's new mental health residential treatment programs. However, despite the BOP's efforts to reduce the number of inmates with mental illness at the ADX, the number of MHCL 2–4 inmates increased. It appears to us that the increase in mental health staff to treat ADX inmates may have contributed to the increase in the MHCLs of inmates at the ADX.

Source: DOJ, *Use of Restrictive Housing,* and OIG observation and analysis.

Other institution mental health staff told us about staffing challenges associated with meeting the requirements established in the new policy. Another Chief Psychologist told us that the new policy has great intentions, but "there are just not enough bodies to carry out the policy." A third Chief Psychologist told us that before the new policy, mental health staff had greater latitude to concentrate resources on inmates with serious mental illness; but, under the new policy, those resources are needed to meet the minimum mental health requirements for inmates who may not clinically need that level of mental health treatment. While many institution mental health staff with whom we spoke described a lack of resources to implement the new requirements, it appears that increased staffing at the ADX may have contributed to the increase in inmate MHCLs at the ADX (see the text box above).[119]

When we asked about the sharp overall decrease in the number of inmates designated at MHCLs 2–4 that our analyses showed BOP-wide, the BOP's Chief of Mental Health Services stated that over time it is difficult to determine whether MHCLs have been "rising or falling" because, since the inception of MHCLs, the BOP has changed its guidance on how to assign them.[120] However, she added, "if [MHCLs have] fallen since the new policy, that's a concern.... If the resources aren't there and a psychologist has to make choices about the amount of service they can provide ... because they don't have enough time to provide services to everyone on their caseload, they may be [an MHCL] 2 instead of [an MHCL] 3. I am very concerned about that." Psychology Services Branch officials told us that they do not believe the BOP has "adequate staffing to fully implement" the new policy.

While the BOP's new policy was intended to enhance care for inmates with mental illness, we believe that the new policy could have unintended consequences that negatively affect some inmates' treatment. During our review, BOP officials and staff acknowledged the concerns revealed by our analysis of MHCL data after the BOP issued its new policy, including the need to consider assigning additional mental health staff to effectively implement the policy's enhanced standards. We believe that the BOP should regularly monitor trends in inmate MHCLs to further assess how the new policy affects the treatment of inmates with mental illness, particularly those in RHUs. Although Psychology Services Branch officials told us that they monitor trends for MHCL 3 and MHCL 4 inmates, they do not monitor MHCL fluctuations at the institution level for all MHCLs. We believe that by monitoring MHCLs and their relation to RHU populations, the BOP Central Office could identify institutions with unusual MHCL fluctuations and further investigate institution or RHU-specific factors that may be influencing these changes.

Mental Health Staffing Does Not Support the Treatment Needs of Inmates with Mental Illness, Including Those in RHUs

The BOP "recognizes that an inmate's mental health may deteriorate during a restrictive housing placement."[121] We found several concerns related to the BOP's mental health staffing that could result in some inmates with mental illness, including those in

[119] A Deputy Chief Psychologist told us that recent litigation caused the BOP to increase its mental health staffing resources for the ADX. An ADX Psychologist stated that BOP institutions have different thresholds for assigning MHCLs. At the ADX, the staff has a lower threshold for raising an inmate's MHCL because of the scrutiny over the use of restrictive housing and the recent litigation.

[120] The RSD Senior Deputy Assistant Director added that mental health staff could have been influenced by program review guidelines that were issued *before* the new policy provided guidance specific to MHCLs. The program review guidance combined treatment standards from the old policy with standards detailed in the new policy, which had not yet been released. For example, under the old policy, MHCL 2 inmates were to be seen at least quarterly; but, under the new policy, they are to be seen monthly. If the staff was influenced by guidance in the old policy, this may have "fuzzied" its understanding of the new policy's guidance on MHCL definitions. However, during our interviews with institution staff, we did not find any evidence to support this concern.

[121] BOP Program Statement 5310.16, 16.

RHUs, not receiving the appropriate treatment for their mental health needs. A lack of or inappropriate level of resources could impact inmates' treatment and contribute to a decline in some inmates' mental health.

First, the numbers of Psychologists within BOP institutions are below the BOP's base staffing guidelines. According to the RSD Senior Deputy Assistant Director, staffing guidelines were "established in 2011 and are based on the mission of the institution and the gender of the inmate."[122] The BOP's FY 2016 budget submission stated that a significant number of institutions are short Psychologists to the point that they do not meet the baseline standard of a 1:500 Psychologist to inmate ratio.[123] We observed this shortfall in six of the seven institutions we visited, which at the time of our visits were understaffed by at least one mental health staff position. A Deputy Chief Psychologist told us that one of those institutions with 1,200 inmates had only a single Staff Psychologist.[124] Based on data provided by the BOP during our fieldwork, we found that an FMC housing some of the BOP's most seriously mentally ill inmates had filled only 12 of its 21 full-time mental health staff positions as of December 2015.

Likewise, we believe that the ratio of SMU Psychologists to inmates at USP Lewisburg does not meet the BOP's staffing guidelines. As noted above, the BOP requires a staffing ratio of no fewer than 1 Psychologist per every 350 inmates for high security institutions. We found that USP Lewisburg was operating with 1 Staff Psychologist per every 582 SMU inmates.[125] This ratio of Staff Psychologists to inmates was more than four times worse than the 1:138 ratio at the ADX, which may well impact treatment for USP Lewisburg SMU inmates with mental illness.[126]

Just as we noted above that increased mental health staffing at the ADX may have led to increased recognition of higher MHCLs for inmates there, we believe that limited SMU staffing may have led to a decrease in MHCL designations for SMU inmates and a possible reluctance to designate new inmates at higher MHCL levels. Based on our sample of 239 SMU inmates with mental illness who had their MHCLs changed at USP Lewisburg during

---

[122] According to Psychology Services Branch officials, as of 2011 the BOP's institutions had the following Psychologist to inmate ratios: Federal Medical Centers (1:100), female institutions (1:250), Detention Centers (1:350), high security institutions (1:350), medium security institutions (1:500), low security institutions (1:600), and camps (1:700).

[123] DOJ, *FY 2016 Performance Budget Congressional Submission,* 80, https://edit.justice.gov/sites/default/files/jmd/pages/attachments/2015/02/02/27._federal_bureau_of _prisons_bop_se.pdf (accessed June 27, 2017).

[124] Based on BOP data, there were 1,548 inmates at this institution as of May 2015. Of these inmates, 95 of were in the SHU, which means that they require more frequent mental health assessments. Six of the 95 SHU inmates were at MHCL 2, which further increases their need for mental health assessments.

[125] Our estimate is based on staff and inmates at USP Lewisburg at the time of our site visit in July 2015. BOP data provided to us showed that the institution housed 1,163 SMU inmates in May 2015. When we visited USP Lewisburg in July 2015, two SMU Staff Psychologists were working primarily with SMU inmates. We were told that the institution had hired a third Staff Psychologist, who had not yet started treating SMU inmates at the time of our visit.

[126] We believe that the ADX is the most appropriate staffing comparison to USP Lewisburg's SMU because both institutions are MHCL 2 facilities that house disproportionately high concentrations of disruptive inmates who are placed in restrictive housing for prolonged periods of time and have been referred from other BOP institutions due to behavioral issues.

our scope, we found that SMU staff made an equal proportion of MHCL increases and decreases among our SMU inmate sample prior to the BOP's new mental health policy. However, after the new policy, no sample SMU inmates at USP Lewisburg had increased MHCLs and the number of SMU inmates with decreased MHCLs nearly doubled. While the numbers are not high, this pronounced trend is consistent with our MHCL analysis for all SMU inmates, which shows a 56 percent reduction (from 70 to 31 inmates) in the total number of inmates who receive regular mental health treatment in the SMU since the BOP's new policy was issued.[127] In fact, while approximately 11 percent of inmates at the ADX were receiving regular mental health treatment as of May 2015, only about 2.5 percent of inmates in the SMU were.[128] Collectively, these analyses are concerning in terms of the impact of staffing on MHCL designations and, therefore, on the treatment of inmates with mental health needs. Table 5 below shows the MHCL changes by SMU staff at USP Lewisburg for our sample of SMU inmates with mental illness.[129]

Second, we are also concerned about the BOP's challenges in recruiting and retaining Psychiatrists. We discussed this concern in detail in our March 2016 *Review of the Federal Bureau of Prisons' Medical Staffing Challenges*.[130] As of October 2015, the BOP had filled only 28 of 49 (57 percent) of its authorized full-time Psychiatrist positions nationwide. The former Assistant Director of the BOP's Health Services Division told us that the BOP does not have a staffing formula to identify its Psychiatrist-to-inmate staffing ratio. The Senior Deputy Assistant Director of the Health Services Division told us that Care Level 4 institutions (FMCs) are given first priority for Psychiatrists, followed by Care Level 3 institutions.[131] However, we found that as of FY 2015, one FMC had only one Psychiatrist position filled out of seven positions authorized and one FCC, which includes an FMC, had only two Psychiatrist positions filled out of eight positions authorized. Our March 2016 report talked about some of the challenges the BOP has faced in filling these positions,

---

[127] We based the percentage on the number of MHCL 2–4 inmates in April 2014 (70) compared to the number of MHCL 2–4 inmates in May 2015 (31). However, during that time in FY 2015, the SMU at USP Florence, which had confined 358 SMU inmates in April 2014, closed. In October 2016, CPD officials told us that some SMU inmates were released from USP Florence's SMU into other institutions' general populations while other inmates were transferred to the SMUs at USP Lewisburg or USP Allenwood. As a result, it appears that the closure of USP Florence's SMU may have contributed to the overall reduction in the total number of SMU inmates who received regular mental health treatment. Although BOP data shows an 11 percent reduction in the overall SMU population during this time, it is important to note that USP Lewisburg's SMU population increased nearly 40 percent (from 844 to 1,163) during this same period.

[128] As of May 2015, we also found that approximately 7 percent of the BOP's SHU population received regular mental health treatment, which is also considerably higher than the rate at USP Lewisburg's SMU.

[129] Based on our sample of SMU inmates with mental illness from October 2009 through August 29, 2015, we also found that SMU staff at USP Allenwood had also increased (four) and decreased a comparable number of inmates' MHCLs (three) prior to the issuance of the May 2014 policy. However, after the new policy was issued, SMU staff did not increase any sample inmates' MHCLs but did decrease the MHCLs of three sample inmates.

[130] DOJ OIG, *Review of the Federal Bureau of Prisons' Medical Staffing Challenges,* Evaluation and Inspections Report 16-02 (March 2016).

[131] Similar to how MHCLs delineate the mental health needs of inmates, the BOP also designates institutional care levels to delineate the varying levels of medical and mental health care that can be provided to inmates at its institutions. For example, an MHCL 4 inmate should be housed only at a Care Level 4 institution because only Care Level 4 institutions have the resources needed to address that inmate's intensive mental health needs.

which is a problem that the BOP should continue to address if inmates are to receive the level of psychiatric care indicated by their MHCLs.

Table 5. MHCL Changes at USP Lewisburg for Our Sample of SMU Inmates with Mental Illness, October 2009 – August 29, 2015

BOP Policies	MHCL Increases	MHCL Decreases	Ratio of MHCL Increases to Decreases
Former Mental Health Treatment Policies (October 2009 – April 30, 2014)	16	16	1:1
New Mental Health Treatment Policy (May 1, 2014 – August 2015)	0	27	0:27

Note: Although the BOP established the MHCL system in December 2009, a few inmates in our sample had MHCLs initiated as early as October 2009, which explains why the scope of this table predates the official establishment of MHCLs. Additionally, our analysis does not account for every MHCL change that may have occurred during these time periods but notes the inmates' MHCL changes, when applicable, from October 2009 through April 2014 and from April 2014 through August 2015. See Appendix 1 for more details.

Source: OIG analysis of BOP data.

Third, as a result of a shortage of Psychiatrists, we found that General Practitioners, without the specialized training normally provided to Psychiatrists, are left to prescribe psychotropic medications to inmates in RHUs. Institution Psychiatrists told us that while General Practitioners have basic training in diagnosing and medicating basic disorders (e.g., depression), they may not be able to manage more complex cases and therefore should consult with a Psychiatrist.[132] One FMC Psychiatrist said that General Practitioners can diagnose and treat depression, and likely have the knowledge and skills to assist with MHCL 1–2 inmates, but that more complex cases may be more difficult for a General Practitioner to manage and treat.

Fourth, the BOP has expanded its use of tele-psychiatry, a form of "direct, patient-to-provider, visual interaction" that occurs in a private setting; but we found that not all institutions are supported by this service. A Chief Psychologist told us that her institution was 25th on the BOP's tele-psychiatry waitlist for about a year before the institution filled its tele-psychiatry vacancy. Though the institution is a Care Level 2 facility, the Chief Psychologist's caseload has about eight or nine MHCL 3 inmates who require more complex treatment and could benefit from this service. Conversely, other staff expressed concerns about the treatment provided through tele-psychiatry and it appears that one SMU institution we visited elected to significantly limit tele-psychiatry services for its inmates.[133] (See the text box.)

[132] The BOP's Chief Psychiatrist told us that there is no issue with general practitioners providing psychotropic medication since it's a practice in the community.

[133] We did not evaluate the effectiveness of tele-psychiatry as part of this review.

USP Lewisburg Has Significantly Limited Tele-Psychiatry Services for SMU Inmates

While the SMU houses inmates with mental illness at MHCL 2, SMU officials told us that, despite having the capability, the institution has rarely, if ever, offered tele-psychiatry services to inmates since 2013 because the mental health needs of its inmates do not necessitate such services. The Medical Officer at USP Lewisburg told us that tele-psychiatry is problematic because tele-Psychiatrists often prescribe medications based on inmates' self-reported conditions in sessions that last only 15 to 20 minutes. He prefers to observe the inmate over extended periods of time. He added that while the institution still has the capability for tele-psychiatry, staff treat inmates themselves. The Medical Officer told us: "We haven't stopped [tele-psychiatry]. It's still available. It's just that since I've come on-board, it's not utilized because I consider myself pretty adept at treating all these conditions." Five SMU inmates told us they were unable to participate in tele-psychiatry at USP Lewisburg, despite having done so while in SMUs at other institutions. The Health Services Division Senior Deputy Assistant Director told us that she would be "very surprised" if an institution had the capability but did not offer tele-psychiatry and that USP Lewisburg would be a "perfect spot" for tele-psychiatry.

Source: OIG interviews.

Finally, inmates told us that they did not think they were receiving the appropriate treatment and care to address their mental health needs. For example, according to the May 2014 policy, individualized treatment plans should be based on collaboration with the inmate and should describe "the inmate's problems and goals, and the interventions planned to assist with goal attainment." Inmates we interviewed indicated that they were generally unaware of their individualized mental health treatment plan, which raises questions as to how collaborative these treatment plans actually are, as well as how they influence the treatment and care of inmates with mental illness in RHUs. Psychology Services Branch officials told us that clinicians have to document that they discussed the treatment plan with the inmate; however, there is no documentation for the inmate to sign acknowledging discussion of his/her treatment.

The May 2014 policy also requires that "all inmates with mental illness in restrictive housing units (i.e., the SHU, SMU, and ADX) will receive, at a minimum, face-to-face mental health contacts consistent with the type and frequency indicated by their care level, to the extent feasible." While our review of case files for inmates at MHCLs 2–4 suggests that contacts occur as frequently as policy requires, the policy also states, "Inmates are removed from their cells for private or extended interviews with Psychology and Psychiatry Services staff as a standard procedure."[134] During our review of inmate case files, we found inconsistent documentation regarding whether inmates were removed from

[134] The May 2014 policy includes exceptions to private critical contacts and mental health treatment in cases in which the inmate is behaving in an aggressive manner or when institutional safety and security require an exception. BOP Program Statement 5310.16, 16.

their cells for private or extended interviews.[135] Specifically, some staff documented the location of private face-to-face interviews with inmates, whereas others did not. One inmate also told us that psychology is "supposed to [make rounds], but whether they do or not is a whole other question... there's no consistency."[136]

According to Psychology Services Branch officials, documenting whether critical contacts occur inside an inmate's cell or outside of a cell in a private setting is a best practice but it is not required by policy.[137] Whether the contact takes place inside or outside an inmate's cell, the officials further explained that the May 2014 policy requires that inmates be treated in a private setting. However, the BOP's inability to track the location in which clinical contacts occur prevents the BOP from assessing the extent to which its policy goal to protect inmate privacy has been achieved and limits its ability to correct practices that are inconsistent with policy, which may limit the appropriate treatment and care afforded to inmates according to MHCL.

Inmates also had concerns regarding their continuity of care. An inmate at an FMC told us that before she was taken to the SHU she had been participating in one-on-one counseling sessions with a Psychologist but that those sessions stopped after she entered the SHU. While the May 2014 policy updated and refined designation, transfer, and release procedures for inmates with mental illness, with an emphasis on continuity of care both across institutions and in the community, we found that it does not discuss the continuity of care for inmates with mental illness in RHUs. According to Psychology Services Branch officials, if an inmate is in group therapy while in general population, the inmate can no longer participate in group sessions during his or her time in restrictive housing. Despite the BOP's efforts to offer group therapy opportunities for inmates in restrictive housing, we found that inmates in restrictive housing may not receive continuous mental health treatment. See below for more information regarding the BOP's secure residential mental health treatment programs.

Mental Health Staffs Disagree on the Diagnoses More Often for Inmates with Mental Illness in RHUs, Which Can Affect the Treatment of Those Inmates

Based on our review, we found that ensuring appropriate mental health treatment for inmates in RHUs is a challenge for the BOP. Specifically, we found that differing clinical

---

[135] The CNA's review and assessment of BOP restrictive housing found that "very few of the monthly mental health assessments occur in private settings on a face-to-face basis." The CNA recommended that BOP psychology and psychiatry staff completely reevaluate inmates' mental health records every 30 days and include a face-to-face interview in a private setting. In the BOP's response to the CNA, the BOP did not specifically address private interviews between Health Services staff and inmates. However, in the CNA's report, the CNA notes that the BOP's 2014 mental health policy addresses critical contacts in a private setting. CNA, *Special Housing Review and Assessment.*

[136] The May 2014 policy also states, "During rounds, all staff will make themselves available for brief conversations that demonstrate concern and their availability to provide assistance." We further discuss institution staff rounds below.

[137] According to policy, all critical contacts, regardless of an inmate's MHCL, will, to the extent possible, be conducted in a private area. BOP Program Statement 5310.16, 15.

opinions among mental health staff, as well as staff not working collaboratively to diagnose mental disorders, could impact continuity of care. These issues raise concerns as to whether inmates with mental illness are receiving appropriate care.

BOP policy states that all inmates must undergo an initial screening when they arrive at their designated BOP institution. The screening is usually conducted by BOP Psychologists and, based on our review of 59 case files from the RHUs that we visited, with a few isolated exceptions, it is generally done in a timely fashion.[138] BOP officials told us that during the screening the mental health staff should identify an inmate's mental health disorders and, based on their evaluation, assess whether the inmate needs regular treatment to determine his or her MHCL.[139] If the mental health staff disagrees with an inmate's previous diagnosis, BOP policy states that the Mental Health Treatment Coordinator or treating Psychologist attempts to reconcile differences; consults with other treatment providers, including the Health Services staff; performs a clinical interview; and observes the inmate's symptoms and behaviors in making a determination.[140] The Chief of Mental Health Services told us that if a Psychologist makes a diagnosis that differs from the inmate's previous mental health diagnosis, that Psychologist must explain both the rationale for the new diagnosis and why it is inconsistent with the previous diagnosis.

According to mental health staff we interviewed, BOP providers disagreed with the prior diagnoses of approximately one out of five inmates. Of the 29 mental health staff we interviewed, 26 (90 percent) told us they have disagreed with inmates' previous diagnoses that were documented by other institution staff.[141] While staff at every institution we visited reported diagnosis disagreements for inmates with mental illness, staff at the ADX, SMU, and secure residential mental health treatment program institutions reported higher rates of diagnosis disagreements for their inmate populations, with an average reported disagreement rate of 24 percent as opposed to 16 percent by staff from the remaining institutions we visited.[142] More frequent disagreements among the staffs for these inmate populations could negatively affect the continuity of care for these inmates.

Our case file reviews also confirmed instances in which mental health staff disagreed on the prior diagnoses of inmates placed in restrictive housing.[143] In one inmate's case file,

---

[138] Program Statement 5310.12, Psychology Services Manual (PSM) (March 7, 1995). In August 2016, the BOP rescinded Program Statement 5310.12 and issued a revised PSM. We did not assess the August 2016 PSM as part of this review. See Appendix 2 for a summary of changes between the March 1995 and August 2016 PSMs.

[139] One Chief Psychologist also told us that she will continue to monitor an inmate for up to 12 months after their initial screening before potentially changing the inmate's mental health diagnosis and that the screening of inmates does not conclude with the initial screening process.

[140] BOP Program Statement 5310.16, 9.

[141] We did not include mental health staff we interviewed who were not qualified to independently diagnose inmates' mental disorders.

[142] From the 29 mental health staff we interviewed, we based our calculations on quantifiable responses from 25 mental health staff. We believe that staff responses from ADX, SMU, and secure residential treatment program institutions (which house many former ADX inmates) may have been influenced by the disproportionately high concentrations of disruptive inmates managed under strict controls for prolonged periods of time.

[143] Although we reviewed inmate case files, we could not use these documents to determine a reliable rate of conflicting diagnoses by mental health staff for several reasons. First, OIG staff are not professionally trained to determine whether diagnoses are conflicting or complementary. Second, there were institutional inconsistencies

the Psychologist had noted that she did not agree that the inmate met the criteria for Bipolar Disorder and reduced the inmate's care level to MHCL 1, thus discontinuing the inmate's treatment. In another inmate's case file, psychology records indicated that the inmate had previously been diagnosed with Psychotic Disorder (Not Otherwise Specified) and Borderline Intellectual Functioning. A different Psychologist did not identify any "significant mental health issues" during a subsequent mental health review and, consequently, reduced the inmate's care level to MHCL 1. Case file documentation for another inmate revealed that although Health Services believed that the inmate should be diagnosed with Schizophrenia (Paranoid Type), Psychology Services found "no evidence" of that disorder at the time and did not adjust the inmate's level of care. However, less than 3 months later, the inmate was transferred to an FMC after Psychology Services elevated the inmate to MHCL 4.[144] We further discuss differences in clinical opinions between Psychology Services and Health Services later in this chapter.

Institution staff members offered a number of reasons that could account for some of the disagreements in diagnosis. A Staff Psychologist said that an inmate's Psychology Services Intake Questionnaire, used to screen the inmate upon arrival at a BOP institution, is not very thorough and can be difficult to confirm because information is self-reported. She added that, generally, BOP clinicians tend to over-diagnose inmates because they are not "unpacking the core" of inmates' mental health issues. She stated that large mental health caseloads prevent staff from screening inmates more comprehensively. A Psychology Services Branch official told us that BOP staff are able to identify inmates "where their symptoms are pretty prevalent" but acknowledged that the BOP does not have the resources to do an in-depth mental health evaluation of each inmate entering the BOP. Another Staff Psychologist told us that because mental health is fluid, even an accurate diagnosis could become inaccurate at a later point in time, which we recognize as contributing to clinical disagreements for inmates with mental illness.

We also found that differing clinical opinions between institutions' Health Services, including General Practitioners, Psychiatrists, and Psychology Services, contribute to conflicting diagnoses for inmates with mental illness.[145] Some Psychologists told us that

---

in the mental health documentation provided to us and diagnostic disagreements may have been noted in documents we did not receive or request, such as diagnostic reconciliations that may have occurred when the inmate was not in restrictive housing. Third, case file documents indicate the current diagnoses for inmates but generally do not show diagnoses that have been subsequently removed. Last, as we discuss in Appendix 1, we focused our review on case files from January 2014, 4 months before the new mental health policy was issued, until the most recent documentation available to us at the time of our site visit. Thus, we did not review these inmates' entire historical records of diagnosis and treatment while in BOP custody.

[144] In response to a working draft of this report, the BOP stated that these are complex cases and that diagnostic discrepancies are common. Additionally, the BOP stated that research on the reliability of the DSM diagnoses finds relatively high rates of diagnostic discrepancies among community treatment providers. Finally, the BOP stated that diagnoses change over time and that modifying a diagnosis is a requirement of good clinical care. Nevertheless, we believe that the level and nature of the discrepancies we found are potentially significant for the BOP in ensuring that it provides an appropriate level of care to inmates.

[145] In the BOP, Psychologists are primarily responsible for diagnosing and treating the mental disorders of inmates. However, Psychologists can share these responsibilities with General Practitioners and Psychiatrists, particularly when an inmate needs medication.

these disagreements may be attributed in part to differences in each profession's education and mental health training.[146] One Psychologist told us that because some Health Services staff may not have extensive mental health training, certain words they hear from an inmate may lead them to conclude that the inmate must have mental illness. Another Psychologist said that Psychologists and Health Services staffs frequently disagree about complicated mental health cases, particularly when inmates are reporting different symptoms to different staff for personal gain (we discuss malingering later in this chapter).

In addition, we were told that Health Services and Psychology Services staffs do not always work collaboratively to diagnose inmates' mental disorders. A Deputy Chief Psychologist said that she disagrees with Health Services' mental health diagnoses up to 60 percent of the time and that her institution's Psychology Services and Health Services staffs were not working collaboratively. A Staff Psychologist at this institution told us, "I don't even know half the time who medical [Health Services] is." The Staff Psychologist added that Health Services was extremely short staffed, which contributed to this problem. A Chief Psychologist at another institution told us that her institution's Psychology Services and Health Services staffs had made no effort to reconcile discrepancies in BEMR-PDS for inmates with conflicting mental health diagnoses.[147] Because the two staffs may disagree on inmates' diagnoses, the treatment that Psychology Services provides may not be complemented with medications that, generally, only a qualified Health Services provider can prescribe. This may result in inmates receiving inadequate care, particularly in RHUs where disagreements may be more prevalent.

While the BOP Has Taken Recent Steps to Mitigate Mental Health Concerns for Inmates in RHUs, Additional Actions Can Be Taken

As discussed above, the BOP's 2014 mental health policy, intended to enhance mental health treatment for inmates, has nevertheless led to additional concerns that inmates in RHUs may not be receiving adequate mental health care. Still, during our review period, we found that the BOP has made efforts to mitigate mental health concerns for inmates in RHUs. The BOP has begun diverting inmates with serious mental illness from traditional

---

[146] Both General Practitioners and Psychiatrists go to medical school and become medical doctors who are licensed to diagnose mental illness and prescribe medications, including psychotropic medications. Psychiatrists generally receive more extensive and specialized mental health training than do General Practitioners. Psychologists are not medical doctors. They go to graduate school and earn a doctorate degree in psychology. They are trained to apply psychological assessments and testing for mental health diagnoses, but they generally are not licensed to prescribe medications without additional, specialized training.

[147] In 2014, the BOP merged the PDS, the system the Psychology Services staff uses, into the BEMR, which the Health Services staff uses. We were told that the BOP merged these systems in part to help facilitate a better working relationship between Psychology Services and Health Services. As a result, both staffs have access to each other's clinical notes and mental health diagnoses for BOP inmates at their institution.

RHUs into alternative programs such as secure residential mental health treatment programs. The BOP also has reduced the use of SHUs and the length of time that inmates are placed in them. While we believe these are positive steps, we found a number of areas that the BOP needs to further improve, such as by developing formal performance metrics to help measure the effectiveness of secure residential mental health treatment programs, improving the mental health training for RHU correctional staff, increasing the use of alternative sanctions to further prevent inmates with serious mental illness from being placed in restrictive housing, and developing guidance and training to discern and document malingering.

The BOP Has Started to Implement Secure Residential Mental Health Treatment Programs as Alternatives to Traditional Restrictive Housing

In October 2013, the BOP began transferring a limited number of inmates with serious mental illness from placement in RHUs, including SHUs, SMUs, and the ADX, to secure residential mental health treatment programs. These programs house inmates in a single-cell, modified therapeutic environment that requires all participants to live on the same unit and engage in treatment together.[148] Inmates have out-of-cell time for recreation or individual and group programming. These programs are generally viewed as being better environments for the treatment of inmates with mental illness than confinement in traditional RHUs. In August 2015, the BOP had two such programs: Secure Mental Health Step Down (Step Down) and Steps Toward Awareness, Growth, and Emotional Strength (STAGES).[149] However, slow inmate progression through these programs and limited resources such as staff and bed space create waitlists and prevent inmates with mental illness from availing themselves of these alternative treatment opportunities.

We found that an inmate with serious mental illness may be on a waitlist for a secure residential mental health treatment program because it could take years for an actively enrolled inmate to complete the program. For example, Step Down was activated in October 2013 at USP Atlanta and currently operates in two facilities, including USP Allenwood, as a residential treatment program for inmates with serious mental illness and a history of violence. As of October 2016, no inmate had completed the program despite its target duration of 18 months.[150] The USP Atlanta staff told us that one of the biggest challenges with the program is identifying the appropriate custodial setting for inmates

[148] Secure residential mental health treatment programs are designed to reduce psychological symptoms, improve functioning, facilitate institutional adjustment, reduce incidents of misconduct, reduce the need for psychiatric hospitalization, and facilitate successful reentry into society. See DOJ, *FY 2016 Performance Budget Congressional Submission,* 38.

[149] BOP Program Statement 5330.11, Psychology Treatment Programs (March 16, 2009), contains policy, procedures, and guidelines for BOP psychological treatment programs, including mental health treatment programs such as Step Down units. The program statement does not discuss secure residential mental health treatment programs. See Appendix 2 for more information on psychological treatment programs established within Program Statement 5330.11. For more information about the secure Step Down and STAGES Programs, see Appendix 3.

[150] The program's 18-month target completion time assumes perfect inmate progress through each phase.

after they complete it. The BOP's Chief of Mental Health Services said that the BOP wants to open a secure open unit into which inmates from the high security mental health Step Down program can transition. Unfortunately, the lack of staffing and resources make it difficult for the BOP to expand this program.

Similarly, the Secure STAGES Program operates at one BOP institution for male inmates with serious mental illnesses and a primary diagnosis of Borderline Personality Disorder. As of October 2016, Psychology Services Branch officials told us that there are currently 30–40 inmates on the waitlists for both Step Down and Secure STAGES. The waitlists for these programs are a treatment concern because inmates awaiting placement are not receiving the level of care they would receive if they were enrolled in a mental health program. BOP officials told us that the BOP's Central Office manages these waitlists on a one-in, one-out basis.

BOP officials told us that the BOP would like to expand its use of residential mental health treatment programs; but, as discussed above, limited numbers of staff and beds — according to BOP, a total of 67 as of November 2016 for the 2 programs — impacts the scalability of these programs. For example, Step Down at USP Atlanta has the capacity for 30 participants but, as of August 2015, had staff available for only 21.[151] Similarly, STAGES has the capacity for 18 participants but as of August 2015 had staff available for only 12. The RSD Senior Deputy Assistant Director told us that the Psychology Services Branch considers a variety of factors in the development of these programs, including the recruitment of enthusiastic, highly skilled coordinators. These programs are staff intensive, which makes it difficult for the BOP to staff them adequately. For example, at the time of our fieldwork, the Step Down Program at USP Atlanta had a ratio of 4 staff to 21 inmates. USP Atlanta had a Psychologist vacancy and only 2 Psychologists for the program's 21 inmates.[152] In addition, a Psychologist told us that inadequate Correctional Officer staffing can affect the scheduling of inmate programming, adding that it is especially problematic due to staffing changes and requirements for many Correctional Officers to move inmates. Nevertheless, according to the BOP, "these programs have demonstrated [their ability] to significantly reduce misconduct among program participants."[153]

Finally, the BOP does not have formal performance metrics for these programs.[154] Staff for the Mental Health Step Down Program told us that measuring and tracking behavioral change is a challenge given that behavior is a human, subjective measurement. BOP officials told us that potential performance measures for the STAGES Program are fewer suicide risk assessments, fewer disciplinary infractions, and a lower number of days of

---

[151] During our visit to USP Allenwood, Step Down was not yet fully activated. As of November 2016, USP Allenwood's program had 30 inmates.

[152] In response to a working draft of this report, the BOP stated that the Step Down Program at USP Atlanta has a ratio of 5 mental health staff to 24 inmates. There is a Program Coordinator, two Program Psychologists, and two Program Treatment Specialists.

[153] DOJ, *FY 2016 Performance Budget Congressional Submission*, 36.

[154] We did not evaluate the effectiveness of the Mental Health Step Down and STAGES Programs as part of this review.

suicide watch. Despite the inherent challenges, BOP officials told us that the BOP is developing a formal evaluation of these programs.

The expansion of these treatment programs is contingent on funding for mental health positions. When we requested the costs associated with these programs, the BOP responded that it was "unable to break down the costs of the various programs within the Psychology Services Department (we do not have the capability to capture the cost to that level of detail)." However, the Department has estimated that it would cost approximately $10 million to expand the programs.[155] According to the BOP's Chief of Mental Health Services, this would enable the BOP to expand these programs to all security levels and to at least one female institution. We believe that, in order to make informed decisions regarding the potential increased use and staffing for these alternative housing programs, the BOP needs to develop and implement metrics to assess their performance and cost.

Residential Mental Health Treatment Programs in State Departments of Corrections May Offer Insights to Help the BOP Improve Its Mental Health Treatment Program

As part of our review of the BOP's mental health treatment program, we researched the programs of eight state correctional systems. We found that six of the eight state systems have developed residential mental health treatment programs as alternatives to housing mentally ill inmates in traditional RHUs. Officials with Pennsylvania's Department of Corrections told us that they have Diversionary Treatment Units, which are secure units that provide expanded or personalized mental health services to inmates with serious mental illness who have committed disciplinary infractions. Inmates are allowed 20 hours of out-of-cell time per week, which can include recreation, group therapy, and private consultations with a Psychologist. Officials from the Massachusetts Department of Corrections told us that inmates with serious mental illness may be housed in a Secure Treatment Unit, which allows inmates 15 hours per week of out-of-cell clinical programming in addition to recreation. Four state officials told us that their programs have out-of-cell group therapy for high security inmates for 10–20 hours per week using "program security chairs or tables," which allow inmates to be safely restrained in a classroom setting.[156] Officials with the Washington State Department of Corrections told us that program security chairs were a "game changer" for providing treatment and programming for inmates. In contrast to the state systems that had security chairs, at BOP

---

[155] The Department's January 2016 report on the use of restrictive housing "estimates that the expansion of these programs would cost in its first year approximately $5.843 million for staff and $4 million for building and facilities and modernization." DOJ, *Use of Restrictive Housing,* 113.

[156] The Department's January 2016 report stated: "In 2016, the Bureau expects to publish a final rule modifying 28 C.F.R. § 552.22(h) (4), thereby permitting the use of secure programming chairs. Once the revised rule is published, the Bureau intends to purchase 610 of these chairs, which would allow inmates to receive in-person educational and mental health programming in a less restrictive manner than currently used. The Bureau estimates that the one-time purchase of security chairs would cost approximately $1.7 million." DOJ, *Use of Restrictive Housing,* 116.

institutions we observed inmates with serious mental illness participating in out-of-cell group therapy using individual metal enclosures to separate them during group treatment.

The BOP Has Reduced Its Use of SHUs

As we discussed above, the frequency, duration, and conditions of confinement of restrictive housing can have significant adverse effects on inmates' mental health. We found that the BOP reduced the overall number of inmates, including but not limited to inmates with mental illness, placed in the SHUs by about 20 percent from FY 2010 to May 2015. The former CPD Deputy Assistant Director told us that the BOP accomplished this reduction through three initiatives. First, the BOP developed an investigative template that reduces the amount of time inmates are held in a SHU pending completion of a protective custody investigation.[157] Second, the BOP developed a daily, automated SHU report to assist BOP officials and institution Executive Staff, such as the Warden, in monitoring SHU inmate totals by institution. Third, the BOP has been training Disciplinary Hearing Officers (DHO) to consider administrative time served when determining sanctions for inmates who have committed a prohibited act.[158] The former CPD Deputy Assistant Director also told us that the BOP is revising its program statement on the Inmate Discipline Program and is considering whether to significantly reduce the maximum sanction for the greatest severity offenses.[159]

We visited FCC Terre Haute, which emphasized diverting inmates, including inmates with mental illness, from the SHU whenever possible.[160] Institution officials told us that if

---

[157] To further reduce the placement of inmates in the SHU for non-punitive reasons, such as protective custody, CPD officials told us that in February 2014 the BOP developed the Reintegration Housing Unit at the Federal Correctional Institution (FCI) in Oakdale, Louisiana, which allows vulnerable inmates to be placed into less restrictive settings through state placement and reintegration into the general population. However, in January 2016, the Department reported that this program does not accept inmates who require "substantial medical or mental health treatment." DOJ, *Use of Restrictive Housing,* 24.

[158] The Department's January 2016 report, *Use of Restrictive Housing,* recommended that the BOP revise its written policies for the Inmate Discipline Program to require that time spent in administrative detention status pending investigation be credited toward any term of disciplinary segregation status imposed for that violation. According to the Department's "180-day Status Report," the BOP revised its internal document to require that all disciplinary investigations be completed within 30 days, absent compelling circumstances.

[159] The BOP stated that this effort was partly in response to the CNA report, which stated that the BOP should "establish by policy that a sanction of restrictive housing time should be issued retroactive to the date of the original admission, providing credit for time served." See CNA, *Federal Bureau of Prisons: Special Housing Unit Review and Assessment* (December 2014).

The Department's January 2016 report, *Use of Restrictive Housing,* also recommended that the BOP reduce its maximum sanction to 60 days for a first offense and 90 days for a subsequent offense. The Department recommended that the BOP provide guidance that, ordinarily, DHOs should impose concurrent sentences for disciplinary violations arising from the same episode and that the BOP should prohibit SHU placement for all low level and first-time moderate level offenses. According to the Department's "180-day Status Report," maximum penalties are codified in the Code of Federal Regulations and any changes would require formal rulemaking. The Department is reviewing a draft Notice of Proposed Rulemaking, which is expected to be issued for public comment in the near future.

[160] According to the BOP's revised SHU policy, the BOP now prohibits SHU placement for inmates whom mental health staff have designated at MHCL 3 or 4, who have a psychology alert in SENTRY (the BOP's primary mission support database), or who have been identified on the monthly SHU advisory (Hot List) unless the inmate presents an immediate or serious danger to self, staff, or the orderly operation of a facility. In the event that an inmate who meets one of these criteria is placed in the SHU, Psychology Services staff should be notified

the Psychology Services staff identifies an inmate with a serious mental illness and a history of self -harming behavior during prior SHU placements, the staff may house the inmate in the general population while the discipline hearing is pending.[161] The institution's DHO said that BOP policy does not restrict him from imposing alternative sanctions if the Psychology Services staff expresses concerns about SHU placement. Rather than placing an inmate in the SHU, the DHO may impose a monetary fine, which he said had been a particularly effective deterrent; confiscate the inmate's property; or restrict the inmate to his cell. At the time of our visit, only five inmates were in the institution's SHU for disciplinary segregation, which the DHO attributed to his use of alternative sanctions.[162] The former CPD Deputy Assistant Director said that DHOs have always had the discretion to deny inmate privileges in lieu of imposing SHU time. Based on our observations and the DHO's statements, we believe that the BOP should consider policies that encourage the use of alternative sanctions when appropriate to further prevent inmates with mental illness from placement in restrictive housing.

Also at FCC Terre Haute, the acting Complex Warden told us that during SHU meetings, which are held to review inmates' continued placement in the SHU, the staff first discusses inmates based on length of time in the SHU rather than in alphabetical order, which is intended and helps to prioritize discussions on whether these inmates can be returned to the general population. The acting Complex Warden also stated that, for transfer inmates who are routinely placed in SHU on "Holdover Status," staff will work to determine which inmates can be safely released to the general population while pending transfer to their designated institution.

By contrast, we found that the BOP routinely places holdover inmates in SHUs as a standard practice, despite the potential mental health concerns attributed to placing inmates in restrictive housing. At FCC Petersburg, we observed that holdover inmates were all housed in its SHU while awaiting transfer.[163] The Chief Psychologist at the time of our visit told us that holdover inmates with mental illness can become particularly problematic for staff and that her institution receives holdover inmates who have serious mental illness. She estimated that they may be single-celled in the SHU for up to 3 weeks. Although the

---

and should conduct a mental health evaluation within 24 hours of placement. See BOP Program Statement 5270.11, Special Housing Units (November 2016), 15–16.

161 During our site visit, the institution's DHO told us that there were approximately 100 inmates pending a disciplinary hearing who were currently placed in the SHU under administrative segregation status.

162 At the time of our site visit, the USP Terre Haute SHU also housed its FCI SHU inmates due to construction. This was also a factor that contributed to the DHO's alternative sanctions because the USP's SHU was normally full with both medium and high security inmates.

We note that as of May 30, 2015, this institution had the most MHCL 3 inmates in its SHU compared to all other BOP institutions. According to BOP policy, MHCL 3 represents inmates with serious mental illness. At the time of our site visit, we also interviewed multiple inmates who had serious mental illness and were currently in the SHU. However, as discussed earlier, because we believe that the BOP's new mental health care policy (BOP Program Statement 5310.16) may have affected some inmates' MHCL designations, it is difficult for us to compare and contrast BOP institutions. We also recognize that FCI inmates placed in the USP's SHU may have skewed the data.

163 At the time of our site visit, the SHU Lieutenant stated that there were approximately 35 holdover inmates housed in the institution's SHU.

staff physically places inmates with serious mental illness at the front of the SHU so they can be monitored more closely, she acknowledged that SHU placement can be detrimental to these inmates' mental health and may also compromise the SHU staff's safety. She added that her institution receives holdover inmates who are new to the BOP and, as a result, the Psychology Services staff has little information about their mental health and generally does not provide intake screenings for inmates in holdover status.[164] We believe that the BOP can improve its handling of holdover inmates to further prevent inmates with mental illness from being placed in restrictive housing when it may not be necessary.

The BOP Has Made Particular Progress in Reducing Lengthy SHU Placements

In addition to reducing overall SHU use by about 20 percent since FY 2010, we found that the BOP has reduced by 58 percent the total number of inmates placed in a SHU for at least 150 consecutive days and these inmates' average number of days housed in the SHU by almost 10 percent. Specifically, 1,862 inmates were housed in SHUs for at least 150 consecutive days, with an average duration of 296 consecutive days, at the end of FY 2010.[165] By the end of FY 2014, the BOP had reduced this population to 780 inmates housed in SHUs for at least 150 consecutive days, with an average stay of 268 consecutive days (See Table 6).

Table 6. Inmates in a SHU for at Least 150 Consecutive Days FY 2010 through FY 2014

	FY 2010	FY 2011	FY 2012	FY 2013	FY 2014	% Change FY 2010 – FY 2014 (+/-)
No. of Inmates in a SHU for at Least 150 Consecutive Days	1,862	1,871	2,072	1,197	780	-58.11%
Average No. of Days in a SHU	296	280	291	285	268	-9.46%

Note: This table includes all inmates who were continuously placed in a SHU for at least 150 days as reported by the BOP's dashboard, which does not specifically identify inmates with mental illness.
Source: OIG analysis of BOP data.

In addition to reducing the overall use of SHUs and the incidence of particularly lengthy SHU stays, the BOP has implemented a number of other actions that are directly targeted at helping monitor and mitigate mental health concerns for inmates in RHUs:

[164] BOP policy states that, for individuals in holdover status, a preliminary screening by a Physician's Assistant is sufficient, unless a significant problem is identified. Inmates referred to Psychology Services following their preliminary medical screening are supposed to be evaluated promptly by a Psychologist. See BOP Program Statement 5310.12, ch. 4, p. 3.

[165] We requested that the BOP apply its SHU dashboard to previous fiscal years to assess inmates who were in comparably prolonged periods of SHU confinement. As mentioned earlier, the BOP developed this dashboard after the new mental health care policy to notify institutions' staff of inmates who may be due for their required Extended Restrictive Housing Placement Review. We were told that inmates, as detailed in Table 6, from FY 2010 through FY 2013, did not receive these reviews because former BOP policies did not require them.

- The Psychology Services staff must conduct a Psychology Services Review after every 30 days of continuous SHU placement for every inmate, regardless of MHCL.[166]
- The Psychology Services staff may also place inmates with mental illness on the monthly advisory (Hot List) in the BOP's SHU Application to alert correctional staff of those who "could potentially cause a problem if placed in SHU."[167]
- If restrictive housing appears to affect an inmate's mental health, the Mental Health Treatment Coordinator is required to work with the CCARE team to "mitigate the negative impact or identify an appropriately secure alternative placement."[168]

The BOP distributes among various staff members the responsibility for monitoring inmates in RHUs.[169] The May 2014 mental health policy states that all staff are required to make themselves available to RHU inmates for brief conversations and demonstrate concern and availability to provide assistance.[170] The former CPD Deputy Assistant Director said that Correctional Officers must make RHU rounds every 30 minutes, a supervisor must visit with each RHU inmate during every shift, and the Captain must visit with each RHU inmate every week.[171] Finally, institution staff told us that the Executive Staff, including the institution's Warden, Associate Wardens, Captain, Chief Psychologist, and Health Services staff, make weekly RHU rounds.[172]

---

166 Based on our case file reviews of inmates with mental illness in RHUs, we found that Psychology Services Reviews were conducted within the timeliness standards detailed by policy. However, contrary to policy, we found that the Psychology Services staff at the ADX did not always document the threat the inmate posed to self, staff, and other inmates. Our case file reviews indicated that the BOP had developed standardized default fields for SHU and SMU reviews to capture this information but ADX reviews did not incorporate these standardized data fields, which we believe contributed to this issue.

167 While only the Psychology Services staff may edit the SHU Application's Hot List, all SHU staff members can see it and become aware of potential issues. Further, the SHU Application includes some information from BEMR-PDS so that the correctional staff can see when the Psychology Services staff last visited with an inmate. We found that the correctional staff with whom we spoke were aware of the Hot List, and they told us that they are required to review it at least monthly. They also stated that the Hot List may be distributed to them in an email and may be posted in the applicable RHU.

168 BOP Program Statement 5310.16.

169 The Department's "180-day Status Report" stated that the BOP is developing a training program called "Core Correctional Communications," which is intended to enhance communications between Correctional Officers and inmates. The BOP is conducting pilot training and plans to expand the program to all of its institutions by the end of 2017.

170 BOP Program Statement 5310.16.

171 We did not review BOP documentation to assess RHU rounds by the correctional staff. However, Correctional Officers told us that they make irregular 30-minute rounds to monitor inmates.

172 Inmates told us that Executive Staff make rounds on a weekly basis. Executive Staff rounds are recorded in a logbook that all staff members must sign as they enter the unit. The RHU logbook records the staff member's name, times of entry and exit, and the reason for the visit. We could not use the logbook to verify whether or not the Executive Staff walked each RHU range and made themselves available to each inmate on that range because these actions can be verified only through observation. As a result, we did not review RHU logbooks.

The BOP Has Taken Steps to Address Mental Health Staffing Shortages

Despite staffing challenges, we found that the BOP has sought to increase the mental health services it provides to inmates, including those in RHUs. BOP officials told us about and we observed some steps that the BOP has taken, or is in the process of taking, to meet inmate treatment requirements, including efforts to increase pay for BOP Psychiatrists, hiring regional health service recruiters, as well as program initiatives (detailed below) intended to improve psychology services throughout the BOP. The BOP's FY 2016 budget submission requested 130 additional mental health positions, mostly Psychologists, to address staffing concerns. However, the BOP did not receive its requested positions and Psychology Services Branch officials told us that the BOP was not anticipating additional funding in FY 2017.[173] Additional steps taken or underway include:

- **SHU Pilot Program.** According to BOP officials, the pilot program was initiated at six high security institutions in which a Restrictive Housing Psychologist will be designated to the SHU. The program was intended "to increase the treatment of SHU inmates and evaluate an inmate's need for placement in SHU" with individualized interventions based on inmate needs. As of October 2016, the BOP had filled five of six pilot program positions.
- **Psychology Internship Program.** The Pre-Doctoral Psychology Internship Program allows Pre-Doctoral students to complete their 1 year of internship at a BOP institution. The program, which the BOP indicates predates and was expanded prior to the May 2014 policy, includes student loan repayment as an incentive for individuals interested in working for the BOP.[174]

Though we acknowledge these positive steps in attempting to address mental health staffing shortages, we believe that the BOP needs to do more to ensure that inmates with mental illness, including those in restrictive housing, receive care consistent with its May 2014 policy.

The BOP Needs to Improve Mental Health Training for Its Correctional Staff

As stated above, various staff members, including correctional staff, monitor inmates in RHUs. During our site visits, BOP Psychology Services staff told us that they provide suicide prevention training to SHU staffs on a quarterly basis, in addition to the annual

---

[173] See DOJ, *FY 2016 Performance Budget Congressional Submission.*

[174] We spoke to a Psychologist who started her career with the BOP as a Pre-Doctoral Psychology Intern. She later became a Staff Psychologist, was promoted to Advanced Care Level Psychologist, and is now an Internship Coordinator. Several Psychologists told us that the internship program is a good recruitment tool for the BOP.

refresher training on mental health that all staff receive.[175] An ADX Correctional Officer told us that the annual refresher training covers erratic behaviors, changes in behavior, and how to report and document these observations. However, a SHU Lieutenant suggested that annual refresher training could be improved by incorporating de-escalation techniques to help the correctional staff learn how to calm inmates with mental illness who become distressed. Further, while all correctional staff we interviewed said they had received annual refresher training, several RHU correctional staff could not speak to any specific information related to the training's mental health content.

According to BOP policy, additional mental health specialty training will be made available in select MHCL 2–4 and administrative institutions.[176] During our site visits, staff at two BOP secure residential mental health treatment program institutions told us that they had received specialized mental health training to better manage inmates with mental illness in restrictive housing.[177] However, we found that staff at other BOP institutions who work with inmates with serious mental illness in RHUs had not received this specialized training. One Correctional Officer who has worked extensively with MHCL 4 inmates in restrictive housing stated that he has been provided with only RHU -specific suicide training in addition to basic SHU training. A Chief Psychologist at a Care Level 3 complex told us that he was unaware of the specialized mental health training referenced in BOP policy. BOP policy states that "to support this specialized training, adequate Psychology Services staffing must be in place" at these institutions. Despite the policy providing for such training in select MHCL 2–4 and administrative institutions, the BOP's inadequate mental health staffing has affected the Psychology Services Branch's ability to provide specialized training to correctional staffs working in RHUs who are responsible for monitoring the behavior of inmates, including many with mental illness.[178] Psychology Services Branch officials told us that due to the lack of additional funding the BOP has not required that specialty training be provided to any institution staff. As of October 2016, specialty training was offered at some FMCs and MHCL 2 and 3 institutions.

---

[175] The BOP's revised SHU policy mandates that correctional staff must complete quarterly SHU trainings prior to each quarter, regardless of prior completions, and includes training content in dealing with inmates who have mental illness. See Program Statement 5270.11, 17.

[176] BOP policy states that the "Mental Health Specialty Training will include 24 hours of specialized mental health training, including suicide prevention, understanding mental illness, cultural diversity and sensitivity, psychiatric medications, behavior management principles, confidentiality, communication skills, de-escalation skills, and building collaborative relationships." See BOP Program Statement 5310.16, 22.

[177] During our site visit to USP Atlanta's secure residential mental health treatment program, a staff member, who had worked in this RHU for nearly 2 years, told us that although additional, specialized mental health training was provided to correctional staff initially assigned to this RHU, this training had not been provided on a recurring basis. As a result, correctional staff who rotate into this RHU did not receive the more extensive, specialized mental health training and, consequently, this staff member did not believe they are adequately trained to work in this RHU.

[178] According to the Department's "180-day Status Report," the BOP has begun training that incorporates the "Guiding Principles," established in the Department's January 2016 report on restrictive housing, into curricula for quarterly and annual training programs for staff assigned to SHUs and to Wardens, Associate Wardens, Captains, Lieutenants, and new Correctional Officers.

The BOP Lacks Guidance and Training for Determining and Documenting When an Inmate's Symptoms May Not Be Genuine, Which May Affect Inmates in Restrictive Housing

We found that the BOP does not have guidance or training for staff in determining and documenting when an inmate's symptoms may not be genuine, a behavior commonly known as malingering.[179] Because malingering is classified as a behavior and not a mental disorder, BOP policy does not require staff to document malingering when they observe it.[180] Consequently, staff use their own discretion to document malingering and inmates with legitimate mental illness may continue to be placed in RHUs for longer periods of time without receiving the treatment they need.

According to BOP data, at the end of FY 2014 there were 430 inmates, or less than 1 percent of the BOP's total inmate population, for whom staff chose to document malingering. But such reporting is not required, as discussed above, and feedback that the OIG received from BOP staff strongly suggests that it may not accurately reflect the prevalence of malingering throughout the BOP. For example, staff at USP Lewisburg told us that malingering is widespread in the SMU inmate population. The text box provides an example of an inmate who staff believed was malingering, who was taken off previously prescribed medications but was later removed from the SMU because of mental health reasons.

Challenges for SMU Staff in Determining When an Inmate's Symptoms May Not Be Genuine

According to an inmate's case file, he was diagnosed with three mental disorders when he arrived at the SMU and was prescribed one antipsychotic medication and one medication to reduce the side effects of antipsychotic treatment. The inmate previously had been diagnosed with five mental disorders and prescribed a variety of medications during his incarceration at other BOP institutions.

Nine months after arriving at the SMU, the inmate was removed from his medications after the SMU Psychologist determined that his behavior was malingering rather than genuine symptoms of mental disorder. The Psychologist's notes state, "Despite the litany of diagnoses and psychiatric medications [the inmate's] contacts with psychology staff indicate a clear history of malingering and feigning symptoms to change conditions of his confinement." The inmate "has not exhibited nor reported any mental health symptoms indicative of an acute mental health disorder, although he has repeatedly engaged in disruptive behaviors as well as malingered

[179] Malingering is the intentional production of false or grossly exaggerated physical or psychological problems and, usually, is the result of an individual's external motivations. Malingering is not considered a mental illness but should be suspected when there is a discrepancy between the individual's claimed distress and the clinician's objective findings, a lack of cooperation during evaluations and in complying with prescribed treatment, or if the individual has been diagnosed with Antisocial Personality Disorder. See Medscape.com, "Malingering Clinical Presentation," http://emedicine.medscape.com/article/293206-clinical (accessed June 7, 2017).

[180] Therefore, we could not use BOP data to determine the prevalence of malingering throughout the BOP or RHUs or to assess BOP or RHU trends of malingering.

suicidality in an attempt to regain his medications." Two months later, two of the inmate's three mental disorders were classified as no longer current. Nevertheless, 3 months after the inmate was removed from his medications, and 1 year after the inmate entered the SMU program, the inmate was transferred out of the SMU for mental health reasons.

Source: BOP inmate case file.

According to the Administrator of the Psychology Services Branch, mental health staff should be "conservative about attaching that label [malingering] to anyone because once it's in the record, it can really color other peoples' judgment about the inmate." Institution staffs told us that they rely on their prior clinical training, correctional experience, or even a "gut feeling" to determine whether an inmate's symptoms are real or the inmate may be malingering. One Clinical Director told us that it would be useful for the BOP to issue guidelines or training that explains how to deal with malingering inmates because it is a "big problem in the institutions" and many inmates are simply seeking medication. Yet, BOP officials cautioned us about the risks of providing guidance to staff to assess malingering. The Chief of Mental Health Services cautioned:

> We want to make sure that our staff [doesn't] find malingering when it's actually not there. If you're working in a stressful environment with difficult inmates, it can be easy to dismiss someone. You could be at risk to dismiss someone as malingering so you can get them off your caseload and not have to deal with them. So, I think what we focus on is making accurate mental health diagnosis for true disorders and recognizing that yes, someone can have a serious mental illness and malinger.

BOP officials offered alternatives to guidance on malingering. A Senior Deputy Assistant Director from the RSD said that the BOP could provide staff with webinar trainings on using a psychology assessment tool known as the Structured Interview of Reported Symptoms to better accurately assess inmates' symptoms.[181] While training to assess whether mental health symptoms are genuine could assist mental health staff, we question whether, without careful guidance and consideration, inmates with legitimate symptoms of mental illness will be dismissed as malingerers by overworked RHU mental health staff.

---

[181] The BOP also employs Forensic Psychologists, who are licensed and have more specialized training in malingering because, as part of their job duties, they screen the mental health of defendants in criminal cases who could have a strong incentive to malinger symptoms of mental illness. However, most BOP Psychologists are not Forensic Psychologists. According to Psychology Services Branch officials, up to 40 percent of BOP Psychologists are unlicensed.

In response to a working draft of this report, the BOP stated that in order to be hired as a BOP Psychologist, an individual must have a doctoral degree in clinical or counseling psychology from an accredited university, which fully qualifies him or her to diagnose mental disorders regardless of licensing status. Nevertheless, we believe that many BOP mental health services staffs, both Health Services and Psychology Services staffs, may benefit from receiving more specialized training in screening inmates for genuine mental illness.

CONCLUSION AND RECOMMENDATIONS

Conclusion

The BOP's mission is to protect society by confining federal offenders in correctional facilities that are safe, humane, cost-efficient, and secure, and to provide reentry programming to ensure inmates' successful return to the community. While in the BOP's custody, inmates at times may have to be placed in Restrictive Housing Units (RHU) to ensure the safety and security of inmates and staff. However, studies show that the frequency, duration, and conditions of confinement of restrictive housing, even for short periods of time, can have a significant impact on inmates' mental health and can be particularly harmful for inmates with mental illness. The BOP has taken some measures to improve the treatment of inmates with mental illness in its institutions and to monitor all inmates who are housed in RHUs. However, we believe that significant additional steps are required to screen, treat, and monitor inmates with mental illness in these restrictive environments, especially those in single-cell confinement. The lack of policies to adequately address conditions of confinement that amount to solitary confinement may result in inmates having limited human contact and out- of-cell opportunities, which research suggests may negatively affect their mental health. We have identified several areas of concern with regard to the frequency, duration, and conditions of confinement for inmates with mental illness in RHUs.

First, BOP data shows, and we observed, inmates with mental illness housed in traditional RHUs, such as Special Housing Units (SHU), Special Management Units (SMU), and the U.S. Penitentiary Administrative Maximum Security Facility (ADX), as well as other forms of restrictive housing, for long periods of time and in conditions that could constitute solitary confinement. We also found that the BOP cannot determine how many of its inmates are placed in single-cell confinement because it does not track this information.

Moreover, although the BOP monitors all inmates' *consecutive* days in RHUs, it does not monitor inmates' *cumulative* time in RHUs, including the SHUs that house over 80 percent of BOP's restrictive housing population. Also, inmates with mental illness spend disproportionately longer periods of time in restrictive housing than do their peers. The OIG's analysis of BOP data shows that inmates with mental illness at both the SMUs and the ADX spent about 14 to 17 months longer in these RHUs than what the BOP reported for all inmates in these RHUs.

Additionally, we found that the BOP does not sufficiently track or monitor inmates with mental illness, including those in RHUs. BOP mental health officials estimated the percentage of inmates who have mental illness as significantly higher than what BOP data indicates. We believe that the prevalence of mental illness throughout the BOP is likely underreported because institution staffs do not always document inmates' mental health diagnoses. Also, because over 90 percent of BOP inmates are designated at Mental Health Care Level 1 and are not required to have a mental health diagnosis, the BOP cannot differentiate between inmates who may have undocumented mental illness and inmates who simply do not have any mental disorders. Consequently, the BOP cannot accurately determine the number of inmates, including those in RHUs, who have mental illness or ensure that it is providing appropriate treatment to all inmates with mental illness.

Although the BOP issued a policy in 2014 intended to enhance mental health treatment for inmates, including inmates in RHUs, it does not appear that the BOP has provided sufficient staffing to implement the new policy effectively. To the contrary, the OIG found that after the new policy was issued, BOP mental health staff reduced the number of inmates required to receive regular mental health treatment by approximately 30 percent. Based on our analysis of BOP data and feedback from institution staffs, we are concerned that the number of inmates required to receive regular treatment decreased substantially following the BOP's adoption of the 2014 policy and, as a result, the treatment for many inmates with mental illness, including those in RHUs, may have been discontinued.

In addition, shortages of Psychologists and Psychiatrists throughout the BOP may also affect the treatment provided to inmates with mental illness, including those in RHUs. Staffing challenges can contribute to conflicting mental disorder diagnoses, which can also affect the continuity of care for inmates.

We identified a number of issues with U.S. Penitentiary (USP) Lewisburg's SMU program in particular, which is concerning since this SMU is the BOP's most populated RHU and, as of June 2016, confined over 1,100 inmates. Among the issues we identified, we found that since the BOP issued its new mental health policy, SMU staff downgraded the level of care for a disproportionate number (56 percent) of SMU inmates and, as a result, some inmates may not receive necessary mental health care. In addition, inmates with mental illness are in the SMU significantly longer than their peers and longer than the program's intended duration. Further, misleading SMU performance metrics may compromise the BOP's oversight of the program and inaccurately reflect the circumstances of inmates who have been in the SMU. Moreover, USP Lewisburg's aged infrastructure, including its undersized cells with poor ventilation that do not meet generally accepted standards, could adversely affect the conditions of confinement for all SMU inmates and may be particularly harmful for inmates with mental illness who can spend years in this SMU.

Finally, while the BOP has taken steps to remove inmates from placement in traditional RHUs and to mitigate mental health concerns for inmates in RHUs, we found a number of areas that continue to need improvement. The BOP needs to develop meaningful performance metrics to help measure the effectiveness of its secure residential mental health treatment programs. We found that some state corrections systems have developed variations of residential mental health treatment programs with potential efficiencies that we believe the BOP should consider. Further, the BOP should improve the mental health training for RHU correctional staff, explore the potential to increase the use of alternative sanctions to further prevent inmates with mental illness from being placed in restrictive housing, and provide additional guidance and training to mental health staff to determine whether mental health symptoms are genuine and to document malingering.

Recommendations

To ensure that inmates, including those with mental illness, are placed in restrictive housing under conditions of confinement that adhere to specific standards that are applied consistently and sustain appropriate mental health care, we recommend that the BOP:

1) Establish in policy the circumstances that warrant the placement of inmates in single-cell confinement while maintaining institutional and inmate safety and security and ensuring appropriate, meaningful human contact and out-of-cell opportunities to mitigate mental health concerns.
2) Define and establish in policy extended placement in measureable terms.

To ensure that inmates receive appropriate mental health care and are sufficiently tracked and monitored during their placement in restrictive housing, we recommend that the BOP:

3) Track all inmates in single-cell confinement and monitor, as appropriate, the cumulative amount of time that inmates with mental illness spend in restrictive housing, including single-cell confinement.
4) Identify all forms of restrictive housing utilized throughout its institutions and ensure that all local policies are updated to reflect standards for all inmates in restrictive housing consistent with established nationwide policies.
5) Evaluate and limit as appropriate the consecutive amount of time that inmates with serious mental illness may spend in restrictive housing.
6) Ensure that the Psychology Services staff documents inmates' mental illness diagnoses in the Bureau's Electronic Medical Record System and Psychology Data System.
7) Reassess the Mental Health Care Level system to ensure that it fully captures the mental health needs of inmates, including inmates in restrictive housing, and that classifications distinguish between inmates who have some form of mental illness and those who do not have any form of mental illness.
8) Regularly monitor, by institution and type of Restrictive Housing Unit, trends in inmates' designated Mental Health Care Levels to further assess the factors that affect the treatment of inmates with mental illness.

9) Determine what additional steps can be taken to prioritize and incentivize the hiring of mental health staff at institutions that have inmates with mental illness in long-term restrictive housing.

To improve the BOP's efforts to mitigate the placement of inmates with mental illness in traditional RHUs and enhance the effectiveness of secure residential mental health treatment programs, we recommend that the BOP:

10) Assess the scalability of secure residential mental health treatment programs and develop alternatives to address their potential limitations.
11) Develop and implement formal performance metrics sufficient to measure the effectiveness of secure residential mental health treatment programs.
12) Survey institutions and/or take other steps to identify alternative practices that reduce the frequency and duration of the placement of inmates with mental illness in restrictive housing, and implement such alternatives when appropriate.
13) Provide additional mental health training to correctional staff who are responsible for monitoring the behavior of inmates in restrictive housing.
14) Provide additional guidance and training to mental health staff on diagnosing mental illness, including guidance on documenting malingering behavior by inmates.

To address concerns regarding inmates with mental illness at USP Lewisburg's SMU, we recommend that the BOP:

15) Conduct a comprehensive review of U.S. Penitentiary Lewisburg's Special Management Unit that addresses the staffing, treatment, conditions of confinement, and performance metrics of the program.

APPENDIX 1. METHODOLOGY OF THE OIG REVIEW

Standards

The OIG conducted this review in accordance with the Council of the Inspectors General on Integrity and Efficiency's *Quality Standards for Inspection and Evaluation* (January 2012).

Data Analysis

Inmates with a History of Mental Illness

The OIG used BOP data from the end of FY 2014 to determine the number of sentenced inmates whom the BOP had diagnosed with mental disorders. The BOP provided us with

inmate mental disorders that were documented in the Bureau's Electronic Medical Record System and Psychology Data System (BEMR-PDS) for every BOP inmate within our scope.[182] Each BOP inmate had one data row with corresponding columns that were populated with as many mental disorders as applicable, since many inmates had multiple mental health diagnoses. Table 7 is a condensed version of actual mental illness data for a sample of four anonymous BOP inmates. Based on BOP data in this table, Inmate A did not have any documented diagnoses while Inmate B had one, Inmate C had three, and Inmate D had two.

Because we asked the BOP to provide all mental illness diagnoses in a sequential order beginning in the "Mental Health Illness 1" data field, we were able to use this data field to filter out all of the inmates who did not have any documented diagnoses and determine the number of inmates with a documented history of mental illness (18,066 inmates).

Table 7. BOP Inmate Mental Illness Data

		Mental Health Illness		
BOP Inmates	MHCL	1	2	3
A	1			
B	2	Bipolar I Disorder – Most Recent Episode Depressed		
C	4	Antisocial Personality Disorder	Psychotic Disorder Not Otherwise Specified	Personality Disorder Not Otherwise Specified
D	2	Mood Disorder Not Otherwise Specified	Psychotic Disorder Not Otherwise Specified	

Notes: MHCL = Mental Health Care Level. The BOP data also included the date the BOP diagnosed the inmate with the mental disorder; the status of the diagnosis (current, remission, or resolved); and the date the inmate's status was documented in BEMR-PDS. We did not include these categories in this table.

Source: BOP data.

In doing so, as discussed in the report, we found that there were 968 inmates who were designated at Mental Health Care Levels (MHCL) 2–4 who did not have any corresponding diagnoses documented in the data.[183] Because these 968 inmates were designated at

[182] We excluded chemical dependency (substance abuse) diagnoses from our data request.

[183] As we discussed above, the BOP's Chief of Mental Health Services told us that these inmates did not have diagnoses in the BOP data provided to us because BOP staff did not enter any mental health diagnoses into BEMR-PDS; staff entered diagnoses into BEMR-PDS with different diagnostic codes that were not provided to

MHCLs 2–4, we knew they had to have a history of mental illness. As a result, we added this inmate total to the 18,066 inmates with a documented history of mental illness to determine that at least 19,034 inmates, or approximately 12 percent of the BOP's total inmate population, had a history of mental illness.[184]

Inmates with a History of Mental Illness by Restrictive Housing Unit Type, FY 2014

We used BOP mental illness data from the end of FY 2014, as well as BOP population snapshot data, to determine the number of sentenced inmates whom the BOP had diagnosed with mental disorders and who were in Restrictive Housing Units (RHU). In addition to the mental illness data discussed above, the BOP also provided us with Special Housing Unit (SHU), Special Management Unit (SMU), and U.S. Penitentiary Administrative Maximum Security Facility (ADX) population snapshot data from the end of FY 2010 through FY 2014, as well as for May 30, 2015. The BOP's mental illness dataset and its SHU, SMU, and ADX population datasets included the inmates' full name, gender, and unique BOP registration number. Using the BOP's inmate registration numbers, we matched all 397 ADX inmates; all 1,248 SMU inmates; and 94 percent of all SHU inmates (8,166 out of 8,667) who were in these RHUs at the end of FY 2014 to BOP mental illness data from the end of FY 2014. Using this methodology, we determined that 37 percent of ADX inmates (146 out of 397); 27 percent of SMU inmates (331 out of 1,247); and 21 percent of SHU inmates (1,651 out of 7,980) had a BOP-documented history of mental illness.[185]

Mental Health Care Level Changes for Sample RHU Inmates

We selected a sample of 688 RHU inmates designated at MHCLs 1–4. This sample included inmates selected from BOP population snapshot data:

- all 239 SMU inmates who were designated at MHCLs 2–4 at the end of FYs 2012, 2013, 2014, and on May 30, 2015;

---

us; or staff manually entered diagnoses as free text rather than selecting diagnoses from a drop-down menu, which resulted in the diagnoses not being captured when the BOP extracted this information.

184 In this report, an inmate with a history of mental illness is defined as any inmate who has at least one BOP diagnosis — either current, in remission, or resolved — documented in BOP data. Also, as discussed in the report, we did not include inmates in our count who had undergone an initial mental health records review, were given a tentative MHCL designation by the BOP's Designation and Sentence Computation Center, but had yet to be examined, in person, by a mental health clinician.

185 Because we were able to match only 94 percent of all SHU inmates (8,166 out of 8,667) at the end of FY 2014, we cannot comment on the prevalence of documented mental illness among the 501 inmates whom we were unable to match. Additionally, while we successfully matched 8,166 SHU inmates with BOP mental illness data, 186 of these inmates had yet to be examined, in person, by a mental health clinician. Thus, we also excluded these inmates from our analysis.

Furthermore, while we successfully matched all 1,248 inmates at the SMU, we excluded 1 inmate from our analysis because this inmate had yet to be examined, in person, by a mental health clinician. We therefore determined the prevalence of documented mental illness among 1,247 SMU inmates.

- 57 ADX inmates who were designated at MHCLs 2–4 or had been at one point during our scope;
- 182 SHU inmates from institutions we visited who were designated at MHCLs 2–4 from the end of FY 2010 through May 30, 2015, or had been at one point during our scope;
- 36 ADX inmates who were designated at MHCL 1 from the end of FY 2010 through May 30, 2015, or had been at one point during our scope; and
- 174 SHU inmates designated at MHCL 1 from the end of FY 2010 through May 30, 2015, or had been at one point during our scope.

In our sample, we included 210 BOP inmates who were designated at MHCL 1 during our scope and who may not have had mental illness. We evaluated whether BOP inmates designated at MHCL 1 may have had their MHCL increased before or after the issuance of the BOP's new mental health policy on May 1, 2014. We believed that if we focused only on inmates who were already designated at MHCLs 2–4, this may have prevented us from recognizing MHCL 1 inmates whose care level may have increased. As mentioned in the report, over 90 percent of BOP inmates, including the majority of inmates with mental illness, are designated at MHCL 1.

Also, as stated in the report, this analysis does not account for every MHCL change that may have occurred for our sample of RHU inmates between FY 2010 and August 29, 2015. Rather, we identified whether or not sample inmates' MHCLs increased or decreased at specific points of time during our scope. More specifically, we assessed sample inmates' initial MHCL assignment (which began in FY 2010 for BOP inmates) and then assessed whether an inmate's MHCL increased, decreased, or remained the same as of April 30, 2014 (the day before the new policy was issued). Likewise, we then again assessed sample inmates' MHCLs as of April 30, 2014, and then assessed whether an inmate's MHCL had increased, decreased, or remained the same as of August 29, 2015 (about 16 months after the new policy was issued).[186] Table 8 below shows BOP data for a sample inmate's MHCL change. Based on the BOP data in this table, we recorded that this inmate's MHCL had increased before the new policy was issued and had decreased after the new policy was implemented.

Table 8. One Sample BOP Inmate's MHCL Data

Inmate's MHCL	Date Inmate's MHCL Was Assigned	Date Inmate's MHCL Stopped
1	July 7, 2010	April 21, 2011
2	April 21, 2011	October 21, 2014
1	October 21, 2014	August 29, 2015

186 For some of our 688 sample RHU inmates, we could not determine whether the change to the inmate's MHCL occurred in restrictive housing, such as those who were placed in institution SHUs, or in the general population.

Note: The inmate in this table was designated at MHCL 1 when the BOP extracted this information on August 29, 2015.

Source: BOP data.

Site Visits

From June 2015 through August 2015, we visited seven BOP institutions designated at Care Levels 2, 3, and 4: U.S. Penitentiary (USP) Allenwood, Pennsylvania; USP Atlanta, Georgia; Federal Medical Center Carswell, Fort Worth, Texas; Federal Correctional Complex (FCC) Florence (ADX), Colorado; USP Lewisburg, Pennsylvania; FCC Petersburg, Hopewell, Virginia; and FCC Terre Haute, Indiana. We selected these seven BOP sites based on their special RHU programs or the large number of inmates with mental illness in their RHUs, as determined by the number of inmates designated at MHCLs 2–4.

Interviews

We interviewed senior officials from the BOP Central Office's Correctional Programs Division, Reentry Services Division, Health Services Division, and Office of Research and Evaluation.

During site visits, we interviewed Executive Staff, including Wardens, Chief Psychologists, Clinical Directors, and a Chief Psychiatrist. We also interviewed mental health staff who worked or had worked in RHUs, including Staff Psychologists, Staff Psychiatrists, General Practitioners, a Psychiatric Nurse, a Physician's Assistant, a Treatment Specialist, and a Recreation Therapist. In addition, we interviewed other institution staff, including RHU Lieutenants and Correctional Officers, as well as unit team officials and Disciplinary Hearing Officers. At the seven institutions we visited, the OIG team had private interviews with 53 inmates with a history of mental illness. Most of the inmates we interviewed were in restrictive housing at the time of our visit or had recently been released from restrictive housing.

We also interviewed officials with the Office of the Deputy Attorney General regarding the development of the Department's January 2016 report on the use of restrictive housing, the project lead and Psychiatrist from the Center of Naval Analysis and Solutions team that conducted the review and assessment of the BOP's use of restrictive housing, as well as officials from the U.S. Government Accountability Office (GAO) for more information related to the two FY 2013 GAO reports issued on the BOP's use of SHUs and the BOP's oversight of its mental health treatment programs. Additionally, we interviewed staff from the Department's Civil Rights Division for more information related to its May 2013 investigation of the Pennsylvania State Institution at Cresson and February 2014 investigation of the Pennsylvania Department of Corrections.

Finally, we interviewed senior officials from eight state departments of corrections that we had selected for their publicized reforms or progressive policy relating to the placement of inmates with mental illness in restrictive housing. These eight states were Massachusetts, Washington, Pennsylvania, New York, Virginia, Mississippi, Maine, and Colorado.

Inmate Case File Review

We analyzed the content of case files for 59 inmates with a history of mental illness, most of whom we interviewed during our site visits. These case files included, but were not limited to, psychology intake screening documents (screening), clinical contacts (treatment), and restrictive housing psychology reviews (monitoring). Due to the size of the inmate case files, we limited our review from January 1, 2014 (4 months before the BOP issued the new mental health policy) to the most recent documents available at the time of our site visits (June 2015 through August 2015). We reviewed these documents to assess BOP mental health staffs' compliance with BOP policy, such as timeliness standards, based on document dates, indications of in-cell or out-of-cell contacts with inmates, or other important notes that are relevant to the BOP's screening, treatment, and monitoring of inmates with mental illness in RHUs.

Our analysis featured several important limitations. The primary limitation was the sample of documents each institution provided. While some institutions, particularly the ADX, provided us with thousands of inmate records, other institutions provided us with substantially less psychology documentation, which hindered the consistency of our analysis of the institutions. Therefore, any conclusions drawn from case file reviews about the screening, treatment, and monitoring of inmates with mental illness could be based only on documentation we received from the institutions we visited. There were also inconsistencies in the psychology forms, such as Psychology Services Reviews, used among the institutions we visited and even within the institutions, which in some cases did not capture all of the information that we had regularly been assessing. This further hindered the consistency of our analysis of psychology documents.

Finally, we learned that the dates we used to assess timeliness standards were entered by mental health staff and were not automated by BEMR-PDS (other than the date and time the form was completed). As a result, the dates we used in our report to assess timeliness standards, such as the date Psychology Services staff conducted an intake screening or a Psychology Services Review, result from staff inputs. Although there are legitimate reasons for this, such as staff not having time to input information into BEMR-PDS for all the clinical contacts they conducted during a single day, we recognize that mental health staff could potentially backdate these documents to artificially meet BOP timeliness standards. We note that mental health staff told us that the BOP has greater transparency in BEMR-PDS; can see when a document was created, edited, and completed; and thus may be able to detect any backdating of documents. Because we did not have access to BEMR-PDS, we were unable to determine whether backdating documents may have occurred for inmates with mental illness in RHUs.

APPENDIX 2. BOP POLICIES GOVERNING RESTRICTIVE HOUSING AND MENTAL HEALTH SCREENING, TREATMENT, AND MONITORING

This appendix contains a brief description of the requirements established through BOP policies for Restrictive Housing Units (RHU) and mental health care, including the screening, treatment, and monitoring of inmates with mental illness. We describe the BOP's national policies for operating its Special Housing Units (SHU) and its Special Management Units (SMU), as well as local policy for the care and treatment of inmates with mental illness at the U.S. Penitentiary Administrative Maximum Security Facility (ADX). We also describe the BOP's new national policy for the care and treatment of inmates with mental illness; national policy for disciplining inmates, including those with mental illness; and national policies, procedures, and operational guidelines for providing psychology services.

Restrictive Housing Units

Program Statement 5270.10, Special Housing Units (August 2011)

SHUs at BOP institutions confine inmates separately from the general population, either alone or with a cellmate. In a SHU, inmates may be confined to their cells for up to an average of 23 hours each day. Inmates may be placed in a SHU as punishment for having committed a prohibited act (disciplinary segregation) or for a non- punitive purpose (administrative detention).[187] While SHUs are not intended for the long-term housing of an inmate, BOP national policy establishes no limit to the number of times an inmate may be placed in disciplinary segregation, nor does it limit the time an inmate, with or without mental illness, may remain in administrative detention. All inmates placed in administrative detention are to receive a review by a Segregation Review Officer within 3 workdays of their placement, and all inmates placed in the SHU are to receive a formal status review within 7 continuous calendar days of their placement, with subsequent reviews conducted at the same interval thereafter. This policy also states that after every

---

[187] Reasons to place an inmate in administrative detention include protective custody; a pending security classification or reclassification; holdover during transfer to another destination; and segregation of an inmate who poses a threat to life, property, self, other inmates, the public, or to the security or orderly operation of the institution.

30 calendar days of continuous placement in the SHU, all inmates are to be examined by mental health staff, including a personal interview. Emergency mental health care must be available to inmates in the SHU.

Program Statement 5270.11, Special Housing Units (November 2016)

On November 23, 2016, the BOP issued a revised SHU program statement in response to recommendations cited in the Department's January 2016 report on the use of restrictive housing. According to the revised policy, the BOP now prohibits SHU placement for inmates whom mental health staff have designated at Mental Health Care Level (MHCL) 3 or 4, have a psychology alert in SENTRY (the BOP's primary mission support database), or have been identified on the monthly SHU advisory (Hot List) unless the inmate presents an immediate or serious danger to self, staff, or the orderly operation of a facility. In the event that an inmate who meets one of these criteria is placed in the SHU, Psychology Services staff should be notified and conduct a mental health evaluation within 24 hours of the inmate's placement. Further, in an effort to enhance inmates' out-of-cell time, the revised SHU policy requires that staff at each BOP institution locally develop plans for increasing recreation and states that institutions with the necessary resources should increase recreation opportunities for inmates. The revised SHU policy also states that, ordinarily, inmates nearing the end of their term of incarceration will not be placed in the SHU, except when their presence in the general population threatens the safety, security, or the orderly operation of an institution, and that every effort will be made to prevent inmates' direct release from the SHU into the community. Last, the SHU policy mandates that correctional staff must complete quarterly SHU trainings prior to each quarter, regardless of prior completions, and includes training content regarding inmates with mental illness.

Program Statement 5217.01, Special Management Units (November 2008)

The SMU Program was established in 2008 to provide close management of and programming for inmates referred to the program from other institutions BOP-wide; to ensure the safety, security, and orderly operation of BOP facilities; and to protect the public. Referral to the SMU program is non-punitive and must be approved by the BOP's Central Office, which may happen when the inmate has:

- participated in or had a leadership role in geographical group/gang-related activity;
- a history of serious and/or disruptive disciplinary infractions;
- committed any 100-Level prohibited act after being classified as a member of a disruptive group;
- participated in, organized, or facilitated any group misconduct that adversely affected the orderly operation of an institution; and/or

- otherwise participated in or been associated with activity such that greater management of interactions with other persons is necessary to ensure the safety, security, or orderly operation of BOP institutions, or to protect the public.[188]

By policy, SMUs consist of four program phases, with each phase differentiated by its conditions of confinement, level of interaction with other inmates, delivery of programming, and expected time frame for inmates' progression to the next level.[189] Inmates are expected to complete a four-phase program within 18 to 24 months. The four phases of the SMU program are:

- **Phase 1:** Expected completion time is 4 months, with an initial progress review within 28 days and subsequently every 90 days. Inmates will normally be restricted to their cells.
- **Phase 2:** Expected completion time is 6–8 months, with a progress review every 90 days. Inmates will normally be restricted to their cells, but out-of-cell activities/programming may be increased on a case-by-case behavioral performance basis.
- **Phase 3:** Expected completion time is 6–8 months, with a progress review every 90 days. Inmates may be housed and participate in activities together, as necessary to protect the safety, security, and good order of the institution. There are also increased privileges for inmates who accomplish unit goals and maintain appropriate conduct.
- **Phase 4:** Expected completion time is 2–4 months, with a progress review every 30 days. Inmates must be able to demonstrate their sustained ability to coexist and interact appropriately with other individuals and groups in the unit.[190]

Conditions of confinement for SMU inmates are much more restrictive than those for general population inmates, but they become less restrictive as an inmate progresses from phase to phase of the program. Minimum SMU standards for conditions of confinement include placement in cells that should ordinarily house only the number of inmates for

---

[188] The BOP staff may impose sanctions on inmates who commit prohibited acts, which are categorized by the Greatest severity (100 Level), High severity (200 Level), Moderate severity (300 Level), and Low severity (400 Level). See Program Statement 5270.09, Inmate Discipline Program (July 8, 2011). The BOP classifies inmates as members of a disruptive group when they belong to or are closely affiliated with, for example, prison gangs, which have a history of disrupting operations and security. This also applies to inmates who may require separation from a specific disruptive group. See BOP Program Statement 5180.05, Central Inmate Monitoring System (December 31, 2007).

[189] Inmates assigned to the SMU are expected to complete the four-phase SMU program in 18 to 24 months, after which they may be designated to another appropriate facility. Inmates at SMU Program Phases 2, 3, or 4 who fail to make satisfactory progress may be returned to any previous phase. If an inmate continues to exhibit disruptive conduct after 6 additional months in the SMU, the inmate may be referred for designation to another appropriate facility, consistent with the orderly operation of BOP institutions.

[190] BOP Program Statement 5217.01, Special Management Units (November 19, 2008).

which the cells were designed and opportunities for exercise outside inmates' individual cells for 5 hours each week, ordinarily in 1-hour periods on different days. Additionally, each inmate in the SMU program is to be evaluated by mental health staff every 30 days, with emergency mental health care always made available either at the institution or from the community.

Program Statement 5217.02, Special Management Units (August 2016)

On August 9, 2016, as a result of recommendations in the Department's January 2016 report on the use of restrictive housing, the BOP issued a revised program statement for the SMU program. The revised SMU policy reduces the phases from four to three and the intended time frame for inmates' completion of the program from an average of 18–24 months to 9–13 months. According to the BOP, the revised SMU policy also requires a greater review of an inmate's mental health records prior to placement in a SMU, as well as at each stage of the program to ensure that mental health needs do not preclude him or her from completing the program. Specifically, the revised SMU policy states that a copy of an inmate's referral to the SMU program will be sent to the Psychology Services Branch, which will review the inmate's mental health record to determine whether mental health concerns preclude SMU program placement. An inmate in the SMU program may be removed if it becomes clear that his or her mental health does not reasonably allow him or her to complete the SMU program. The recommendation is forwarded to the Administrator, Psychology Services Branch, Central Office. If the recommendation is approved, the Psychology Administrator notifies the Warden. Upon successful completion of the SMU program, inmates are placed in the general population or designated to another appropriate facility.

U.S. Penitentiary, Administrative Maximum, Institution Supplement FLM 5310.16A, Treatment and Care of Inmates with Mental Illness (July 2015)

This policy supplements BOP national policy and provides institution-specific guidelines for the treatment and care of inmates with mental illness housed at the ADX at Florence, Colorado.[191] The ADX houses inmates who have a history of violent, disruptive behavior, both before and after their incarceration, and/or were escape prone in other correctional institutions. Ordinarily, inmates diagnosed with a serious mental illness will be diverted or removed from the ADX. The placement or continued housing of an inmate with serious mental illness at the ADX may occur only if extraordinary security needs are identified that cannot be managed elsewhere. If an inmate is identified as suffering from a serious mental illness while housed at the ADX, and the Chief Psychologist or ADX psychiatric services provider determines that the inmate does not need inpatient

---

[191] The local policy supplements BOP Program Statement 5310.16, Treatment and Care of Inmates with Mental Illness (May 1, 2014).

hospitalization, the Mental Health Treatment Coordinator will convene a multidiscipline committee to determine whether extraordinary security needs exist that prevent the inmate from being managed elsewhere.[192] Inmates who are newly identified as suffering from a serious mental illness while at the ADX, but who do not have extraordinary security needs, will be referred to an appropriate treatment program or other setting outside the ADX. Inmates at MHCL 4 are not to be housed at the ADX.

Upon arrival, Health Services staff will conduct inmates' initial intake screenings and assessments and identify whether newly transferred inmates have a current prescription for psychotropic medication. The Health Services intake screening seeks to identify inmates' mental health care problems and needs, which include, but are not limited to psychosis, hallucinations, suicidality, history of self-injury, mood disorders, disturbance, sexual victimization, and psychotropic medication use. In addition, a psychology intake evaluation of each inmate will follow within 7 business days of the inmate's arrival at the facility. At this intake evaluation, a Psychologist conducts a clinical interview of the inmate in a private setting and evaluates the accuracy of the inmate's designated MHCL. Psychology Services and Health Services staffs ensure that every inmate with a clinically identified need for psychological treatment has access to mental health care. An inmate's housing status does not affect the level of care he receives. Inmates will ordinarily have access to in-cell therapeutic activities, including psychology programming, through closed-circuit television.

A Psychologist makes weekly rounds in each ADX housing unit to identify and address mental health and behavioral concerns and conducts a psychological review of each ADX inmate at 30-day intervals. For inmates designated at MHCL 2 or 3, inmates who have been referred for mental health services, or inmates who demonstrate changes in functioning, both the weekly and 30-day rounds will consist of a face-to-face interaction with the inmate's outer cell door opened and a correctional staff member present, if required. If clinically indicated, the inmate will be removed from the cell to be interviewed in a private interview space. Consistent with BOP national policy, inmates also receive Extended Restrictive Housing Placement Reviews when continuously housed in the ADX's SHU for 6 months or elsewhere at the ADX for 12 months, with update placement reviews conducted at the same intervals thereafter.

All inmates are to have reasonable access to "Inmate Request to Staff Member" forms to request mental health services, although such requests are to be accepted in any format. When a request or referral for mental health services relating to an ADX inmate is received at the Psychology Services Branch, the staff evaluates the referral or request on the same day; classifies it as emergent, urgent, or routine; and responds to it within 4 hours, 24 hours,

---

[192] The multidiscipline committee will ordinarily consist of the Warden, Associate Wardens, Captain, Special Investigative Agent, Case Management Coordinator, Unit Manager, Psychology Services, psychiatric services provider(s), Assistant Health Services Administrator/Supervisory Nurse, Psychiatric Nurse, and Supervisory Attorney. The Warden makes the final determination regarding extraordinary security needs.

or no more than 10 business days, respectively. Tele-psychiatry services are available to ADX inmates as needed when in-person psychiatry services are unavailable. To ensure continuity of tele-psychiatry care, tele-Psychiatrists will make intermittent onsite visits to the ADX to see inmates in person. At a minimum, inmates receiving psychiatric medications will be seen by a Psychiatrist, psychiatric midlevel provider, or other qualified provider every 90 days, or more often as clinically indicated, for at least the first year.

The ADX Care Coordination and Reentry (CCARE) team meets weekly to review inmate cases and identify strategies to mitigate the potentially negative effects of the correctional environment on inmates with mental illness. Each ADX inmate's case is reviewed at least monthly, and the CCARE team reviews and updates inmates' individual treatment plans at 6-month and annual intervals. The CCARE team, along with the treating clinician, identifies any proposed changes to inmates' treatment plans, and the treating clinician discusses them with the inmate. For inmates with mental illness who are scheduled for release within the following 12 months, staff members involved in their pre-release planning attend CCARE team meetings. Inmates with mental illness who are pending release into the community, to home detention, or to a Residential Reentry Center are provided reentry services.

Mental Health Screening, Treatment, and Monitoring

BOP Program Statement 5310.16, Treatment and Care of Inmates with Mental Illness (May 2014)

The BOP issued this national policy to ensure that inmates with mental illness are identified and receive treatment to assist their progress toward recovery while reducing or eliminating the frequency and severity of symptoms and associated negative outcomes of mental illness, such as placement in restrictive housing. The new policy redefines inmate MHCLs and incorporates diagnostic, impairment, and intervention-based criteria that substantially increased the work expected of BOP mental health care staff for inmates at MHCLs 2–4.

Prior to May 2014, Program Statement 5310.13, Institutional Management of Mentally Ill Inmates (1995), and a BOP policy memorandum that defined the BOP's MHCLs (2009) prescribed the BOP's policies and guidance for the care and treatment of inmates with mental illness.[193] Table 9 compares the BOP's former and revised mental health treatment standards.

All inmates at MHCLs 2–4 are to have an individualized mental health treatment plan, which identifies individual and/or group programming needs and describes the inmate's

---

[193] Former mental health treatment policies include Program Statement 5310.13, Institution Management of Mentally Ill Inmates (March 31, 1995), and the Assistant Director of the Correctional Programs Division, policy memorandum, December 16, 2009, which established the BOP's MHCL system.

mental health problems and goals, as well as the interventions planned to help the inmate meet those goals. These plans are to be reviewed and updated at a frequency determined by the inmate's MHCL.[194]

Inmates also receive psychosocial interventions with mental health staff, normally Psychologists, at a frequency determined by their MHCL.[195] However, any BOP staff member who observes inmate behaviors that may indicate mental illness is to report these observations to the Chief Psychologist or Mental Health Treatment Coordinator at the institution, which may result in an unscheduled psychosocial intervention with mental health staff. The Psychology Services staff conducts an Extended Restrictive Housing Placement Review when an inmate is housed continuously in the SHU for 6 months, in the ADX for 12 months, or in the SMU for 18 months, to determine whether the inmate has mental health issues that should preclude placement in that setting.

Table 9. The BOP's Mental Health Treatment Standards

Inmate Designations	Former Mental Health Treatment Policies (FY 2010 – April 30, 2014)	New Mental Health Treatment Policy (May 1, 2014 – Present)
MHCL 1	No required recurring mental health services after the intake screening	No required recurring mental health services after the intake screening
MHCL 2	Treatment interventions at least once every 3 months after the intake screening	Treatment interventions at least once per month after the intake screening
	CCARE meetings not established	CCARE meetings at least once per year
	No required updates for individual treatment plans	Individual treatment plans updated at least once per year
MHCL 3	Treatment interventions provided at least once per month after the intake screening	Treatment interventions provided at least once per week after the intake screening
	CCARE meetings not established	CCARE meetings at least once every 6 months
	No required updates for individual treatment plans	Individual treatment plans updated at least once every 6 months
MHCL 4	No detailed timelines standards for treatment interventions	Treatment interventions at least once per week after the intake screening
	CCARE meetings not established	CCARE meetings on a case-by-case basis
	No required updates for individual treatment plans	Individual treatment plans updated at least once every 3 months

Source: OIG analysis of BOP policies.

[194] Individualized mental health treatment plans are to be reviewed and updated every 12 months for inmates at MHCL 2, every 6 months for inmates at MHCL 3, and every 90 days for inmates at MHCL 4.

[195] As described in BOP Program Statement 5310.16, psychosocial intervention consists of a face-to-face mental health contact between an inmate and a Psychologist, in a manner that protects the inmate's privacy to the extent that it does not compromise the safety and security of staff. The contact should be consistent with the goals of the inmate's treatment plan.

Program Statement 5270.09, Inmate Discipline Program (July 2011)

The BOP's inmate discipline program helps ensure the safety, security, and orderly operation of correctional facilities and the protection of the public. It allows BOP staff to impose disciplinary sanctions on inmates who commit prohibited acts, and to do so in an impartial and consistent manner that is neither capricious nor retaliatory. Prohibited acts are divided into four categories based on their respective levels of severity: Greatest (100), High (200), Moderate (300), and Low (400). Each category of prohibited acts includes a range of disciplinary sanctions that may be imposed upon determination of the inmate's guilt. The discipline process starts when the staff becomes aware of an inmate's involvement in a prohibited act. A staff member completes an incident report describing the inmate's behavior and provides a copy to the inmate.[196] The Warden or a delegated authority appoints a BOP staff officer to investigate the incident. The investigating officer provides an investigative report to the Unit Discipline Committee, which may impose sanctions or refer the case to a Disciplinary Hearing Officer (DHO) to conduct a hearing.[197] The DHO may conduct a hearing on an incident report only if it is referred by the Unit Discipline Committee.[198] Disciplinary segregation is among the sanctions that may be imposed — up to 12 months for a Greatest Level severity prohibited act or up to 6 months for a High Level severity prohibited act. Loss of recreation privileges (exercise periods) may not be imposed on inmates in the SHU. An inmate may be removed from any program or group activity for a specified period of time as a sanction. Finally, consecutive disciplinary sanctions may be imposed on inmates found to have committed multiple prohibited acts.

If it appears at any stage of the discipline process that an inmate is mentally ill, the inmate will be referred to a mental health professional to determine whether the inmate is responsible for his or her conduct and whether he or she is competent. When an inmate is found to be mentally incompetent, the incident report will show as a finding that the inmate should not be disciplined for the prohibited act because he/she was found not mentally competent. If evidence, to include evidence presented by mental health staff, indicates that an inmate cannot understand the nature of the disciplinary proceedings or cannot participate in his or her own defense, disciplinary proceedings may be postponed until the inmate is competent enough to understand the proceedings and assist in his/her defense.

Program Statement 5310.12, Psychology Services Manual (March 1995)

The BOP's Psychology Services Manual (PSM) established policies, procedures, and operational guidelines for psychology services within the BOP. The PSM pre-dated the

---

[196] The incident report should note anything unusual about the inmate's behavior.

[197] All 100 and 200 Level severity charges must be referred to the DHO.

[198] The DHO is an independent officer who conducts hearings and imposes sanctions for incidents of misconduct referred by the Unit Discipline Committee. The DHO is an impartial decision maker who was not a victim, witness, investigator, or otherwise significantly involved in the incident.

BOP's new program statement for the care and treatment of inmates with mental illness by 19 years. Consequently, the PSM did not reflect current BOP policy and procedures to designate inmates by MHCL. Further, the PSM's definition of mental illness reflected the criteria of an earlier version of the American Psychiatric Association's *Diagnostic and Statistical Manual for Mental Disorders.*[199] The PSM implemented a stratified approach for providing mental health services to inmates with mental illness. Severely disturbed individuals are cared for at inpatient treatment facilities, and less disturbed inmates most often receive ongoing care in less restrictive environments.

According to the PSM, psychology services at each BOP institution should be sufficient to ensure that every inmate with a documented need and/or interest in psychological treatment has access to a level of care comparable to that available in the community and consistent with the overall mission of the institution. All inmates are to have access to direct clinical services from Psychology Services staffs. These include crisis intervention, brief counseling focused on a specific issue or problem, individual and/or group psychotherapy, and psycho-educational group programs. Though the provision of psychology services within an institution may vary depending on its mission, security level, staff and inmate characteristics, and availability of resources, the PSM placed the highest priority on the treatment of mentally ill inmates, initial psychological screening evaluations of newly admitted inmates, and detention/segregation unit visits and psychological reporting.

A Physician's Assistant medically screens each inmate for signs of psychological disturbance with 24 hours of arrival at a BOP facility. When psychological disturbance is suspected, the Physician's Assistant refers the inmate to Psychology Services for prompt and appropriate evaluation. Psychological Services staff conduct psychological screening of an inmate within the first 14 days of arrival at the facility (30 days for transferred inmates). This screening includes the inmate's voluntary completion of a Psychology Services Inmate Questionnaire, an interview by Psychology Services staff qualified to conduct a clinical interview, and psychological testing if judged necessary by the Psychologist.[200] When an inmate's responses to the Psychology Services Inmate Questionnaire indicate suicidal thoughts or feelings or when an inmate requests psychological services, a member of the Psychology Services staff will promptly meet with the inmate. For an inmate in holdover status, a preliminary screening by a Physician's Assistant is sufficient, unless a significant problem is identified. An individual referred to

---

[199] The PSM (Program Statement 5310.12) defines mental illness using criteria of the American Psychiatric Association, *Diagnostic and Statistical Manual for Mental Disorders,* 4th ed. (Arlington, Va.: American Psychiatric Association, 1994) (DSM-4). The current version, as of the issuance of this report, is DSM-5, which was published in 2013 and reflects a different definition.

[200] As time and resources permit, the BOP may enhance the psychological screening through behavioral observations, review of available historical information found in the Central File or through SENTRY (the BOP's primary mission support database), and psychological testing when deemed appropriate by a Psychologist.

Psychology Services as a result of this preliminary medical screening should be evaluated promptly by a Psychologist.

Each Chief Psychologist is responsible to assess the treatment needs of the inmate population on an annual basis and to determine what methods of treatment will best meet these needs. A treatment plan is to be formulated and executed for each inmate diagnosed with significant mental disturbance. The PSM refers to the Health Services Manual in recommending that each institution without a full-time Psychiatrist employ a consultant to meet the needs of inmates requiring medication. Psychotropic medication is not designed for, nor should it be used as, a method of chemical restraint to control behaviors unrelated to mental illness.

The BOP recognizes that extended periods of confinement in the SHU may have an adverse effect on the overall mental status of some individuals. Therefore, any inmate confined in the SHU for 30 consecutive days or longer will be psychologically evaluated. At least one member of the Psychology Services staff will visit the SHU on a weekly basis and document this visit in the SHU visitor's log. An inmate housed in the SHU for 30 days or longer will receive a psychological assessment at 30-day intervals.

Program Statement 5310.17, Psychology Services Manual (August 2016)

In August 2016, the BOP rescinded its March 1995 PSM and issued a revised PSM that establishes general procedures, guidelines, and priorities for psychological services.[201] The revised PSM includes a revised mission statement and psychology services priorities, including an increased emphasis on reentry services. The revised PSM also includes previously issued guidance regarding Transfer Intake Screenings, strategies to assess and support the core clinical skills of correctional Psychologists, and guidance for the operation of graduate student practicum programs in psychology services. The revised PSM removes duplicative content addressed in other psychology services program statements and updates guidance regarding the creation and maintenance of professional clinical documentation. Finally, the revised PSM references other psychology services program statements that provide more detailed procedures and guidelines for specific program areas.

In addition, the revised PSM establishes enhanced psychological services offered in restrictive housing settings. For example, restrictive housing Psychologists are assigned to provide direct clinical services such as screenings, evaluations, pre-treatment, and treatment services for inmates in restrictive housing settings, including the ADX, SMU, or at the six institutions participating in the SHU pilot program (discussed in the Results of the Review). A Psychologist also reviews the psychological status of any inmate confined

[201] The U.S. Government Accountability Office (GAO) recommended that the BOP Director develop and implement updated program statements to ensure that these statements reflect currently accepted treatment practices and standards related to inmate mental health care. See GAO, *Bureau of Prisons: Timelier Reviews, Plan for Evaluations, and Updated Policies Could Improve Inmate Mental Health Services Oversight,* GAO-13-1 (July 2013).

in a SHU, SMU, the ADX, or any other similar housing for more than 30 consecutive calendar days using data from multiple sources, including contact with the inmate, input from unit Correctional Officers, and documentation contained in the Bureau's Electronic Medical Record System and Psychology Data System (BEMR-PDS). The results of the psychological review are documented in BEMR-PDS using an appropriate note, such as ADX Review, SHU Review, or SMU Contact. The revised PSM also describes prevention, diversion, mitigation, intervention, transition, and oversight strategies employed by the Psychology Services Branch to intervene with inmates in restrictive housing settings.

Program Statement 5330.11, Psychology Treatment Programs (March 2009)

This program statement establishes policy, procedures, and guidelines for psychology treatment programs and serves as a training device for new Psychologists and treatment specialists, as well as a reference for more experienced Psychologists and treatment specialists. The program statement, also known as the BOP's Psychology Treatment Programs Manual, establishes guidelines for five treatment programs: (1) drug abuse programs; (2) "Resolve" trauma programs for women; (3) the Bureau Rehabilitation and Values Enhancement Program; (4) the Challenge Program; and (5) mental health treatment programs, including the Habilitation Program, Skills Program, Axis II Program, and Mental Health Treatment Units (or Step-Down Units).

APPENDIX 3. BOP RESIDENTIAL MENTAL HEALTH TREATMENT PROGRAMS

Table 10.

Mental Health Step Down Program	The Mental Health Step Down Program is a residential treatment program offering an intermediate level of care for male and female inmates with serious mental illness. The program is designed specifically to serve inmates who do not require impatient treatment but lack the skills to function in a general population prison setting. The program uses an integrative model that includes an emphasis on a modified therapeutic community cognitive behavioral therapies and skills training. The goal of the Step Down Program is to provide evidence-based treatment to chronically mentally ill inmates in order to maximize their ability to function and minimize relapse and the need for inpatient hospitalization.
	Mental Health Step Down Programs operate as modified therapeutic communities and utilize cognitive behavioral treatments, cognitive rehabilitation, and skills training. Criminal thinking is addressed through the identification of criminal thinking errors and engagement in pro-social interactions with staff and peers. The programs work closely with Psychiatry Services to ensure participants receive appropriate medication and have the opportunity to build a positive relationship with the treating Psychiatrist. Program content is designed to promote successful reentry into society at the conclusion of an inmate's term of incarceration, and program staff collaborates with community partners to facilitate reentry.

	Inmates with serious mental illnesses, who would benefit from intensive residential treatment, are considered for the program. Male inmates with a primary diagnosis of Borderline Personality Disorder are referred to the STAGES Program (see below). Mental Health Step Down Program participants must volunteer for the program and must not be acutely mentally ill (i.e., they must not meet criteria for inpatient mental health treatment).
	The Mental Health Step Down Program is conducted over 12–18 months. Inmates may participate in the program at any point in their sentence. Formal programming is facilitated half-days, 5 days a week with the remaining half-day dedicated to an institution work assignment or other programming, as participants are able.

Notes: The Step Down Program is available at Federal Correctional Institution (FCI) Butner, North Carolina (medium security); U.S. Penitentiary (USP) Atlanta, Georgia (high security); and USP Allenwood, Pennsylvania (high security). BOP Psychology Services Branch officials told us that a female Step Down Program had been available at FCI Danbury; however, since FCI Danbury is no longer a female institution, the BOP no longer has a Step Down Program for females.

Source: BOP, A Directory of Bureau of Prisons' National Programs, May 22, 2015.

Table 11.

Steps Toward Awareness, Growth, and Emotional Strength (STAGES) Program	The STAGES Program is a residential treatment program for male inmates with serious mental illnesses and a primary diagnosis of Borderline Personality Disorder. The program uses an integrative model that includes a modified therapeutic community, cognitive behavioral therapies, and skills training. The program is designed to increase the time between disruptive behaviors, foster living within the general population or community setting, and increase pro-social skills.
	The program curriculum is derived from Dialectical Behavior Therapy and takes place in a modified therapeutic community. There is also an emphasis on basic cognitive-behavioral skills consistent with other BOP treatment programs; for example, criminal thinking is addressed through the identification of criminal thinking errors and engagement in pro-social interactions with staff and peers. Program content is designed to prepare inmates for transition to less secure prison settings and promote successful reentry into society at the conclusion of their term of incarceration. Program staff collaborate with community partners to facilitate reentry.
	Inmates referred to the STAGES Program have a primary diagnosis of Borderline Personality Disorder and a history of unfavorable institutional adjustment linked to this disorder. Examples of unfavorable institutional adjustment include multiple incident reports, suicide watches, and/or extended placement in restrictive housing. Inmates designated to the STAGES Program must volunteer for treatment and be willing to actively engage in the treatment process. Willingness to engage in the treatment is addressed through a brief course of pre-treatment in which the inmate learns basic skills at the referring institution.
	The STAGES Program is conducted over 12–18 months. Inmates may participate in the program at any time during their sentence. Formal programming is facilitated half -days, 5 days a week, with the remaining half-day dedicated to an institution work assignment or other programming.

Notes: The STAGES Program is available at FCI Terre Haute, Indiana (medium security), and USP Florence, Colorado (high security).

Source: BOP, A Directory of Bureau of Prisons' National Programs.

APPENDIX 4. THE BOP'S RESPONSE TO THE DRAFT REPORT

U.S. Department of Justice
Federal Bureau of Prisons
Office of the Director

Washington DC 20534

June 23, 2017

Memorandum for Nina S. Pelletier
Assistant Inspector General
Office of Inspector General
Evaluation and Inspections Division

FROM: Thomas R. Kane, Acting Director

SUBJECT: Response to the Office of Inspector General's (OIG)

FORMAL DRAFT Report: OIG Review of the Federal Bureau of Prisons' Use of Restrictive Housing for Inmates with Mental Illness, Assignment Number A-2015-004

The Bureau of Prisons (BOP) appreciates the opportunity to respond to the open recommendations from the draft report entitled OIG Review of the Federal Bureau of Prisons' Use of Restrictive Housing for Inmates with Mental Illness. Please find the Bureau's response to the recommendations below:

Recommendations

Recommendation 1: Establish in policy the circumstances that warrant the placement of inmates in single-cell confinement while maintaining institutional and inmate safety and security and ensuring appropriate meaningful human contact and out-of-cell opportunities.

Response: The BOP agrees with this recommendation and will establish in policy factors to be considered when placing/retaining mental health inmates in single-cell confinement.

Recommendation 2: Define and establish in policy extended placement in measureable terms.

Response: The BOP agrees with this recommendation and will define and establish extended placement in measureable terms.

Recommendation 3: Track all inmates in single-cell confinement and monitor, as appropriate, the cumulative amount of time that inmates with mental illness spend in restrictive housing, including single-cell confinement.

Response: The BOP agrees with this recommendation as it pertains to mental health inmates, and we will track and monitor inmates with mental health care levels 2, 3, and 4.

Recommendation 4: Identify all forms of restrictive housing utilized throughout its institutions and ensure that all local policies are updated to reflect standards for all inmates in restrictive housing consistent with established nation-wide policies.

Response: The BOP agrees with this recommendation and will review all forms of restrictive housing, and ensure local, or national, policies are in place to direct their operation.

Recommendation 5: Evaluate and limit as appropriate the consecutive amount of time that inmates with serious mental illness may spend in restrictive housing.

Response: The BOP agrees with this recommendation and will establish limits, as appropriate, on consecutive placements in restrictive housing as it pertains to mental health inmates.

Recommendation 6: Ensure that the Psychology Services staff documents inmates' mental illness diagnoses in the Bureau's Electronic Medical Record System and Psychology Data System.

Response: The BOP agrees with this recommendation. The Psychology Services Branch will ensure Psychology Services staff document inmates' mental illness diagnoses in the Bureau's Electronic Medical Record and Psychology Data System.

Recommendation 7: Reassess the Mental Health Care Level system to ensure that it fully captures the mental health needs of inmates, including inmates in restrictive housing, and that classifications distinguish between inmates who have some form of mental illness and those who do not have any form of mental illness.

Response: The BOP agrees with this recommendation. The Psychology Services Branch will reassess the Mental Health Care Level system to ensure that it fully captures the mental health needs of inmates, including inmates in restrictive housing, and that there is a method to distinguish between inmates who have some form of mental illness and those who do not have any form of mental illness.

Recommendation 8: Regularly monitor, by institution and type of Restrictive Housing Unit, trends in inmates' designated Mental Health Care Levels to further assess the factors that affect the treatment of inmates with mental illness.

Response: The BOP agrees with this recommendation. The Psychology Services Branch will monitor trends in inmates' designated mental health care levels by institution and type of restrictive housing unit. This will be used to further assess the factors that affect the treatment of inmates with mental illness.

Recommendation 9: Determine what additional steps can be taken to prioritize and incentivize the hiring of mental health staff at institutions that have inmates with mental illness in long-term restrictive housing.

Response: The BOP agrees with this recommendation. The Psychology Services Branch and Health Services Division will determine what additional steps can be taken to prioritize and incentivize the hiring of mental health staff at institutions that have inmates with mental illness in long-term restrictive housing.

Recommendation 10: Assess the scalability of secure residential mental health treatment programs and develop alternatives to address their potential limitations.

Response: The BOP agrees with this recommendation. The Psychology Services Branch will assess the scalability of secure residential mental health treatment programs and develop alternatives to address their potential limitations.

Recommendation 11: Develop and implement formal performance metrics sufficient to measure the effectiveness of secure residential mental health treatment programs.

Response: The BOP agrees with this recommendation. The Psychology Services Branch will develop and implement formal performance metrics sufficient to measure the effectiveness of secure residential mental health treatment programs.

Recommendation 12: Survey institutions and/or take other steps to identify alternative practices that reduce the frequency and duration of the placement of inmates with mental illness in restrictive housing, and implement such alternatives when appropriate.

Response: The BOP agrees with this recommendation. The Psychology Services Branch and Correctional Programs Division will survey institutions and/or take other steps to identify alternative practices that reduce the frequency and duration of the placement of inmates with mental illness in restrictive housing, and implement such alternatives when appropriate.

Recommendation 13: Provide additional mental health training to correctional staff who are responsible for monitoring the behavior of inmates in restrictive housing.

Response: The BOP agrees with this recommendation, though we note it appears to be based on the opinions of a few staff, instead of any adverse event or incident caused by insufficient training. Correctional staff responsible for monitoring the behavior of inmates in restrictive housing currently receive a substantial amount of training, of which OIG may not be aware, but we will identify opportunities to provide additional training, including remedial training.

Recommendation 14: Provide additional guidance and training to mental health staff on diagnosing mental illness, including guidance on documenting malingering behavior by inmates.

Response: The BOP agrees with this recommendation. The Psychology Services Branch will provide additional guidance and training to mental health staff on diagnosing mental illness, including guidance on documenting malingering behavior by inmates.

Recommendation 15: Conduct a comprehensive review of U.S. Penitentiary Lewisburg's Special Management Unit that addresses the staffing, treatment, conditions of confinement, and performance metrics of the program.

Response: The BOP agrees with this recommendation. A multi-discipline group from various geographic locations is being assembled to conduct a comprehensive review of U.S. Penitentiary Lewisburg's Special Management Unit that addresses the staffing, treatment, conditions of confinement, and performance metrics of the program.

APPENDIX 5. OIG ANALYSIS OF THE BOP'S RESPONSE

The OIG provided a draft of this chapter to the Federal Bureau of Prisons (BOP). The BOP's response is included in Appendix 4. The BOP agreed with all of the OIG's recommendations. Below, we discuss the OIG's analysis of the BOP's response and actions necessary to close the recommendations.

Recommendation 1: Establish in policy the circumstances that warrant the placement of inmates in single-cell confinement while maintaining institutional and inmate safety and security and ensuring appropriate, meaningful human contact and out-of-cell opportunities to mitigate mental health concerns.

Status: Resolved.

BOP Response: The BOP agreed with this recommendation and will establish in policy the factors to be considered when placing/retaining mental health inmates in single-cell confinement.

OIG Analysis: The BOP's actions are at least partially responsive to our recommendation. By October 27, 2017, please clarify whether all inmates, including those with mental illness, will be included in policy, and how it will maintain institutional and inmate safety and security while ensuring appropriate, meaningful human contact and out-of-cell opportunities to mitigate mental health concerns, and provide a copy of the proposed policy language.

Recommendation 2: Define and establish in policy extended placement in measureable terms.

Status: Resolved.

BOP Response: The BOP agreed with this recommendation and will define and establish extended placement in measureable terms.

OIG Analysis: The BOP's actions are responsive to our recommendation. By October 27, 2017, please provide the BOP's definition for extended placement in measurable terms and describe how it will be established in policy.

Recommendation 3: Track all inmates in single-cell confinement and monitor, as appropriate, the cumulative amount of time that inmates with mental illness spend in restrictive housing, including single-cell confinement.

Status: Resolved.

BOP Response: The BOP agreed with this recommendation as it pertains to mental health inmates and will track and monitor inmates with Mental Health Care Levels (MHCL) 2, 3, and 4.

OIG Analysis: The BOP's actions are partially responsive to our recommendation. By October 27, 2017, please clarify whether the BOP will track all inmates in single-cell confinement or only those inmates who have previously needed recurring treatment interventions with mental health staff, as reflected by MHCLs 2, 3, and 4 or otherwise. Also, please describe how the BOP will track inmates in single-cell confinement and monitor, as appropriate, the cumulative amount of time that inmates with MHCLs 2, 3, and 4 spend in restrictive housing, including single-cell confinement. Further, please detail how the BOP will use this information in reviewing the placement of all inmates in Restrictive Housing Units (RHUs), including whether this information will be used as an additional metric that can trigger an Extended Restrictive Housing Placement Review.

Recommendation 4: Identify all forms of restrictive housing utilized throughout its institutions and ensure that all local policies are updated to reflect standards for all inmates in restrictive housing consistent with established nationwide policies.

Status: Resolved.

BOP Response: The BOP agreed with this recommendation and will review all forms of restrictive housing and ensure that local or national policies are in place to direct their operation.

OIG Analysis: The BOP's actions are responsive to our recommendation. By October 27, 2017, please provide the OIG with a list of all forms of restrictive housing, per institution, and describe how the BOP identified these RHUs. Also, please describe how the BOP will ensure that local or national policies are in place to direct the operation of all RHUs.

Recommendation 5: Evaluate and limit as appropriate the consecutive amount of time that inmates with serious mental illness may spend in restrictive housing.

Status: Resolved.

BOP Response: The BOP agreed with this recommendation and will establish limits, as appropriate, on consecutive placements in restrictive housing as it pertains to mental health inmates.

OIG Analysis: The BOP's actions are responsive to our recommendation. By October 27, 2017, please provide the OIG with proposed limits for the placement of inmates with serious mental illness in RHUs and describe how these limits will be implemented. Also, please describe the circumstances that would allow the BOP to exceed these limits in the placement of inmates with serious mental illness in RHUs and how these circumstances will be communicated to institution staff.

Recommendation 6: Ensure that the Psychology Services staff documents inmates' mental illness diagnoses in the Bureau's Electronic Medical Record System and Psychology Data System.

Status: Resolved.

BOP Response: The BOP agreed with this recommendation. The Psychology Services Branch will ensure that Psychology Services staff document inmates' mental illness diagnoses in the Bureau's Electronic Medical Record System and Psychology Data System (BEMR-PDS).

OIG Analysis: The BOP's actions are responsive to our recommendation. By October 27, 2017, please describe how the BOP will ensure that Psychology Services staff document inmates' mental illness diagnoses in BEMR-PDS.

Recommendation 7: Reassess the Mental Health Care Level system to ensure that it fully captures the mental health needs of inmates, including inmates in restrictive housing, and that classifications distinguish between inmates who have some form of mental illness and those who do not have any form of mental illness.

Status: Resolved.

BOP Response: The BOP agreed with this recommendation. The Psychology Services Branch will reassess the MHCL system to ensure that it fully captures the mental health needs of inmates, including inmates in restrictive housing, and that there is a method to distinguish between inmates who have some form of mental illness and those who do not have any form of mental illness.

OIG Analysis: The BOP's actions are responsive to our recommendation. By October 27, 2017, please describe how the BOP will ensure that the MHCL system fully captures the mental health needs of inmates and distinguishes inmates who have some form of mental illness.

Recommendation 8: Regularly monitor, by institution and type of Restrictive Housing Unit, trends in inmates' designated Mental Health Care Levels to further assess the factors that affect the treatment of inmates with mental illness.

Status: Resolved.

BOP Response: The BOP agreed with this recommendation. The Psychology Services Branch will monitor trends in inmates' designated MHCLs by institution and type of RHU. This will be used to further assess the factors that affect the treatment of inmates with mental illness.

OIG Analysis: The BOP's actions are responsive to our recommendation. By October 27, 2017, please describe how the BOP will monitor trends in inmates' MHCLs by institution and type of RHU, and how this information will be used to further assess the factors that affect the treatment of inmates with mental illness.

Recommendation 9: Determine what additional steps can be taken to prioritize and incentivize the hiring of mental health staff at institutions that have inmates with mental illness in long-term restrictive housing.

Status: Resolved.

BOP Response: The BOP agreed with this recommendation. The Psychology Services Branch and Health Services Division will determine what additional steps can be taken to prioritize and incentivize the hiring of mental health staff at institutions that have inmates with mental illness in long-term restrictive housing.

OIG Analysis: The BOP's actions are responsive to our recommendation. By October 27, 2017, please describe the additional steps that the BOP can take to incentivize the hiring of mental health staff at institutions that have inmates with mental illness in long-term restrictive housing, including the length of time that the BOP considers as "long-term restrictive housing" for this purpose.

Recommendation 10: Assess the scalability of secure residential mental health treatment programs and develop alternatives to address their potential limitations.

Status: Resolved.

BOP Response: The BOP agreed with this recommendation. The Psychology Services Branch will assess the scalability of secure residential mental health treatment programs and develop alternatives to address their potential limitations.

OIG Analysis: The BOP's actions are responsive to our recommendation. By October 27, 2017, please describe how the BOP assessed the scalability of these programs, the outcomes of the assessment, and the BOP's plan to address any limitations that may exist.

Recommendation 11: Develop and implement formal performance metrics sufficient to measure the effectiveness of secure residential mental health treatment programs.

Status: Resolved.

BOP Response: The BOP agreed with this recommendation. The Psychology Services Branch will develop and implement formal performance metrics sufficient to measure the effectiveness of secure residential mental health treatment programs.

OIG Analysis: The BOP's actions are responsive to our recommendation. By October 27, 2017, please provide the OIG with formal performance metrics for the secure residential mental health treatment programs. Also, please describe how the performance metrics were implemented and how the BOP will apply these performance metrics in evaluating the effectiveness of these programs.

Recommendation 12: Survey institutions and/or take other steps to identify alternative practices that reduce the frequency and duration of the placement of inmates with mental illness in restrictive housing, and implement such alternatives when appropriate.

Status: Resolved.

BOP Response: The BOP agreed with this recommendation. The Psychology Services Branch and Correctional Programs Division will survey institutions and/or take other steps to identify alternative practices that reduce the frequency and duration of the placement of inmates with mental illness in restrictive housing, and implement such alternatives when appropriate.

OIG Analysis: The BOP's actions are responsive to our recommendation. By October 27, 2017, please provide the OIG with the results of the survey to institutions and/or describe other steps BOP has taken to identify alternative practices that reduce the frequency and duration of the placement of inmates with mental illness in restrictive housing. Additionally, please describe how the BOP plans to assess, communicate, and implement alternative practices that can be replicated across its institutions.

Recommendation 13: Provide additional mental health training to correctional staff who are responsible for monitoring the behavior of inmates in restrictive housing.

Status: Resolved.

BOP Response: The BOP agreed with this recommendation, noting that it appears to be based on the opinions of a few staff, instead of any adverse event or incident caused by insufficient training. Correctional staff responsible for monitoring the behavior of inmates in restrictive housing currently receive a substantial amount of training. The BOP believes that the OIG may not be aware of this training; but the BOP will identify opportunities to provide additional training, including remedial training.

OIG Analysis: The BOP's actions are responsive to our recommendation. By October 27, 2017, please detail all of the BOP's current training for correctional staff responsible for monitoring the behavior of inmates in restrictive housing. Please also describe additional training opportunities for correctional staff who are responsible for monitoring such inmates, including remedial training, and provide copies of training materials for these identified opportunities.

Recommendation 14: Provide additional guidance and training to mental health staff on diagnosing mental illness, including guidance on documenting malingering behavior by inmates.

Status: Resolved.

BOP Response: The BOP agreed with this recommendation. The Psychology Services Branch will provide additional guidance and training to mental health staff on diagnosing mental illness, including guidance on documenting malingering behavior by inmates.

OIG Analysis: The BOP's actions are responsive to our recommendation. By October 27, 2017, please provide copies of training materials and guidance for mental health staff in diagnosing mental illness and documenting malingering. Also, please describe how and when the guidance and training materials will be delivered to mental health staff.

Recommendation 15: Conduct a comprehensive review of U.S. Penitentiary Lewisburg's Special Management Unit that addresses the staffing, treatment, conditions of confinement, and performance metrics of the program.

Status: Resolved.

BOP Response: The BOP agreed with this recommendation. A multidiscipline group from various geographic locations is being assembled to comprehensively review U.S. Penitentiary (USP) Lewisburg's Special Management Unit (SMU) and address the staffing, treatment, conditions of confinement, and performance metrics of the program.

OIG Analysis: The BOP's actions are responsive to our recommendation. By October, 27, 2017, please provide the OIG with an update regarding the BOP's review of USP Lewisburg's SMU, including a description of the review's objectives, scope, and methodology.

Office of the Inspector General
U.S. Department of Justice
www.justice.gov/oig

INDEX

#

A

B

C

D

E

F

G

H

I

J

K

L

M

N

Q

R

S

W

Y

The Impact of Severe Mental Illness on Quality of Life: Challenges for Research and Practices

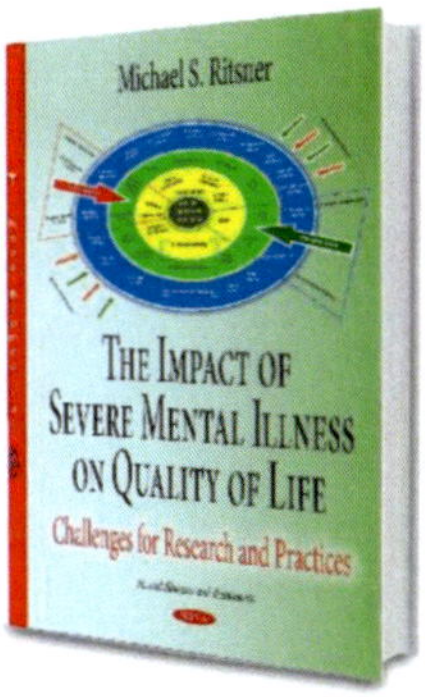

Author: Michael S Ritsner (Rappaport Faculty of Medicine, Israel Institute of Technology (Technion), The National Insurance Institute, Haifa, Israel)

Series: Mental Illnesses and Treatments

Book Description: This monograph deals with the health-related quality of life deficit (QOL) of people with severe mental disorders, focusing on issues related to its concept, characteristic profile, on developing the Distress/Protection Vulnerability Quality of Life Model including vulnerability (neurobiological and genetic), primary, and secondary factors, as well as on challenges for research and practice.

Hardcover ISBN: 978-1-53612-168-1
Retail Price: $310

Federal Programs Supporting People with Serious Mental Illness: An Assessment

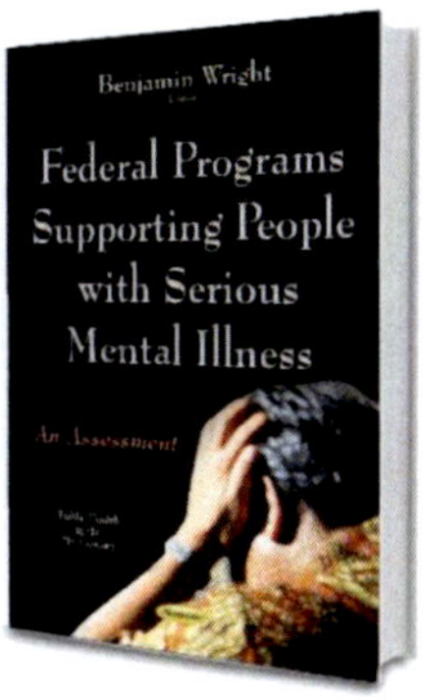

Editor: Benjamin Wright

Series: Public Health in the 21st Century

Book Description: This book briefly describes the methodology and results of three large surveys that provide national prevalence estimates of diagnosable mental illness.

Softcover ISBN: 978-1-63483-043-0
Retail Price: $69

Mental Health: Services, Assessment and Perspectives

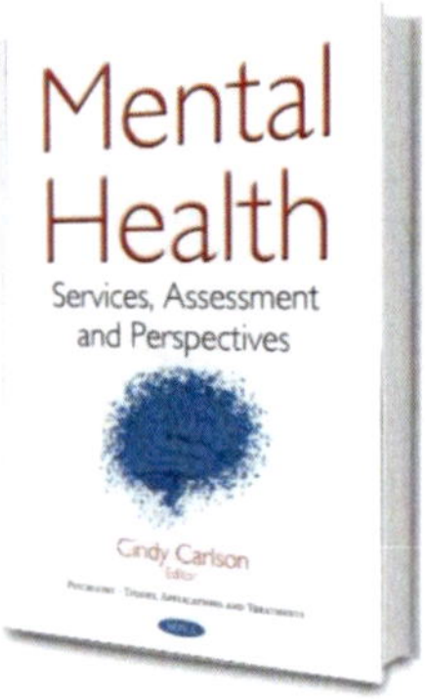

Editor: Cindy Carlson

Series: Psychiatry – Theory, Applications and Treatments

Book Description: Research from health psychology and medical science has shown that a considerable number of cancer patients tend to rely on meaning while coping with stress caused by their illness.

Softcover ISBN: 978-1-53612-209-1
Retail Price: $82

The Role of Emotions in Mental Illness

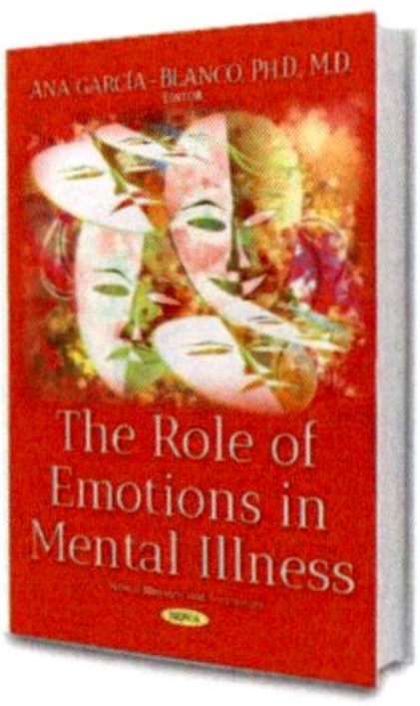

Editor: Ana García-Blanco, M.D., Ph.D. (Neonatal Research Unit, Health Research Institute La Fe, Valencia, Spain)

Series: Mental Illnesses and Treatments

Book Description: This book has attempted to highlight the importance of emotions in mental illness. Emotional experiences have an important effect on child development and to determine emotional organization. This emotional organization influences the perception of the self, others, and the world.

Softcover ISBN: 978-1-53612-628-0
Retail Price: $82